## a CORE Curriculum for Diabetes Education
### Fourth Edition

# Diabetes Management Therapies

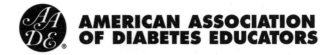

**AMERICAN ASSOCIATION OF DIABETES EDUCATORS**

# a CORE Curriculum for Diabetes Education
## Fourth Edition

# Diabetes Management Therapies

**Editor**
*Marion J. Franz, MS, RD, LD, CDE*
**Associate Editors**
*Karmeen Kulkarni, MS, RD, BC-ADM, CDE*
*William H. Polonsky, PhD, CDE*
*Peggy Yarborough, MS, RPh, BC-ADM, CDE*
*Virginia Zamudio, MSN, RN, CDE*

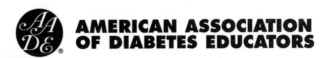

**AMERICAN ASSOCIATION OF DIABETES EDUCATORS**

**a CORE Curriculum for Diabetes Education, 4th Edition**
Diabetes Management Therapies
Published by the American Association of Diabetes Educators

©2001, American Association of Diabetes Educators, Chicago, Illinois.
ISBN 1-881876-06-3 (Volume Two)
ISBN 1-881876-09-8 (Four-Volume Set)

Library of Congress Control Number: 2001091524

Printed and bound in the United States of America.

**a CORE Curriculum for Diabetes Education**

# Diabetes Management Therapies

## In this Volume:

## Table of Contents

Introduction/Acknowledgements . . . . . . . . . . . . . . . . . . . . . . . . . . . . . . . . . . vii

Editors . . . . . . . . . . . . . . . . . . . . . . . . . . . . . . . . . . . . . . . . . . . . . . . . . . . . ix

Authors . . . . . . . . . . . . . . . . . . . . . . . . . . . . . . . . . . . . . . . . . . . . . . . . . . . x

Reviewers . . . . . . . . . . . . . . . . . . . . . . . . . . . . . . . . . . . . . . . . . . . . . . . . . xii

## Diabetes Management Therapies

**1** Medical Nutrition Therapy for Diabetes . . . . . . . . . . . . . . . . . . . . . . . . . 3

**2** Exercise . . . . . . . . . . . . . . . . . . . . . . . . . . . . . . . . . . . . . . . . . . . . . . . . 57

**3** Pharmacologic Therapies . . . . . . . . . . . . . . . . . . . . . . . . . . . . . . . . . . 91

**4** Monitoring . . . . . . . . . . . . . . . . . . . . . . . . . . . . . . . . . . . . . . . . . . . . 153

**5** Pattern Management of Blood Glucose . . . . . . . . . . . . . . . . . . . . . . . 175

**6** Insulin Pump Therapy and Carbohydrate Counting for Pump Therapy:

Carbohydrate-to-Insulin Ratios . . . . . . . . . . . . . . . . . . . . . . . . . . . . 203

**7** Hypoglycemia . . . . . . . . . . . . . . . . . . . . . . . . . . . . . . . . . . . . . . . . . 231

**8** Illness and Surgery . . . . . . . . . . . . . . . . . . . . . . . . . . . . . . . . . . . . . 263

Index . . . . . . . . . . . . . . . . . . . . . . . . . . . . . . . . . . . . . . . . . . . . . . . . . . .285

*Other Volumes in Core Curriculum, 4th Edition:*

## Diabetes and Complications

1 Pathophysiology of the Diabetes Disease State

2 Hyperglycemia

3 Chronic Complications of Diabetes: An Overview

4 Diabetic Foot Care and Education

5 Skin and Dental Care

6 Macrovascular Disease

7 Eye Disease and Adaptive Diabetes Education for
   Visually Impaired Persons

8 Nephropathy

9 Diabetic Neuropathy

## Diabetes Education and Program Management

1 Applied Principles of Teaching and Learning

2 Psychosocial Assessment

3 Behavior Change

4 Cultural Competence in Diabetes Education and Care

5 Teaching Persons With Low Literacy Skills

6 Psychological Disorders

7 Management of Diabetes Education Programs

8 Payment for Diabetes Education

## Diabetes in the Life Cycle and Research

1 Diabetes During Childhood and Adolescence

2 Pregnancy: Preconception to Postpartum

3 Gestational Diabetes

4 Diabetes in Older Adults

5 Lifestyle for Diabetes Prevention

6 Biological Complementary Therapies in Diabetes

7 The Importance of Research and Outcomes

# Introduction/Acknowledgements

It is a very exciting and challenging time for diabetes educators. Exciting because of the many advances that help people with diabetes to better manage their diabetes—new medications, technologies, research that makes lifestyle recommendations easier to understand and apply, the empowerment approach to education—to name just a few. The challenges and frustrations are the difficulties of sharing this information with individuals with diabetes, the lack of opportunities to individualize care, and the lack of time to assist in facilitating behavior changes. Resources—personnel, payment for services, training new educators—are other challenges. Although for years the person with diabetes has been acknowledged as the center of the diabetes team and the person who makes the final decision on what he/she is willing and able to do, often the individual with diabetes is still left out of the decision-making process. The Core Curriculum, 4th Edition cannot solve all the challenges but it can update the educator's knowledge and provide suggestions for skills to assist in facilitating necessary behavior changes for persons with diabetes.

The Core Curriculum was originally planned to help educators prepare for the Certified Diabetes Educator (CDE) exam. This has continued to be a goal for subsequent editions; however, the use and the scope of the Core Curriculum has expanded. It is a key reference for the Advanced Diabetes Management credential exam. Furthermore, the Core Curriculum has evolved into being a diabetes educator's authoritative source of information for diabetes education and management. One of the objectives of this edition is to move this goal one step further ahead. Just as all medicine is moving toward evidence-based practice, this must also be a goal for education. Chapters must have appropriate and adequate references and as a reader you have the right to question statements in the Core Curriculum that do not have adequate documentation. As all of us continue this focus, the Core Curriculum will truly become an evidence-based document.

As with all projects of this magnitude, there are many individuals to whom we are indebted. It begins with the chapter authors who have been willing to share their expertise and provide up-to-date information and management skills for the reader. It continues to the chapter reviewers who provide suggestions to make the chapters stronger. The authors and reviewers are listed in each volume of the Core Curriculum. As an educator, when you see these individuals please extend your thanks to them for the valuable service they have provided. The Associate Editors—Karmeen Kulkarni, William Polonsky, Peggy Yarborough, Virginia Zamudio—have provided valuable assistance in moving the process along efficiently and synthesizing the reviewers' comments to the chapter authors. Dr. Lois Book, RN, Director of Professional Relations, and Kaitrin Hall at the AADE National Office have also provided valuable suggestions for core content and support for the process of writing and editing of the Core Curriculum. We have all been fortunate to work with very competent editorial and publishing professionals. Mary Beach and Jim West at Stenson Bauer Communications have kept the process moving efficiently. Karen Lloyd has provided editorial assistance for the new chapters. Nancy Williams has used her copyreader and editing skills to make sure small details and mistakes were not missed and Michele Montour at Montronics made sure text was accurately typeset. To all these fine professionals, the AADE owes a great deal of gratitude.

But this fourth edition of the Core Curriculum with the new four-volume format would not have been possible without the contributions of previous Core editors. I am proud to join this elite group of educators beginning with Diana Guthrie, Julie Meyer, Kathryn Godley, Virginia Peragallo-Dittko, and continuing to Martha Funnell, editor of the third edition. Each edition has moved the professionalism of the Core forward and, hopefully, we have continued this process. There is still work ahead to make the Core truly evidence-based, and I look forward to future editions.

As authors, reviewers, and editors we have done our best to make this edition of the Core Curriculum a valuable resource for all diabetes educators. We welcome suggestions from you, the reader and professional, who will be using the Core as to how we can continue to make the Core Curriculum better and stronger. But for today, I personally am very proud of this edition. Please use this edition to improve the education and care that you provide for people with diabetes. That ultimately is the final goal, to enrich the lives of persons with diabetes who have been, for all of us, our best educators!

Marion J. Franz, MS, RD, LD, CDE
Editor, Core Curriculum, 4th Edition

## Editor

Marion J. Franz, MS, RD, LD, CDE
Nutrition Concepts by Franz, Inc.
Minneapolis, Minnesota

## Associate Editors

Karmeen Kulkarni, MS, RD, BC-ADM, CDE
St. Marks Hospital Diabetes Center
Salt Lake City, Utah

William H. Polonsky, PhD, CDE
Department of Psychiatry
University of California
San Diego, California

Peggy Yarborough, MS, RPh, BC-ADM, CDE
Campbell University and Wilson Community Health Center
Wilson, North Carolina

Virginia Zamudio, RN, MSN, CDE
Alamo Diabetes Team
San Antonio, Texas

## Authors

Jessie H. Ahroni,
PhD, ARNP, CDE
Veterans Affairs Puget Sound
Health Care System
School of Nursing, University
of Washington
Seattle, Washington

Robert M. Anderson, EdD
Michigan Diabetes Research
and Training Center
University of Michigan
Ann Arbor, Michigan

James D. Anderst, MD
Medical College of Wisconsin
Milwaukee, Wisconsin

Mindy Andrus,
RD, LDN, CDE
East Carolina University
Brody School of Medicine
Greenville, North Carolina

Susan L. Barlow, RD, CDE
Amylin Pharmaceuticals, Inc.
Indianapolis, Indiana

Marla Bernbaum, MD
St. Louis University Health
Sciences Center
Division of Endocrinology
St. Louis, Missouri

Jean Betschart,
MSN, MN, CPNP, CDE
Children's Hospital
of Pittsburgh
Pittsburgh, Pennsylvania

Susan A. Biastre,
RD, LDN, CDE
Women & Infants' Hospital
Providence, Rhode Island

Ann Marie Brooks, RN, CDE
St. Marks Hospital
Diabetes Center
Salt Lake City, Utah

R. Keith Campbell,
RPh, MBA, CDE
Washington State University
Spokane, Washington

Belinda P. Childs, RN, MN,
ARNP, CDE
Mid-America Diabetes
Associates
Wichita, Kansas

Beth Ann Coonrod, PhD,
MPH, RN, CDE
Heritage Valley Health
System
Beaver and Sewickley,
Pennsylvania

Angela D'Antonio, RD
University of South Carolina
Norman J. Arnold School of
Public Health
Columbia, South Carolina

Mayer B. Davidson, MD
Charles R. Drew University
Los Angeles, California

Kristina L. Ernst,
BSN, RN, CDE
Atlanta, Georgia

James A. Fain,
PhD, RN, FAAN
University of Massachusetts
Worcester
Graduate School of Nursing
Worcester, Massachusetts

Eva L. Feldman, MD, PhD
Department of Neurology
University of Michigan
Medical School
Ann Arbor, Michigan

Marion J. Franz,
MS, RD, LD, CDE
Nutrition Concepts
by Franz, Inc.
Minneapolis, Minnesota

Martha Mitchell Funnell,
MS, RN, CDE
Michigan Diabetes Research
and Training Center
University of Michigan
Medical Center
Ann Arbor, Michigan

Patti Geil, MS, RD, CDE
Lexington, Kentucky

Linda Gonder-Frederick, PhD
University of Virginia
Behavioral Medicine Center
Charlottesville, Virginia

Diana W. Guthrie,
RN, ARNP, FAAN, CDE
Professor Emeritus
University of Kansas School
of Medicine
Wichita, Kansas

Richard A. Guthrie,
MD, CDE
Mid-America Diabetes
Associates
Via Christi Regional
Medical Center
University of Kansas School
of Medicine
Wichita, Kansas

Deborah Hinnen,
RN, MN, ARNP,
BC-ADM, CDE
Via Christi Regional
Medical Center
Wichita, Kansas

Carol Homko,
RN, PhD, CDE
Temple University Hospital
Philadelphia, Pennsylvania

Cheryl Hunt,
RN, MSEd, CDE
Health Education
and Resources
Alexandria, Virginia

Donna Jornsay,
BSN, RN, CPNP, CDE
MiniMed
Great Neck, New York

Elaine Boswell King,
MSN, RN, CS, CDE
Vanderbilt Diabetes Research
and Training Center
Nashville, Tennessee

Karmeen Kulkarni,
MS, RD, BC-ADM, CDE
St. Marks Hospital
Diabetes Center
Salt Lake City, Utah

Janie Lipps,
MSN, RN, CS, CDE
Vanderbilt Diabetes Research
and Training Center
Nashville, Tennessee

Nancy Leggett-Frazier,
RN, MSN, CDE
East Carolina University
Brody School of Medicine
Greenville, North Carolina

Elizabeth J. Mayer-Davis,
PhD, RD
University of South Carolina
Norman J. Arnold School of
Public Health
Columbia, South Carolina

Stephania Miller, PhD
Diabetes Research and
Training Center
Vanderbilt University
School of Medicine
Nashville, Tennessee

Catherine A. Mullooly,
MS, RCEPsm, CDE
Joslin Clinic
Boston, Massachusetts

Kathryn Mulcahy,
RN, MSN, CDE
Fairfax Hospital INOVA
Diabetes Center
Fairfax, Virginia

Joseph P. Napora,
PhD, LCSW-C
The Johns Hopkins
University School of Medicine
The Johns Hopkins
Diabetes Center
Baltimore, Maryland

Anne T. Nettles,
RN, MS, CDE
Healthcare Consultant
Minneapolis, Minnesota

Jan Norman, RD, CDE
Washington Department
of Health
Diabetes Control Program
Olympia, Washington

Virginia Peragallo-Dittko,
RN, MA, CDE
Diabetes Education Center
Winthrop-University Hospital
Mineola, New York

Michael A. Pfeifer,
MD, FACE, CDE
East Carolina University
Brody School of Medicine
Greenville, North Carolina

James W. Pichert, PhD
Diabetes Research and
Training Center
Vanderbilt University
Nashville, Tennessee

Robert E. Ratner, MD, CDE
Medstar Research Institute
Washington, DC

Lynne S. Robbins, PhD
University of Washington
Department of
Medical Education
Seattle, Washington

Richard R. Rubin, PhD, CDE
The Johns Hopkins
University School of Medicine
Departments of Medicine
and Pediatrics
Baltimore, Maryland

Laura Shane-McWhorter,
PharmD, BCPS, FASCP, CDE
College of Pharmacy
University of Utah
Salt Lake City, Utah

Tamara Stich,
RN, MSN, CDE
Washington University School
of Medicine
Department of Metabolism
St. Louis, Missouri

Catrine Tudor-Locke, PhD
University of South Carolina
Norman J. Arnold School of
Public Health
Columbia, South Carolina

Frank Vinicor, MD, MPH
Centers for Disease
Control and Prevention
Division of Diabetes
Translation
Atlanta, Georgia

John R. White, Jr.,
RPh, PharmD, PA-C
Washington State University
Spokane, Washington

Peggy C. Yarborough,
RPh, MS, BC-ADM, CDE
Campbell University and
Wilson Community
Health Center
Wilson, North Carolina

## Reviewers

Barbara J. Anderson, PhD
Joslin Diabetes Center
Harvard University School
of Medicine
Boston, Massachusetts

Gary M. Arsham, MD, PhD
Arsham Consultants, Inc.
San Francisco, California

Anita K. Austin, RPh, CDE
University of Pittsburgh
Physicians
Pittsburgh, Pennsylvania

David W. Bartels,
PharmD, CDE
University of Illinois at
Chicago College of Pharmacy
Department of Pharmacy
Practice and College of
Medicine at Rockford
Department of Family and
Community Medicine

David S. Bell, MD
University of Alabama
Medical School
Birmingham, Alabama

Kathy J. Berkowitz,
RNC, FNP, CDE
Diabetes Unit, Grady
Health System
Atlanta, Georgia

Liz Blair, ANP, CDE
Joslin Diabetes Center
Boston, Massachusetts

Barbara H. Bodnar,
RN, MS, CDE
West Virginia University
Morgantown, West Virginia

John B. Buse, MD, PhD, CDE
University of North Carolina
Diabetes Care Center
Durham, North Carolina

Denise Charron-Prochownik,
PhD, RN, CPNP
University of Pittsburgh
School of Nursing/
Health Promotion
Pittsburgh, Pennsylvania

Belinda Childs, RN, MN,
ARNP, CDE
Mid-America Diabetes
Associates, PA
Wichita, Kansas

Beth Ann Coonrod,
PhD, MPH, RN, CDE
Heritage Valley Health
System
Beaver and Sewickley,
Pennsylvania

Alicia Correa,
RN, BSN, MBA
Texas Diabetes Institute
San Antonio, Texas

Marjorie Cypress,
MSN, C-ANP, CDE
Lovelace Medical Center
Endocrinology/Diabetes
Department
Albuquerque, New Mexico

Anne Daly,
MS, RD, LD, BC-ADM, CDE
Springfield Diabetes and
Endocrine Center
Springfield, Illinois

Mary Ellinger, RD, CDE
Diabetes Self Care,
Matria Healthcare
Centreville, Virginia

Janine Freeman,
RD, LD, CDE
Diabetes Nutrition Specialist
Atlanta, Georgia

Sandra J. Gillespie,
MMSc, RD, LD, CDE
Diabetes Resource Center
Piedmont Hospital
Atlanta, Georgia

Russell E. Glasgow, PhD
AMC Cancer Research
Center
Denver, Colorado

Kathryn Godley,
MS, RN, CDE
Albany Medical College
Albany, New York

Marilyn R. Graff,
RN, BSN, CDE
MiniMed Professional
Education Department
Sylmar, California

Richard A. Guthrie,
MD, FCAP, CDE
Mid-America Diabetes
Associates, Inc.
Wichita, Kansas

Leo E. Hendricks,
PhD, LICSW, CDE
LHCA's Diabetes Self-
Management Skills
Training Center
Silver Springs, Maryland

Rosetta T. Hendricks,
PhD, RN, CS, FNP, CDE
Veterans Affairs
Medical Center
Washington, DC

Lea Ann Holzmeister,
RD, CDE
Nutrition Consultant
Tempe, Arizona

David Holtzman
Director of
Government Affairs
American Association of
Diabetes Educators
Chicago, Illinois

Bonnie Irvin,
MS, RD, LD, CDE
Iredell Memorial Hospital
Health Care System
Diabetes Center for Learning
Statesville, North Carolina

Timothy J. Ives,
PharmD, MPH
Department of
Family Medicine
University of North Carolina
Chapel Hill, North Carolina

Scott J. Jacober, DO, CDE
Eli Lilly & Co.
Indianapolis, Indiana

Dennis Janisse, CPed
National Pedorthic Services
Milwaukee, Wisconsin

Jane Kadohiro,
DrPH, APRN, CDE
University of Hawaii School
of Nursing and
Dental Hygiene
Honolulu, Hawaii

Ginger Kanzer-Lewis,
RNC, EdM, CDE
GKL Associates
Pomona, New York

Wahida Karmally,
MS, RD, CDE
The Irving Center for Clinical
Research, Columbia
University
New York, New York

Julienne K. Kirk,
PharmD, CDE, BCPS
Department of Family
Medicine
Wake Forest University
School of Medicine
Winston-Salem,
North Carolina

Davida F. Kruger,
MSN, RN, BC-ADM, CDE
Henry Ford Health Systems
Endocrinology/Metabolism
Detroit, Michigan

Andrea J. Lasichak,
MS, RD, CDE
Michigan Diabetes Research
Training Center
University of
Michigan Hospital
Ann Arbor, Michigan

Daniel Lorber,
MD, FACP, CDE
Diabetes Control Foundation
Flushing, New York

Melinda D. Maryniuk,
MEd, RD, FADA, CDE
Joslin Diabetes Center
Boston, Massachusetts

Susan McLaughlin, RD, CDE
On-Site Health &
Wellness, LLC
Omaha, Nebraska

Arlene Monk, RD, LD, CDE
International Diabetes Center
Minneapolis, Minnesota

Arshag D. Mooradian, MD
St. Louis University Medical
Center Division of
Endocrinology
St. Louis, Missouri

Charlotte Reese Nath,
MSN, RN, EdD, CDE
West Virginia University
Department of Family
Medicine
Robert C. Byrd Health
Sciences Center
Morgantown, West Virginia

Jan Nicollerat,
MSN, RN, CS, CDE
Duke University Adult
Diabetes Education Program
Cary, North Carolina

Jan Norman, RD, CD, CDE
Washington State
Department of Health
Olympia, Washington

Belinda O'Connell,
MS, RD, CDE
International Diabetes Center
Minneapolis, Minnesota

Joyce G. Pastors,
RD, MS, CDE
Virginia Center for Diabetes
Professional Education
Charlottesville, Virginia

Teresa L. Pearson,
MS, RN, CDE
Health Partners Center for
Health Promotion
Minneapolis, Minnesota

Suzanne Pecoraro,
RD, MPH, CDE
Diabetes Education Society
Denver, Colorado

Martha Price,
DNSc, ARNP, CDE
Group Health Cooperative
Diabetes Clinical Roadmap
Seattle, Washington

Diane M. Reader, RD, CDE
International Diabetes Center
Minneapolis, Minnesota

Dawn Satterfield,
RNC, MSN, CDE
Centers for Disease Control
and Prevention
Division of Diabetes
Translation
Atlanta, Georgia

J. Terry Saunders, PhD
Virginia Center for Diabetes
Professional Education
Charlottesville, Virginia

Pamela Scarborough,
PT, MS, CDE, CWS
Education 2000 Plus
Dallas, Texas

Gary Scheiner, MS, CDE
Integrated Diabetes Services
Wynnewood, Pennsylvania

Barbara Schreiner,
RN, MN, BC-ADM, CDE
Texas Children's Hospital
Diabetes Care Center
Houston, Texas

Michelle Burdette-Taylor
BT & T Health Education
with a Purpose
San Diego, California

Christine Tobin,
RN, MBA, CDE
Health Care Consultant
Atlanta, Georgia

Elizabeth A. Walker,
RN, DNSc, CDE
Albert Einstein College
of Medicine
Diabetes Research and
Training Center
Bronx, New York

Hope S. Warshaw,
MMSc, RD, CDE
Hope Warshaw Associates
Alexandria, Virginia

Madelyn L. Wheeler,
MS, RD, FADA, CDE
Diabetes Research and
Training Center
Indiana University School
of Medicine
Indianapolis, Indiana

Neil H. White, MD, CDE
Pediatric Endocrinology and
Metabolism
Washington University
St. Louis, Missouri

Ann Sawyer Williams,
MSN, RN, CDE
Cleveland Heights, Ohio

Donald N. Zettervall,
RPH, CDE
The Diabetes Center
Old Saybrook, Connecticut

# A Core Curriculum for Diabetes Education
## Diabetes Management Therapies

## Medical Nutrition Therapy for Diabetes  1

*Marion J. Franz, MS, RD, LD, CDE*
*Nutrition Concepts by Franz, Inc.*
*Minneapolis, Minnesota*

# Introduction

**1** Diabetes is a chronic progressive disease that often requires lifestyle changes, especially in the areas of nutrition and physical activity. The goal of medical nutrition therapy (MNT) is to assist persons with diabetes in making self-directed behavior changes that will improve their overall health and the management of their diabetes.

**2** Achieving optimal nutrition through healthy food choices is the underlying principle of the American Diabetes Association (ADA) nutrition recommendations for people with diabetes.[1] However, in addition to concerns related to improved health through healthy food choices and physical activity, MNT for diabetes focuses on goals and strategies for the treatment and prevention of diabetes and on achieving optimal metabolic outcomes related to glycemia, lipid profiles, and blood pressure levels.[1-3]

   **A** The ADA nutrition recommendations for health are similar to the nutrition recommendations for the prevention of chronic diseases from other major health organizations (eg, US Department of Agriculture and US Department of Health and Human Services,[4] American Heart Association,[5] American Institute for Cancer Research[6]).

   **B** Although many studies have focused on the role of single nutrients, foods, or food groups in disease prevention or promotion, emerging research suggests health benefits from certain food patterns that include a mixture of foods containing multiple nutrients and nonnutrients.[4,7-12]

   • A healthy diet consists of multiple servings of fruits and vegetables, whole grains, low-fat dairy products, fish, lean meats, and poultry.

**3** Persons with diabetes report that making changes in their lifestyle is one of the greatest challenges they face in managing their diabetes.[13,14] Therefore, it is essential that recommendations take into account lifestyle changes the individual with diabetes is willing and able to make and maintain. This requires the person with diabetes to be involved in the decision-making process. Cultural and ethnic preferences also must be taken into consideration.

**4** MNT is an essential component of successful diabetes management.[15-18]

**5** *Medical nutrition therapy* (or nutrition therapy) is the preferred term and replaces other terms such as diet, diet therapy, and dietary management. MNT involves the use of specific nutrition services to treat an illness or condition and incorporates the process or system for providing individualized nutrition care and specific lifestyle recommendations for that care. The process of providing care includes assessment, intervention/education, goal setting, and evaluation of outcomes; lifestyle recommendations concern food/nutrition and physical activity.

**6** Every individual with diabetes needs a comprehensive treatment approach, which includes

   **A** An individualized food/meal plan appropriate for his/her lifestyle and diabetes management goals.

   **B** Education related to diabetes and nutrition therapy and food/meal planning.

   **C** Mutually agreed-upon short-term and long-term goals for lifestyle changes.

**D** Evaluation of lifestyle change outcomes with appropriate recommendation for changes in medication.

**E** Ongoing education and nutrition care, with regular review and modification, as necessary, of the meal plan, management goals, and self-management education.

**7** For persons requiring insulin therapy, the goal of MNT is to provide a food/meal plan that integrates an insulin regimen into usual eating and activity patterns.[1,2] For persons with type 2 diabetes, the goal of MNT is to normalize metabolic outcomes. This goal can be achieved through improving eating habits; restricting energy intake; achieving moderate weight loss; having consistent carbohydrate intake at meals and for snacks; decreasing fat intake, especially saturated and trans fats and cholesterol; increasing physical activity levels; and adopting new behaviors and attitudes.[1,2]

## Objectives

Upon completion of this chapter, the learner will be able to

**1** Identify medical nutrition therapy goals for diabetes management.

**2** Describe nutrition recommendations for the treatment and prevention of diabetes.

**3** State the goal of MNT for persons with type 1 diabetes.

**4** State the goal of MNT for persons with type 2 diabetes and 5 nutrition-related strategies for achieving that goal.

**5** Describe the role of carbohydrate in food/meal planning for persons with diabetes.

**6** State guidelines for the use of sucrose and fiber.

**7** Explain how the term acceptable daily intake (ADI) relates to the use of nonnutritive sweeteners.

**8** State guidelines for the role of protein in food/meal planning for persons with diabetes.

**9** List nutrition recommendations for the amount and type of fat appropriate in the food/meal plan for persons with diabetes.

**10** State general principles related to the role of certain vitamins and minerals in diabetes management.

**11** List guidelines for the use of alcohol.

**12** Describe how assessment, implementation/education, goal setting, and evaluation apply to nutrition services for diabetes.

**13** Individualize a food/meal plan.

**14** Describe the rationale for carbohydrate counting and how to implement this method for food and meal planning.

**15** Explain the concept of exchange lists including the nutritive values for each list and their use in assessing eating habits.

**16** Implement nutrition recommendations at acute-care and long-term healthcare facilities.

## Goals of Diabetes Medical Nutrition Therapy for Persons With Diabetes

**1** Assist in attaining and maintaining optimal metabolic outcomes, including

**A** Blood glucose levels in the normal range, to the greatest extent possible. Balance food intake, physical activity, and diabetes medications (when needed) to prevent the complications of diabetes.[19,20]

## Table 1.1. Risk for Macrovascular Disease Based on Lipoprotein Values in Adults With Diabetes

| Risk | LDL Cholesterol Levels | HDL Cholesterol* Levels | Triglyceride Levels |
|---|---|---|---|
| High | ≥130 mg/dL (3.36 mmol/L) | <35 mg/dL (0.9 mmol/L) | ≥400 mg/dL (4.40 mmol/L) |
| Borderline | 100-129 mg/dL (2.59-3.34 mmol/L) | 35-45 mg/dL 0.9-1.17 mmol/L) | 200-399 mg/dL (2.20-4.39 mmol/L) |
| Low | <100 mg/dL (2.59 mmol/L) | >45 mg/dL (1.17 mmol/L) | <200 mg/dL (2.20 mmol/L) |

* For women, the HDL cholesterol values should be increased by 10 mg/dL.
*Source:* Reprinted with permission from the American Diabetes Association.[21]
The National Cholesterol Education Program (NCEP) Adult Treatment Panel III (JAMA 285:2486-2497) defines HDL cholesterol <40 mg/dL* as high risk and ≥60 mg/dL as low risk. Triglycerides <150 mg/dL are defined as normal and >200 mg/dL as high.

## Table 1.2. Recommended Lipoprotein Values for Children and Adolescents[22]

| | Cholesterol Levels | LDL Cholesterol Levels | Triglyceride Levels |
|---|---|---|---|
| Desirable | ≤170 mg/dL (4.40 mmol/L) | ≤110 mg/dL (2.85 mmol/L) | *Child, first decade* ≤100 mg/dL (1.13 mmol/L) *Child, second decade* ≤120 mg/dL (1.35 mmol/L) |
| Borderline | 170-199 mg/dL (4.40-5.15 mmol/L) | 110-129 mg/dL (2.85-3.34 mmol/L) | |
| High | ≥200 mg/dL (5.17 mmol/L) | ≥130 mg/dL (3.36 mmol/L) | |

**B** Lipid and lipoprotein profiles that are associated with a decreased risk for cardiovascular disease. Recommended values are shown in Table 1.1[21] and Table 1.2.[22]

**C** Blood pressure levels that are associated with a decreased risk for vascular disease. Optimal blood pressure for adults with respect to cardiovascular risk is <130/80 mm Hg.[23]

**2** Improve health through healthy food choices and physical activity. Nutrition guidelines and nutrient needs are outlined and illustrated in *Dietary Guidelines for Americans*[4] and the diabetes version from the American Diabetes and the American Dietetic Association, *The First Step in Diabetes Meal Planning.*[24]

**3** Individualize nutrition care to achieve health-related goals with attention to personal preferences, cultural appropriateness, and the need/willingness to change lifestyle habits.

## Goals of Diabetes Medical Nutrition Therapy for Specific Populations and Conditions

**1** For youth with type 1 diabetes, provide adequate calories to ensure normal growth and development. The meal plan is not a restriction of calories but is intended to ensure reasonably consistent food intake and a nutritionally balanced eating pattern. Insulin needs to be adjusted to cover the amount of food consumed.

**2** For youth with type 2 diabetes, recommend changes in lifestyle to decrease the risks associated with diabetes. Achieving and maintaining a healthy weight through healthy eating habits and exercise can delay the progression of diabetes. Changes in eating and exercise habits are important for the entire family.[25]

**3** For pregnancy and lactation, provide adequate calories and nutrients. By monitoring glucose levels, urine ketones, appetite, and weight gain, appropriate nutrient and energy adjustments can be made.

**4** For the prevention and treatment of acute complications of diabetes treated with insulin or glucose-lowering agents (eg, hypoglycemia, acute and catabolic illnesses, exercise-related blood glucose problems), provide appropriate nutrition guidelines.

**5** For the prevention and treatment of chronic complications associated with diabetes (eg, nephropathy, hypertension, cardiovascular disease, gastropathies, obesity), provide appropriate nutrition guidelines.

**6** For individuals at risk for diabetes, recommend ways to decrease the risk by improving lifestyle factors. Becoming physically active and maintaining activity[26-29] or sustained weight loss[30] can prevent or delay the onset of type 2 diabetes.

## Nutrition-Related Strategies for Achieving Metabolic Goals for Type 1 Diabetes

**1** The food/meal plan is based on the individual's appetite, preferred foods, and usual schedule of food intake and activities. The insulin regimen can then be integrated into usual eating habits.[1,2,31]

**2** Individuals using intensive insulin therapy consisting of background insulin (basal) and premeal (bolus) insulin doses or insulin pumps have more flexibility in timing and frequency of meals, amount of carbohydrate eaten at meals, and timing of physical activity (see Chapter 4, Monitoring, and Chapter 5, Pattern Management of Blood Glucose, in Diabetes Management Therapies).

   **A** The total carbohydrate content of meals (and snacks, if desired), not the source, is the first priority. The amount is based on the individual's preference.

   **B** The amount of carbohydrate in the meal determines the premeal doses of rapid-acting insulin (lispro or aspart) or short-acting (regular) insulin and is adjusted accordingly.[32,33]

**3** Individuals taking fixed doses of insulin, which often consists of injections of rapid-acting or short-acting insulin and NPH insulin before breakfast and the evening meal, need to eat similar amounts of carbohydrate at consistent times that are synchronized with the time actions of their insulin(s). Consistency in the amount of day-to-day carbohydrate intake is associated with improved blood glucose control.[34]

**4** Improved glycemic control with intensive insulin therapy is often associated with increased body weight. Although it is important to try to prevent weight gain, the benefits of improved blood glucose control outweigh concerns about added pounds.[35] However, because of the potential for weight increases to adversely affect lipids and blood pressure, it is desirable to prevent weight gain.[36,37]

**A** To prevent weight gain and hypoglycemia, insulin therapy should be integrated into usual eating and exercise habits, and insulin doses should be adjusted accordingly.

**B** Overtreatment of hypoglycemia should be avoided. In general, treatment for blood glucose levels <70 mg/dL (3.88 mmol/L) consists of consuming 15 g of carbohydrate. Individuals should retest their blood glucose levels 15 minutes after consuming the carbohydrate to see if additional carbohydrate is needed (see Chapter 7, Hypoglycemia, in Diabetes Management Therapies).

**C** Adjustments in insulin and possibly carbohydrate intake should be made for exercise. In general, it may be more helpful to decrease the dose of rapid-acting or short-acting insulin during the time of the exercise. If additional carbohydrate is needed, 15 g to 30 g can be ingested (depending on the intensity of the exercise), either before or after an hour of exercise (see Chapter 2, Exercise, in Diabetes Management Therapies).

**D** Although the carbohydrate content of the meal determines the premeal insulin dose, meat, meat substitutes, and fat servings cannot be ignored. To prevent weight gain, attention also needs to be given to the total number of calories ingested.

## Nutrition-Related Strategies for Achieving Metabolic Goals for Type 2 Diabetes

**1** MNT for persons with type 2 diabetes focuses on lifestyle strategies that can assist in improving and maintaining normal/optimal metabolic parameters: optimal glucose control, improved lipid profile, and control of blood pressure.[1,2,38]

**2** Several strategies are available to assist individuals in accomplishing these goals. MNT must be individualized, and goals must be based on what the individual with diabetes chooses to focus on.

**A** As research continues to clarify why weight loss,[39,40] and particularly maintaining weight loss,[41,42] is difficult for many persons to achieve, the emphasis for persons with type 2 diabetes needs to shift from weight loss to achieving and maintaining metabolic goals. Both energy restriction and moderate weight loss decrease insulin resistance and are especially helpful early in the course of the disease.[16,43] Energy restriction, independent of weight loss, is associated with increased insulin sensitivity; significant improvements in glycemia generally occur before much weight is lost.[44,45]

• Energy restriction is, therefore, an independent factor for improved glycemic control. Glycemic control improves within 24 hours of caloric restriction and before any weight loss occurs.

• One of the major lessons learned from the United Kingdom Prospective Diabetes Study (UKPDS)[16] is that type 2 diabetes is a progressive disorder and therapy needs to be intensified over time. Early in the course of the disease, when insulin resistance is most prominent, MNT alone may maintain adequate metabolic control. As the disease progresses and the pancreatic beta cells fail, insulin deficiency becomes more of a factor. Oral medication(s) and, for many individuals, insulin eventually need to be combined with MNT to maintain adequate metabolic control.

- In the UKPDS study, the greatest reduction in HbA$_{1c}$ was approximately 2% during the first 3 months with intensive diet and 5% weight loss. The initial glucose response was related more to the decrease in energy intake than to weight loss; the decrease in body weight was a secondary response.
- Fasting plasma glucose levels (FPG) of 110 mg/dL (6.11 mmol/L) were only maintained in patients who continued a restricted caloric intake. In patients who increased their caloric intake, FPG levels increased even if the weight loss was maintained.

**B** Moderate weight loss of 10 to 20 lb (5 to 9 kg), irrespective of starting weight, has been shown to improve hyperglycemia, dyslipidemia, and hypertension.[46-48] However, if glycemia has not improved after a weight loss of approximately 10 lb (5 kg), oral glucose-lowering agents or insulin (alone or in combination) are generally needed.[47]

- *Body mass index* (BMI, in kg/m$^2$) defines overweight and obesity and is based on weight/height squared.[49] To determine BMI, a chart such as Figure 1.1 can be used. In adults, a BMI >25 but <30 is defined as an overweight state, a BMI >30 but <40 is classified as obesity, and a BMI >40 is considered extreme obesity. In children and adolescents, a BMI between the 85th and 95th percentiles indicates an increased risk for overweight, and a BMI >95th percentile is used to define obesity.
- When BMI is excessive (>30, or >25 with comorbidities), energy intake should be less than the energy expended in physical activity to reduce BMI. Energy restriction sufficient to produce weight reductions between 5% and 10% reduces the risk for heart disease and stroke.
- As body adiposity increases so does insulin resistance. A BMI of approximately 27 kg/m$^2$ appears to be the threshold at which insulin resistance begins to impair glucose disposal and thereby aggravates hyperglycemia.[50]
- Target weights for persons with diabetes are based on a reasonable or healthy body weight, which is not the same as the traditionally defined desirable or ideal body weight. *Reasonable body weight* is the weight an individual and health professional acknowledge as achievable and maintainable, both short-term and long-term.
- The type of obesity associated with metabolic diseases (glucose intolerance, hypertension, and lipid abnormalities) is the android or abdominal distribution of adipose tissue. Intra-abdominal obesity is associated with insulin resistance and hyperinsulinemia, which are both risk factors for metabolic disease.[51,52] Waist circumference (>40 in [102 cm] for men, >35 in [88 cm] for women) indicates risk for metabolic disease.[49]
- Energy restriction results in early improvements in glycemia, whereas moderate weight loss results in later improvements in glycemia. Reducing abdominal fat improves insulin sensitivity as well as lipid profiles.[43]

**C** Consistent day-to-day carbohydrate intake at meals and snacks is important because carbohydrate is the macronutrient with the greatest impact on postprandial glucose levels. Individuals need to be provided with basic guidelines for the amount of carbohydrate to eat at meals and/or snacks.

# Figure 1.1. Determining Body Mass Index (BMI)

How to use this chart:

1 Find height (in feet and inches) in the left column.
2 Look across the row to find weight (in pounds).
3 Find the number at the top of the column to determine the BMI.

| BMI | 19 | 20 | 21 | 22 | 23 | 24 | 25 | 26 | 27* | 28 | 29 | 30 | 35 | 40 |
|-----|----|----|----|----|----|----|----|----|-----|----|----|----|----|----|
| | | | | | | | Weight | | | | | | | |
| 4'10" | 91 | 96 | 100 | 105 | 110 | 115 | 119 | 124 | 129 | 134 | 138 | 143 | 167 | 191 |
| 4'11" | 94 | 99 | 104 | 109 | 114 | 119 | 124 | 128 | 133 | 138 | 143 | 148 | 173 | 198 |
| 5' | 97 | 102 | 107 | 112 | 118 | 123 | 128 | 133 | 138 | 143 | 148 | 153 | 179 | 204 |
| 5'1" | 100 | 106 | 111 | 116 | 122 | 127 | 132 | 137 | 143 | 148 | 153 | 158 | 185 | 211 |
| 5'2" | 104 | 109 | 115 | 120 | 126 | 131 | 136 | 142 | 147 | 153 | 158 | 164 | 191 | 218 |
| 5'3" | 107 | 113 | 118 | 124 | 130 | 135 | 141 | 146 | 152 | 158 | 163 | 169 | 197 | 225 |
| 5'4" | 110 | 116 | 122 | 128 | 134 | 140 | 145 | 151 | 157 | 163 | 169 | 174 | 204 | 232 |
| 5'5" | 114 | 120 | 126 | 132 | 138 | 144 | 150 | 156 | 162 | 168 | 174 | 180 | 210 | 240 |
| 5'6" | 118 | 124 | 130 | 136 | 142 | 148 | 155 | 161 | 167 | 173 | 179 | 186 | 216 | 247 |
| 5'7" | 121 | 127 | 134 | 140 | 146 | 153 | 159 | 166 | 172 | 178 | 185 | 191 | 223 | 255 |
| 5'8" | 125 | 131 | 138 | 144 | 151 | 158 | 164 | 171 | 177 | 184 | 190 | 197 | 230 | 262 |
| 5'9" | 128 | 135 | 142 | 149 | 155 | 162 | 169 | 176 | 182 | 189 | 196 | 203 | 236 | 270 |
| 5'10" | 132 | 139 | 146 | 153 | 160 | 167 | 174 | 181 | 188 | 195 | 202 | 207 | 243 | 278 |
| 5'11" | 136 | 143 | 150 | 157 | 165 | 172 | 179 | 186 | 193 | 200 | 208 | 215 | 250 | 286 |
| 6' | 140 | 147 | 154 | 162 | 169 | 177 | 184 | 191 | 199 | 206 | 213 | 221 | 258 | 294 |
| 6'1" | 144 | 151 | 159 | 166 | 174 | 182 | 189 | 197 | 204 | 212 | 219 | 227 | 265 | 302 |
| 6'2" | 148 | 155 | 163 | 171 | 179 | 186 | 194 | 202 | 210 | 218 | 225 | 233 | 272 | 311 |
| 6'3" | 152 | 160 | 168 | 176 | 184 | 192 | 200 | 208 | 216 | 224 | 232 | 240 | 279 | 219 |
| 6'4" | 156 | 164 | 172 | 180 | 189 | 197 | 205 | 213 | 221 | 230 | 238 | 246 | 287 | 328 |

BMI = weight/height$^2$.
* A BMI of approximately 27 appears to be the threshold at which insulin resistance begins to impair glucose disposal.

- Foods containing carbohydrate (fruits, vegetables, whole grains, low-fat dairy products) are important components of a healthy diet. These healthy foods should not be eliminated from the diet because of concerns of elevated glycemia.
- With the help of blood glucose monitoring, the amount of carbohydrate eaten at a particular meal or snack from day to day can be evaluated and adjustments can be made accordingly to find the amount of carbohydrate that can be tolerated by an individual (ie, carbohydrate load).

**D** The total amount of dietary fat consumed, regardless of the type (saturated or polyunsaturated), is associated with insulin resistance.[53-55] Therefore, both the amount and type of fat recommended in the food/meal plan is based on treatment goals and the individual's ability to make lifestyle changes.

- Low-fat diets can assist with weight maintenance[56,57] while high-fat diets may contribute to insulin resistance. A high intake of saturated fat is associated with elevated LDL cholesterol levels.[58]
- Lean individuals with elevated triglyceride levels may benefit from substituting monounsaturated fats for saturated fats and carbohydrates.[59]

**E** The benefits of physical activity are well documented. Physical activity is known to improve insulin sensitivity and enhance cellular glucose uptake by the muscle during or shortly after exercise[60-63] (see Chapter 2, Exercise, in Diabetes Management Therapies).

**F** Eating frequency (eg, having 3 meals per day or smaller but more frequent meals and snacks) is not associated with long-term differences in glucose, lipid, or insulin responses.[64] Therefore, the division of food intake should be based on individual preferences. However, due to a slowed first-phase insulin release, spacing meals and distributing food intake throughout the day may be beneficial.[65,66]

**G** It is important to help the person with diabetes focus on behaviors and attitudes that assist with long-term lifestyle changes.[67]

**H** Testing blood glucose levels premeal and postmeal provides tangible information to assist the person with diabetes in taking a more active role in evaluating food choices.

- If the person with diabetes has made all of the changes that he/she is able or willing to make and the target goals have not been achieved, a change in therapy (addition or changes in medication and/or doses) is needed.[68]
- Persons with diabetes need to be reminded that while food has a significant impact on glucose levels, other variables such as stress, physical activity, and illness also affect blood glucose levels and may be the reason, not food, for variances.

**3** The results of lifestyle changes are evident by 6 weeks to 3 months. Decisions regarding the success of MNT or the need to change therapy (nutrition and/or medical) should be made at this time.[18]

**A** The need to add or change medications should not be viewed as a "diet failure," but rather reflects the usual progression of type 2 diabetes due to beta cell dysfunction. As the disease progresses, therapy must also change. Therapy progresses from MNT alone to MNT combined with oral glucose-lowering agents and/or insulin.

## Nutrients, Food Sources, and Insulin

**1** The therapeutic goals of diabetes care include not only striving toward euglycemia, but also the accompanying return of normal carbohydrate, protein, and fat metabolism.

**2** Insulin is a hormone essential for the use and storage of these nutrients. The action of insulin is both anticatabolic (prevents breakdown) and anabolic (promotes storage), and it facilitates cellular transport of nutrients.

**A** Insulin suppresses hepatic glycogenolysis and gluconeogenesis and inhibits lipolysis and proteolysis. Insulin also stimulates glycogen synthesis and facilitates the transport of glucose into muscle cells.

**B** The effects of insulin are balanced by the effects of the counterregulatory hormones: glucagon, growth hormone, cortisol, epinephrine, and norepinephrine.

**3** Carbohydrate is the body's primary source of energy.

**A** Carbohydrate provides 4 kcal per gram.

**B** The following terminology is recommended for referring to the 3 types of carbohydrates: sugars, starch, and fiber. Terms such as complex carbohydrate, simple carbohydrates or sugars, and fast-acting carbohydrate should not be used because they are imprecise and have never been defined.[69]

- *Monosaccharides* and *disaccharides* (glucose, fructose, sucrose, lactose) are classified as sugars. Food sources include fruit, some vegetables, milk, and sweets. Fructose and galactose (from lactose) are primarily metabolized by the liver and converted into glycogen (and possibly triglycerides, in the case of fructose). Only a small amount is converted to glucose to cause increases in postprandial blood glucose levels. As a result, sugars (fructose, lactose, sucrose) produce a lower blood glucose response than starches and glucose.[70]

- *Polysaccharides* are classified as starch (amylopectin and amylose) or fiber. Nondigestible carbohydrate components of plants are commonly referred to as *food fiber*; however, a more accurate term for these components would be nonstarch polysaccharides. Food sources containing starch include cereal, grains, starchy vegetables (potato, winter squash, peas, corn), and legumes (peas, beans, lentils). The rate and completeness of digestion of starch depends on the structure of the starch, how it is packaged in the plant source, and how the starch-containing food is processed or cooked.[70]

- The glucose that is absorbed after digestion of the carbohydrate-containing foods is largely responsible for raising the blood glucose concentration; other food constituents play only a minor role in this process. However, the response is modified by the gastric emptying rate, intestinal motility, and factors that affect glucose removal from the circulation, such as the insulin response and/or insulin resistance. Usual intake of food fiber has little effect on the plasma glucose response, although it may result in a decrease in LDL cholesterol.[70]

**C** In the metabolism of carbohydrate, insulin facilitates entry of glucose into cells, stimulates glycogen synthesis in liver and muscle cells, and increases triglyceride stores by facilitating the entry of glucose into adipose tissue and its conversion to triglycerides. Without insulin, glucose production by the liver (*gluconeogenesis*) is accelerated and liver and muscle glycogenolysis occurs.

**4** Protein is necessary for growth and tissue maintenance and is a potential secondary source of energy.

**A** Protein contributes 4 kcal per gram.

**B** Dietary sources of protein are both animal (meat, milk, other dairy products) and vegetable (legumes, starches, nuts, seeds, vegetables). The source of the protein is not a concern. Vegetarian diets can easily meet protein needs, and specific food combinations at meals are not necessary.

**C** Ingested protein has minimal, if any, effect on blood glucose levels in people with mild type 2 diabetes. In people with type 1 diabetes who are adequately treated with insulin, ingested protein also has only a minimal effect on blood glucose concentration.[71] (See section on protein.)

**D** In the metabolism of protein, insulin lowers blood amino acids while reducing blood glucose levels, facilitates incorporation of amino acids into tissue protein, and decreases gluconeogenesis. Without adequate insulin, gluconeogenesis increases and proteolysis and amino acid release occurs in muscle.

**5** Fat in the form of free fatty acids (FFA) is used as an energy source.

**A** Fat contributes 9 kcal per gram.

**B** Dietary sources of fat are animal sources (meat, egg yolk, dairy-fat containing foods) and vegetable sources (margarine, oils, nuts, seeds, certain fruits [coconut, avocado]).

**C** Fats in foods are broken down into triglycerides (3 fatty acids attached to glycerol). *Triglycerides* are the form of fat that travels through the bloodstream and are stored in adipose tissue.

**D** In the metabolism of fat, insulin promotes lipogenesis by activating *lipoprotein lipase*, the enzyme that facilitates transport of triglycerides into adipose tissue for storage. Insulin also inhibits lipolysis and stimulates hepatic lipogenesis. Without adequate insulin, ketogenesis occurs in the liver, and lipolysis and fatty acid release occurs rapidly in adipose tissue, leading to excessive production of ketones and eventually ketoacidosis. Triglyceride levels also increase due to a decrease in cellular uptake of triglycerides.

**6** Vitamins and minerals are involved in a wide range of vital body functions. For example, vitamins are involved in the processing of other nutrients (such as carbohydrate, protein, fat, and minerals); minerals are components of many enzyme systems. They do not contribute calories or require insulin to be metabolized, although many micronutrients are intimately involved in carbohydrate and/or glucose metabolism as well as with insulin release and sensitivity.

**7** Water is also considered an essential nutrient and is an important component of body tissue, accounting for between one half to three fourths of body weight.

**A** Water is important in regulating body temperature and carrying nutrients to and waste products away from the cells.

**B** Water is involved in all of the chemical reactions in metabolism.

**C** Daily water losses need to be replaced from dietary sources such as water, beverages, and water in food.

## Carbohydrate in the Diabetes Food/Meal Plan

**1** A number of factors influence glycemic responses to foods, including the amount of carbohydrate, nature of the monosaccharide components, nature of the starch, cooking and food processing, and other food components. Blood glucose levels at the start of the meal also affect the glycemic response. In persons with type 1 diabetes, hyperglycemia has been shown to slow the gastric emptying rate[72] while hypoglycemia increases the gastric emptying rates.[73] In persons with type 2 diabetes, the form of the food[74] and the severity of glucose intolerance,[75] insulin resistance, or insulin deficiency alter postmeal glycemic responses.

**2** A commonly held belief was that sugars, both added and naturally occurring, are rapidly absorbed and lead to hyperglycemia. However, sucrose and other sugars do not have more of a deleterious effect on blood glucose levels and are not absorbed more rapidly than starches. Research has consistently shown that sucrose and other sugars do not have a greater impact on blood glucose levels than other carbohydrates when consumed separately or as part of a meal or snack.[75-79]

   **A** The ADA recommends that sucrose can be used as part of the total carbohydrate in the meal plan, not additive carbohydrate, and in the context of an otherwise healthful eating plan.[1,2]

   **B** Because many factors, often unpredictable, affect the glycemic responses to different carbohydrates in persons with diabetes, the total carbohydrate content of meals and snacks should be the first priority.

     • Evidence from studies on healthy subjects supports the importance of including carbohydrate such as fruits, vegetables, grains, and milk in the diet.

     • Foods containing significant amounts of added sugars (eg, regular soft drinks, syrups, desserts) not only contribute large amounts of carbohydrate to the diet but may be high in calories and/or fat as well.

**3** Recommendations for fiber intake are the same for persons with diabetes as for the general population. In persons with type 2 diabetes, a diet containing 50 g per day of food fiber, compared with 24 g per day, improved glycemia and lipids.[80] Diets containing more typical amounts of food fiber (approximately 15 to 20 g) have not been shown to be beneficial.[81,82] In persons with type 1 diabetes and normal HbA$_{1c}$ levels, a daily intake of 56 g of fiber had no beneficial effect on glycemic control or insulin requirements.[33] However, in persons with type 1 diabetes, a daily intake of approximately 17 g of fiber had beneficial effects on lipid levels and decreased the risk of cardiovascular disease.[83] A dose relationship between fiber and the glycemic response would be expected; however, no such study has been done to evaluate this relationship.

   **A** The average dietary fiber intake for adults is 10 to 30 g per day, with men averaging 19 g and women averaging 13 g.

   **B** It is recommended that all Americans choose a variety of fiber-containing foods, such as whole grains, fruits, and vegetables, because they provide vitamins, minerals, fiber, and other substances important for good health.[4] This would also apply to persons with diabetes.

**4** The *glycemic index* represents the blood glucose area above the fasting glucose concentration following the ingestion of a 50-g carbohydrate portion of food compared with the blood glucose area obtained with a 50-g carbohydrate portion of either glucose or white bread as an index food. The glucose area response to the index food is considered to be 100%. The response to other foods is given as a percentage of that obtained from the index food.

   **A** In people with type 1 and type 2 diabetes, several studies have reported improvements in glycemic control after incorporating low glycemic index foods into the diet, while other studies have reported no differences in long-term glycemic control or insulin requirements from a low glycemic index diet.[2] It is therefore not warranted at this time to make any specific recommendations concerning the use of low glycemic index foods.

   **B** Although the glycemic response is often unpredictable and variable, the glycemic index may be used with preprandial and postprandial glucose results for fine-tuning postmeal hyperglycemia.

**5** Nutritive (caloric) sweeteners are included in the carbohydrate total for meals and/or snacks.

   **A** Scientific evidence does not support the widely held belief that sugars should be avoided based on the assumption that sucrose and other sugars are more rapidly digested and absorbed than starch-containing foods, thereby aggravating hyperglycemia. Sucrose should be substituted for other carbohydrate sources in the food/meal plan or, if added, adequately covered with insulin or other glucose-lowering agents.

   **B** Fructose produces a lower postprandial glucose response than sucrose or starch.[84] This potential benefit may be offset by the concern that fructose may have adverse effects on plasma lipids.[85] However, there is no reason to recommend that persons with diabetes avoid naturally occurring fructose in fruits, vegetables, and other foods.

   **C** *Sugar alcohols* such as sorbitol, mannitol, xylitol, and starch hydrolysates may also produce a lower glucose response than sucrose or glucose and are lower in calories (average, 2 kcal/g) than other sugars (4 kcal/g).[86] No evidence exists that these sweeteners have advantages or disadvantages over sucrose in decreasing the amount of carbohydrate or calories in the diet or in improving overall diabetes control. Consuming amounts greater than 10 g per day of some polyols, such as sorbitol, may cause diarrhea.

**6** *Nonnutritive (low-calorie) sweeteners* currently available include saccharine, aspartame, acesulfame K, and sucralose. Approval is being sought from the US Food and Drug Administration (FDA) for alitame and cyclamates. All FDA-approved nonnutritive sweeteners undergo rigorous testing and are not allowed on the market unless they are safe for the general public to consume, including people with diabetes and pregnant women.

   **A** The *acceptable daily intake* (ADI) is defined as the amount of a food additive that can be safely consumed on a daily basis over a person's lifetime without any adverse effects. This determination includes a 100-fold safety factor and is determined by the FDA.

     • The ADI for aspartame is 50 mg/kg/body weight/day. Aspartame consumption (14-day average) in persons with diabetes has been found to be 2 to 4 mg/kg/day.[87]

The average amount of aspartame is 200 mg per 12-oz diet soft drink and 35 mg per packet of tabletop sweetener.[88]

- The ADI for acesulfame K is 15 mg/kg/body weight/day. The average amount of acesulfame K is 40 mg per 12-oz diet soft drink (based on the most typical blend with 90 mg aspartame) and 50 mg per packet of tabletop sweetener.[88]
- The ADI for sucralose is 5 mg/kg/body weight/day. The average amount of sucralose is 70 mg per 12-oz diet soft drink and 5 mg per packet of tabletop sweetener.[88]
- The US does not have an ADI for saccharin because it is not a food additive, but the World Health Organization's Joint Expert Committee of Food Additives (JECFA) has set an ADI of 5 mg/kg/body weight/day. The average amount of saccharin is 140 mg per 12-oz diet soft drink and 40 mg per packet of tabletop sweetener.[88]

**B** Nonnutritive sweeteners are safe to use during pregnancy. Aspartame use has shown no risk to the fetus when ingested in amounts at least 3 times the ADI.[89] Multigenerational studies on rats with acesulfame K and sucralose have shown no adverse effects on fertility, number of offspring, birth weight, mortality, or fetal development.[90] Although saccharin can cross the placenta to the fetus, there is no evidence that this compound is harmful if consumed during pregnancy.

## Protein in the Diabetes Food/Meal Plan

**1** In the United States, protein intake is between 15% and 20% of the average adult caloric intake. Protein intake is fairly consistent across all ages from infancy to older age.[91]

**A** There is no evidence to suggest a change in usual protein intake. Although consuming 20% of calories from protein is approximately double the adult recommended daily allowance (RDA) for protein, there is limited evidence that protein intake at this level correlates with the development of nephropathy.[91]

**B** One gram of protein per kilogram of body weight will meet the protein needs of most adults, and 1.2 g of protein per kilogram of body weight will meet the protein needs for most children, adolescents, and athletes.

**C** *Protein foods* such as lean meats, low-fat dairy products, and/or low-fat plant protein foods should be selected for a low-fat diet.

**2** The rate of protein degradation and conversion of protein to glucose in individuals with diabetes depends on the state of insulinization and degree of glycemic control.

**A** In persons with poorly controlled diabetes, gluconeogenesis can occur rapidly and adversely affect glycemic control.[92]

**B** In persons with controlled type 2 diabetes, ingested protein does not increase plasma glucose levels. However, in individuals still able to secrete insulin, protein ingestion is just as potent as glucose in stimulating insulin. Furthermore, the peak response to consuming carbohydrate alone or carbohydrate plus protein is similar.[93]

**C** In persons with well-controlled type 1 diabetes, the addition of protein did not slow the absorption of carbohydrate, change peak glucose response, or affect glucose levels at 5 hours.[94] Furthermore, the addition of protein for the treatment of hypoglycemia did not prevent recurrent hypoglycemia.[95]

**D** Persons with diabetes are often taught that because 50% to 60% of protein can be converted to glucose, protein will have half the effect on glucose levels as carbohydrate, and this effect will occur 3 hours to 4 hours after ingestion, thus preventing hypoglycemia. However, the available evidence suggests this is not true.[2] Although approximately 50% to 60% of protein can be converted to glucose, this glucose does not increase the rate of glucose release from the liver and enter the general circulation.[91] What happens to the glucose is unknown, but it is speculated that this glucose is stored in the liver (or muscle) as glycogen.

**3** Individuals with diabetes have traditionally been taught to have a food source of protein before bedtime, or to include protein with other snacks or even before exercise. It is doubtful, however, that the added protein has any beneficial effect.

    **A** To prevent overnight hypoglycemia in insulin users, the following approaches can be used, although it is unknown which is most helpful: adjusting insulin doses appropriately, ingesting carbohydrate alone, or adding protein to the carbohydrate snack.

**4** Although there is an interest in the role of low-carbohydrate, high-protein diets in both glycemic and weight control, carbohydrate foods are still important in a healthful diet. It is unknown whether individuals with diabetes can follow a diet high in protein and low in carbohydrate for an extended time. It is also unknown whether weight loss and/or improvements in glycemia are maintained better on these diets in the long-term than with more conventional low-calorie diets.[91] *or long-term health risks*

**5** Currently recommended treatment for nephropathy focuses on methods that might reverse microalbuminuria or slow the rate of decline in macroalbuminuria and includes reducing blood pressure with angiotension-converting enzyme (ACE) inhibitors, improving glycemia, or reducing protein intake.[96]

    **A** There is no clear evidence to make specific nutrition recommendations for people with diabetes who have either microalbuminuria or clinical nephropathy, based on a small number of clinical studies with some methodological problems.

      • There is supportive evidence for reducing protein intake with microalbuminuria. A protein reduction of 0.8 to 1 g/kg/day is associated with renal improvement. However, the first priority for individuals with microalbuminuria should be to maintain near normal glycemic control and normal blood pressure.

      • With the onset of clinical nephropathy, there is supportive evidence that lowering protein intake to 0.8 g/kg/day or lower may slow the progression toward end-stage renal disease. Protein status should be monitored closely so that the patient's nutritional status is not compromised.[1,2]

    **B** The differing effects of animal and vegetable protein on renal function are currently under investigation. Longer term controlled clinical trials are needed to determine whether a certain type of protein (plant versus animal, different plant or animal proteins) has a beneficial effect on reducing the risk or slowing the progression of early or late diabetes-related renal disease.

## Fat in the Diabetes Food/Meal Plan

**1** Several diabetes-related diet factors influence the risk of developing macrovascular disease (see Chapter 6, Macrovascular Disease, in Diabetes and Complications).

**A** *Saturated fats* raise blood cholesterol levels.[58] Food sources of saturated fats are animal fats (meat, butterfat, lard, bacon); coconut, palm, and palm kernel oils; dairy-fat-containing foods (whole milk, cheese); and hydrogenated vegetable oils. *Trans fatty acids* are found in processed foods (boxed cakes, candy bars, cookies, doughnuts, fried foods, pastries, microwave pastries), hard margarines, and shortenings. Saturated fats account for 12% to 14% of total calories while *trans fatty acids* account for only 2% to 3% of total calories.

**B** *Polyunsaturated fats (n-6 or omega-6)* have been shown to lower cholesterol levels but have a heterogeneous effect on HDL cholesterol levels. Food sources of polyunsaturated fats are vegetable oils (corn, safflower, soybean, sunflower, cottonseed) and walnuts.

**C** *Monounsaturated fats* lower total cholesterol but do not lower HDL cholesterol levels. Food sources of monounsaturated fats are canola, olive, and peanut oils; olives; and nuts (except walnuts).

**D** *N-3 or omega-3 polyunsaturated fats (fish oils)* have an antiplatelet clotting effect and have been shown to lower serum triglycerides. Food sources of omega-3 polyunsaturated fats are fish from cold, deep water; fatty fish such as salmon, herring, albacore tuna, mackerel, and sardines; and plant sources such as flax, walnuts, and canola oil.

**E** *Dietary cholesterol* affects the LDL cholesterol concentration by competing for the cell receptors for LDL cholesterol. Dietary cholesterol is found only in animal food sources. Some individuals are more sensitive to the cholesterol-raising effects of dietary cholesterol than others. Food sources that contribute cholesterol in the American diet include egg yolks, organ meats (especially liver), dairy-fat-containing food products, and meats.

**F** A diet high in total fat can increase chylomicron levels leading to atherogenic remnant particles. (*Chylomicrons* carry food cholesterol and triglycerides from the intestinal mucosa to the liver.)

**2** Saturated fat is the principal dietary determinant of LDL cholesterol levels. There is evidence that persons with diabetes, compared with nondiabetic persons, have an increased risk of coronary heart disease with a higher intake of dietary cholesterol.[97] The debate about this topic is not whether saturated fat and cholesterol be restricted, but what is the best alternative energy source for the person with diabetes.[2]

**A** Diets enriched with monounsaturated fat and low-fat, high-carbohydrate diets improve glucose tolerance and lipid levels compared with diets high in saturated fat.[2]

**B** A diet high in polyunsaturated fat compared with a diet high in monounsaturated fat results in a higher total and LDL cholesterol concentration in persons with type 2 diabetes.[98]

**3** Because 15% to 20% of usual daily calories are from protein, approximately 10% from saturated fat and 10% from polyunsaturated fat, the combined carbohydrate and monounsaturated fat intake will be about 60% to 70% of total daily calories. The division of calories depends on treatment goals such as identified lipid problems; glucose, lipid, and weight goals; and patient preferences.

**A** Less than 10% of total daily calories should be from saturated fats; some individuals may benefit from lowering their intake of saturated fats to less than 7% of daily calories. Dietary cholesterol intake should be 300 mg or less per day; some individuals may benefit from lowering their intake to 200 mg or less per day. Trans fatty acids should also be restricted.[1,2]

**B** To lower LDL cholesterol concentration, saturated fats in the diet can be replaced with either monounsaturated fats or carbohydrate depending on patient preferences (eg, some ethnic groups may prefer monounsaturated fats while other groups may prefer carbohydrate replacements for saturated fat).

- In weight maintenance diets, both high carbohydrate and high monounsaturated fat diets lower LDL cholesterol levels. However, the high carbohydrate diet may modestly increase fasting triglyceride levels.[59] In energy restricted diets, both low fat (high carbohydrate) and high monounsaturated fat diets have been shown to have beneficial effects on lipids, including triglycerides.[99]

**C** Polyunsaturated fat should be limited to less than 10% of calories.

**4** To lower triglyceride levels, efforts at improving glycemic control, achieving moderate weight loss, and increasing physical activity have all been shown to be beneficial. Persons with treated diabetes and with triglyceride levels greater than 1000 mg/dL (11 mmol/L) should have acute restriction of all types of dietary fat and treatment with medications to reduce the risk of pancreatitis.

**5** Although controversial, higher intake of total dietary fat in persons with type 2 diabetes, regardless of the type (saturated, monounsaturated, or polyunsaturated), has been associated with insulin resistance.[54,55]

**A** Fat intake should be individualized. With maintenance isoenergic intake, weight balance is the same on high-carbohydrate or high-monounsaturated fat diets.

**B** Low-fat diets, however, have been shown to assist with weight loss and weight maintenance.[56,57]

**6** Eating two to three servings of fish per week provides dietary n-3 polyunsaturated fat and is encouraged. Effects on LDL cholesterol should be monitored with the use of n-3 supplements, but glucose metabolism is not likely to be adversely affected. N-3 supplements may be beneficial in the treatment of severe hypertriglyceridemia.[100]

**7** The FDA regulatory process provides reasonable assurance that current fat replacers/substitutes are safe to use in food.[88,101]

**A** These substitutes are generally classified according to the nutrients from which they are made.

- Carbohydrate sources of fat replacements are dextrins, maltodextrins, modified food starches, polydextrose, cellulose, and gums.
- Protein sources of fat substitutes are microparticulated proteins from egg whites or milk and texturized proteins.
- Several sources of fat replacements from fat (eg, caprenin, salatrim, and olestra) currently are available in foods that are on the market, and others are under development.

**B** Overt use of foods with fat replacers may help reduce dietary fat but may not reduce total energy intake or weight. People with diabetes need to be aware of the macronutrient content and energy consumption of foods containing fat replacers to determine how these foods impact their individualized treatment goals.

**C** Some fat substitutes such as olestra inhibit the absorption of fat-soluble nutrients, and even if replaced with known lost nutrients, the long-term effects are currently unknown.[102]

## Vitamins and Minerals in Diabetes Management

**1** People differ in their sensitivity to sodium; however, people with type 2 diabetes are more sodium-sensitive than the general public.[103] Moderate sodium intake is recommended. In general, sodium intake should be limited to less than 2400 mg/day.[4,104] The DASH sodium study provides strong support for reducing sodium intake.[105]

**A** A teaspoon of salt (5 g) contains 2300 mg of sodium. The amount of sodium in food products is listed on the nutrition label as mg per serving.

**B** Single servings of foods that contain more than 400 mg of sodium, or entrees with more than 800 mg of sodium, are considered significant sources of sodium in the diet.

**C** The FDA defines a *low-sodium food* as having 140 mg or less of sodium per serving.

**2** Evaluating the micronutrient status of people with diabetes involves a comprehensive clinical history and physical examination. In addition, a comprehensive food/nutrition history should be done, including use of health foods; over-the-counter vitamins, minerals, and herbal supplements; and methods of preparing foods.[1,2]

**A** Persons with diabetes should be educated about the importance of obtaining daily vitamin and mineral requirements from natural food sources as well as the potential toxicity of megadoses of vitamin and mineral supplementation.

**B** Persons who may benefit from vitamin and mineral supplements include those on extremely low-calorie diets, strict vegetarians, the elderly, pregnant or lactating women, those taking medications known to alter micronutrient metabolism, persons in poor metabolic control (with glycosuria), or persons in critical care environments.[106]

**3** Vitamin supplementation in pharmacological doses should be viewed as a therapeutic intervention and, therefore, should be subjected to stringent placebo-controlled trials to demonstrate safety and efficacy.

**4** The following supplements are of special interest for persons with diabetes:

**A** Deficiency of certain minerals such as potassium, magnesium, and possibly zinc and chromium may aggravate carbohydrate intolerance. Potassium and magnesium assessment can be done, but the need for zinc and chromium in persons with diabetes has not been established.[1,2]

**B** Daily intake of 1000 mg to 1200 mg of elemental calcium, especially in older persons with diabetes, appears to be safe and likely will reduce the incidence of metabolic bone disease. However, the value of calcium supplementation in younger age groups is uncertain.[107]

**C** The role of folate in preventing birth defects is widely accepted. However, the association between homocysteine levels and cardiovascular disease and the role of folate supplementation in reducing cardiovascular events is unclear.[108]

**D** The potential benefits of chromium supplementation in persons with diabetes have not been conclusively demonstrated. Until larger clinical trials are conducted in countries similar to the United States and where chromium deficiency is not of concern, it is prudent to avoid chromium supplementation. Long-term benefits from pharmacological doses of chromium (1000 mg) on glycemia and lipids are unknown.[2]

**E** Large observational epidemiological studies have shown a correlation between antioxidants and clinical outcomes. However, large placebo-controlled intervention clinical trials have failed to show benefits, and in some studies an increase in complications was observed. The Heart Outcomes Prevention Evaluation Study (HOPE) included 9451 subjects, 38% of whom had diabetes. Supplementation with 400 IU of vitamin E for 4.5 years did not result in any significant benefits.[109] Because of the uncertainties as to the efficacy or safety of long-term supplementation, it is advisable to discourage routine supplementation with antioxidant vitamins.[1,2]

**5** The impact of herbal medicines on glycemia and lipids requires long-term, placebo-controlled clinical trials to demonstrate efficacy and safety. At present, there is no evidence to suggest benefits. (See Chapter 6, Biological Complementary Therapies in Diabetes, in Diabetes in the Life Cycle and Research).

## Alcohol and Diabetes Management

**1** The same precautions regarding the use of alcohol that apply to the general public also apply to persons with diabetes. Abstaining from alcohol should be advised for people with a history of alcohol abuse, during pregnancy, and for people with other medical conditions such as pancreatitis, advanced neuropathy, and elevated triglycerides. Alcohol also may potentiate or interfere with the action of other medications.[1,2]

**2** The effect of alcohol on blood glucose levels is dependent on the amount of alcohol ingested as well as the relationship to food intake.[110]

**A** Alcohol is absorbed from the stomach and small intestine and, because of its toxicity, is metabolized in the liver before other nutrients are metabolized.

**B** Alcohol does not require insulin to be metabolized even though it is used as an energy source.

**C** Alcohol is not converted to glucose; excessive amounts of alcohol can potentially be converted to fats.

**3** Alcohol blocks *gluconeogenesis* (the release of glucose from the liver) and interferes with the counterregulation to insulin-induced hypoglycemia.

**A** Because alcohol cannot be used as a source of glucose, hypoglycemia can result when alcohol is consumed without food.

**B** Hypoglycemia can occur at blood alcohol levels that do not exceed mild intoxication, and the hypoglycemic effect may persist from 8 to 12 hours after the last drink.

**4** When alcohol is ingested in moderation and with food, blood glucose levels are not affected by the ingestion of moderate amounts of alcohol.[111]

**A** Daily intake should be limited to no more than 1 drink for adult women and 2 drinks for adult men and should be ingested with food.[1]

**B** Alcoholic drinks are an addition to the meal plan. No food should be omitted because of the possibility of alcohol-induced hypoglycemia.

**C** The type of drink does not make a difference. One drink is defined as 12 oz beer, 5 oz wine, or 1½ oz hard liquor (distilled spirits).

**5** Epidemiological evidence in nondiabetic persons suggests that light-to-moderate alcohol ingestion in adults is associated with increased insulin sensitivity and decreased risk of type 2 diabetes, coronary heart disease, and stroke. Several population-based prospective studies[112-114] have reported a decreased risk of coronary heart disease with light-to-moderate alcohol consumption in adult men and women with diabetes. Additional prospective long-term studies are needed to confirm these observations in persons with diabetes.

## Translating Diabetes Nutrition Recommendations Into Clinical Practice

**1** MNT includes recommendations for food/nutrition and physical activity and the process or system for providing nutrition care.

**2** There are 4 steps for assisting persons with diabetes in acquiring and maintaining the knowledge, skills, attitudes, behaviors, and commitment to meet the challenges of daily diabetes self-management successfully.

**A** Assess the individual's food/nutrition and diabetes self-management knowledge and skills.

**B** Conduct intervention/education involving a careful match of a food/meal planning approach and educational materials to meet the individual's needs, keeping the plan flexible to make it doable for the individual.

**C** Identify and negotiate mutually designed goals.

**D** Evaluate outcomes and ongoing monitoring and education.

**3** The process of providing nutrition therapy for diabetes has shifted from nutrition prescriptions based on formulas for caloric requirements and percentage of calories from macronutrients to individualized recommendations based on assessment and mutual goal setting. Furthermore, a system for providing ongoing nutrition care is essential.[68,115]

**4** The following outcomes can be expected from MNT.

**A** In newly diagnosed persons with type 2 diabetes, the United Kingdom Prospective Diabetes Study reported an average decrease in HbA$_{1c}$ of 2% from intensive nutrition therapy provided by dietitians.[16]

**B** In persons with type 2 diabetes with an average duration of 4 years, a clinical trial using nutrition practice guidelines (NPG) for type 2 diabetes reported an average decrease in HbA$_{1c}$ of 1% from intensive nutrition therapy provided by dietitians who followed the NPG.[18]

**C** In newly diagnosed persons with type 1 diabetes, a clinical trial using the NPG for type 1 diabetes reported an average decrease in HbA$_{1c}$ of 1% from intensive nutrition therapy provided by dietitians who followed the NPG.[17]

**D** In persons participating in the intensive therapy arm of the Diabetes Control and Complications Trial, those who reported following their meal plan approximately 90% of the time had HbA$_{1c}$ levels 1% lower than those who reported following their meal plan only approximately 40% of the time.[15]

**E** Depending on the duration of diabetes and previous eating habits, nutrition therapy can be expected to lower HbA$_{1c}$ levels by an average of 1% to 2%. The outcomes of nutrition therapy will be known by 6 weeks to 3 months.[18]

**5** Certain assessments are needed to develop a MNT plan.[63,108]

**A** The following minimum referral data are needed before beginning a nutrition assessment:
- Diabetes treatment program
- Laboratory data (HbA$_{1c}$ levels, fasting/nonfasting plasma glucose, cholesterol and fractionations, fasting triglycerides, and microalbumin [when appropriate])
- Blood pressure
- Medical history
- Medications that affect nutrition therapy
- Medical clearance and/or limitations for exercise

**B** The following patient parameters need to be assessed:
- Anthropometric measures
- Biochemical indices and laboratory data
- Clinical signs
- Food/nutrition history
- Learning style, cultural heritage, religious practices, food-related beliefs, attitudes and concerns, and socioeconomic status

**C** A complete food/nutrition history is needed. Two methods that can be used to assess eating patterns and food choices are a food history taken by the dietitian or food records (for 1 to 3 days) kept by the individual.

**D** A preliminary meal plan can be designed using the food history and the food/nutrition assessment information. The nutrition history form shown in Figure 1.2 can be used to record and modify usual food intake; calculations for the meal plan can then be done based on these data (Figure 1.3).
- A registered dietitian has the major responsibility for working with the patient to develop an appropriate meal plan. Although the nutrition history form in Figure 1.2 is based on the exchange system, the use of exchanges is not necessarily the preferred meal planning approach. The advantage of this form is that it allows the meal plan to be based on the modification of usual eating habits instead of beginning with a predetermined calorie level that is usually not appropriate and then calculating the percentages of calories for macronutrients.
- Nutrient values from the exchange lists (Table 1.3) are useful for evaluating the nutrition assessment and making calculations for the meal plan.[116,117] However, after completing an assessment, the dietitian may determine that the blood glucose goals and meal planning can be best achieved by using basic nutrition or diabetes nutrition guidelines or by using carbohydrate counting.
- Adult calorie needs vary depending on the level of activity, age, and desired weight change. The most accurate method for estimating caloric needs is with a detailed nutrition history of usual food intake that is completed by a dietitian. General guidelines for estimating adult energy requirements are shown in Table 1.4.
- Energy should be prescribed to provide for normal growth and development in children and adolescents. To determine normal growth and weight profiles, the growth of children and adolescents should be monitored on a weight and height growth grid at a minimum of every 3 to 6 months. Children's calorie requirements should be based on a food/nutrition history. The meal plan is not intended to restrict calories but to ensure a reasonably consistent food intake and nutritionally balanced eating pattern. Several methods can be used to evaluate

the adequacy of energy intake (Table 1.5). Parents of young children and adolescents need to be taught to adjust the insulin dose rather than restrict food intake to control blood glucose levels.

- For persons requiring insulin therapy, once the food/meal plan has been mutually determined, insulin regimens can be planned and adjusted to match the individual's customary food intake and activity schedule. For persons on fixed insulin regimens, meals (and snacks) still need to be synchronized with the time actions of the insulins that the patient is injecting. Intensive insulin therapy or use of insulin pumps provides more flexibility in timing and choices of food.
- For persons with type 2 diabetes, having smaller meals and snacks spaced throughout the day may assist in controlling postmeal hyperglycemia.

**E** The preliminary food/meal plan can be evaluated by asking the following questions.

- Is the food/meal plan appropriate for reaching blood glucose and other metabolic goals?
- Does the food/meal plan take into account personal preferences, cultural background, and religious practices?
- Does the food/meal plan encourage healthful eating?
- Are the calories appropriate?

**6** A patient-centered or empowerment approach can improve adherence to MNT. Successful nutrition therapy involves a process of problem solving, adjustment, and readjustment.[118] Nutrition self-management and education occurs in 2 phases.

**A** Initial education provides the information needed at the time of diagnosis, when the patient's treatment program or lifestyle changes, or at the time of initial contact with a patient. Initial skill topics provide information about basic nutrition, diabetes nutrition guidelines, and beginning strategies for altering eating patterns; these are considered basic nutrition therapy survival skills for all persons with diabetes. Basic educational tools are used to discuss initial changes in eating habits (eg, making better food choices, spreading carbohydrate-containing foods throughout the day, eating less fat).

- Identify and monitor outcomes after the second or third visit (approximately 6 weeks after the initial nutrition consult) to determine whether the individual is making progress toward personal goals.
- If no progress is evident, the individual and educator need to reassess and consider making possible revisions to the nutrition plan.
- If the patient has done all that he/she can do or is willing to do and blood glucose levels are not in the target range, notify the provider that medications need to be added or adjusted.
- Food diaries can be helpful for all phases of self-management and education. Food diaries have been shown to be an effective strategy for helping patients make positive changes in their eating patterns as well as reach and maintain weight goals. Patients write down everything they eat, including approximate amounts and the circumstances under which the food was eaten, over a specified time. Food diaries can be kept for 1 day each week, a few days each month, or longer periods (Table 1.6).

# Figure 1.2. Example of Nutrition History Form

| Food Group | MEAL/SNACK/TIME Breakfast | Snack | Lunch | Snack | Dinner | Snack | Total servings/day | CHO (g) | Protein (g) | Fat* (g) | Calories |
|---|---|---|---|---|---|---|---|---|---|---|---|
| Starch | | | | | | | | 15 | 3 | 1 | 80 |
| Fruit | | | | | | | | 15 | | | 60 |
| Milk, Skim | | | | | | | | 12 | 8 | 1 | 90 |
| Vegetables | | | | | | | | 5 | 2 | | 25 |
| Meats/Substitutes | | | | | | | | | 7 | (8)(5)(3)(1) | (100)(75)(55)(35) |
| Fats | | | | | | | | | | 5 | 45 |
| Carbohydrate Choices | | | | | | | | | | | |
| TOTAL | | | | | | | | | | | |
| Calories | | | | | | | | × 4 = | × 4 = | × 9 = | Total = |
| Percent Calories | | | | | | | | | | | |

*Calculations are based on medium-fat meats and skim/very-low-fat milk. If diet consists predominantly of lean meats, use the factor 3 g fat instead of 5 g fat; if predominantly very lean meats, use 1 g fat; if predominantly high-fat meats, use 8 g fat. If low-fat (2%) milk is used, use 5 g fat; if whole milk is used, use 8 g fat.
Source: Adapted from Franz M. A new era in nutrition therapy for diabetes. On the Cutting Edge [Newsletter]. 1995;16(2):6.

# Figure 1.3. Example of Completed Nutrition History Form

| Food Group | MEAL/SNACK/TIME Breakfast | Snack | Lunch | Snack | Dinner | Snack | Total servings/ day | CHO (g) | Protein (g) | Fat* (g) | Calories |
|---|---|---|---|---|---|---|---|---|---|---|---|
| Starch | | | | | | | | 15 | 3 | 1 | 80 |
| Fruit | | | | | | | | 15 | | | 60 |
| Milk, Skim | | | | | | | | 12 | 8 | 1 | 90 |
| Vegetables | | | | | | | | 5 | 2 | | 25 |
| Meats/Substitutes | | | | | | | | | 7 | (8)(5)(3)(1) | (100)(75)(55)(35) |
| Fats | | | | | | | | | | 5 | 45 |
| Carbohydrate Choices | | | | | | | | | | | |

| TOTAL | | | |
|---|---|---|---|
| Calories | × 4 = | × 4 = | × 9 = |
| Percent Calories | | | Total = |

*Calculations are based on medium-fat meats and skim/very-low-fat milk. If diet consists predominantly of lean meats, use the factor 3 g fat instead of 5 g fat; if predominantly high-fat meats, use 8 g fat. If low-fat (2%) milk is used, use 5 g fat; if whole milk is used, use 8 g fat.
*Source:* Adapted from Franz M. A new era in nutrition therapy for diabetes. On the Cutting Edge [Newsletter]. 1995;16(2):6.

## Table 1.3. Macronutrient and Caloric Values per Serving for 1995 Exchange List

| Groups/Lists | Carbohydrate (g) | Protein (g) | Fat (g) | Calories |
|---|---|---|---|---|
| *Carbohydrates* | | | | |
| Starch | 15 | 3 | 1 or less | 80 |
| Fruit | 15 | — | — | 60 |
| Milk | | | | |
|   Skim | 12 | 8 | 0-3 | 90 |
|   Low-fat | 12 | 8 | 5 | 120 |
|   Whole | 12 | 8 | 8 | 150 |
| Other Carbohydrates | 15 | Varies | Varies | Varies |
| *Vegetables* | 5 | 2 | — | 25 |
| *Meat and substitutes* | | | | |
|   Very lean | — | 7 | 0-1 | 35 |
|   Lean | — | 7 | 3 | 55 |
|   Medium-fat | — | 7 | 5 | 75 |
|   High-fat | — | 7 | 8 | 100 |
| *Fat* | — | — | 5 | 45 |

## Table 1.4. Estimating Maintenance Calories for Adults

Approximate caloric requirements for adults based on actual weight

10 kcal/lb (20 kcal/kg) = kcal for obese or very inactive persons and chronic dieters
13 kcal/lb (25 kcal/kg) = kcal for persons over age 55, active women, and sedentary men
15 kcal/lb (30 kcal/kg) = kcal for active men or very active women
20 kcal/lb (40 kcal/kg) = kcal for very active men or athletes

**B** Continuing/in-depth self-management education is the comprehensive level of education that includes both management skills and lifestyle changes (Table 1.7). Continuing education provides essential education for ongoing nutrition self-management. Topics emphasized or chosen are based on the patient's choice; lifestyle; level of nutrition knowledge; and experience in planning, purchasing, and preparing food and meals. During this second phase, which is ongoing, individuals are taught to make adjustments in meal planning for a number of situations. Flexibility in meal planning is also addressed.

## Table 1.5. Estimating Calorie Requirements for Youth

- Base calories on nutrition assessment
- Validate calorie needs using one of the following formulas:

Method 1
- 1000 kcal for 1st year
- Add 100 kcal/y up to age 10 years
- Girls 11 to 15 years old: add 100 kcal or less per year after age 10 years
- Girls >15 years old: calculate as an adult
- Boys 11 to 15 age years old: add 200 kcal/y after age 10 years
- Boys >15 years old: 23 kcal/lb (50 kcal/kg) very active; 18 kcal/lb (40 kcal/kg) usual; 15 to 16 kcal/lb (30 to 35 kcal/kg) sedentary

Method 2
- 1000 kcal for 1st year
- Add 125 kcal x age for boys; 100 kcal x age for girls; up to 20% more kcal for activity
- For toddlers 1 to 3 years old: 40 kcal per inch length

## Table 1.6. Using Food Diaries

*Patients who might benefit from keeping food diaries*
- Those starting a new food/meal plan
- Those initiating intensive insulin therapy or insulin pumps
- Those having problems with blood glucose control
- Those needing motivation to follow their food/meal plan
- Those wanting to lose weight
- Those needing help in setting short-term and long-term goals

*What can be learned from food diaries*
- How much carbohydrate is usually eaten at meals or for snacks
- Portion sizes
- Unconscious eating or nibbling patterns
- Eating from boredom, being tired, being under stress, etc
- Skipping planned meals and/or snacks
- Eating food in places other than at the table
- Food choices, such as foods high in fat, foods with hidden fats, excessive sweets, etc
- Level of exercise

*How information from food diaries can be used*
- To determine what, where, and how much food was eaten
- To identify improvements that can be made
- To identify progress made toward short-term goals
- To determine the effect of food intake and activity on blood glucose levels (correlations can be made between foods eaten and blood glucose records)

## Table 1.7. Topics for Continuing/In-Depth Education

**Management Skills** *(Information required to make decisions to achieve management goals)*
- Food sources of carbohydrate, protein, fat
- How to use nutrition facts on food labels
- Meal planning and insulin adjustments for
    Illness
    Delay or changes in meal times
    Drinking alcoholic beverages
    Eating sugar-containing foods
    Exercise
    Travel
    Competitive athletics
    Holidays
- Treatment and prevention of hypoglycemia
- Nutritional management during short-term illness
- How to use blood glucose monitoring for problem solving and identifying blood glucose patterns
- Behavior change strategies
- Working rotating shifts, if needed

**Improvement of Lifestyle** *(Problem-solving skills)*
- Eating away from home
- Eating lunch in school cafeterias
- Brown bag lunches
- Special occasions, birthdays, holidays
- Grocery shopping
- New ideas for snacks
- Recipe modifications, menu ideas, cookbooks
- Reducing and modifying fat intake
- Reducing salt intake
- Vegetarian food choices
- Ethnic foods
- Use of convenience food
- How to fit foods with fat replacers and sugar substitutes into the meal plan
- Canning and freezing

**7** Appropriate documentation of nutrition self-management and education includes short-term and long-term goals, food/meal plan, educational topics addressed, assessment of patient acceptance and understanding, behavior changes, additional skills or information needed, additional recommendations, and plans for ongoing care. Effectiveness (outcomes) of nutrition interventions also need to be documented.

**8** Follow-up and ongoing/continuing education and care are essential parts of MNT.
　**A** Patients and team members need to understand that persons with diabetes need follow-up and ongoing, long-term nutrition care.

**B** It is recommended that persons with diabetes be seen periodically for continuing education, updating of the food/meal plan, and support.
- Adults should be seen every 6 months to 1 year or if there is any major change in work schedule, activity level, type of diabetes medication (especially insulin), blood glucose control, or medical status (development of complications). Weight management may require more frequent visits.[68]
- Children should be seen a minimum of every 6 months, preferably every 3 months. Calories need to be adjusted to accommodate growth and development requirements.[115]

## Translating Diabetes Nutrition Recommendations for Use in Healthcare Facilities

**1** Standardized calorie-level meal patterns based on exchange lists have traditionally been used to plan meals for hospitalized patients.

**A** The nutrition prescription was usually determined by a physician and ordered as an ADA diet with a specified calorie level and percentage of carbohydrate, protein, and fat.

**B** The term *ADA diet* is no longer appropriate since the American Diabetes Association does not endorse any single meal plan or specified percentages of macronutrients.[119,120]

**2** A number of alternative meal planning systems are available, each with various advantages and disadvantages. A preferred method of meal planning is to implement a *consistent day-to-day carbohydrate diabetes meal plan*. This method uses meal plans that incorporate consistent carbohydrate intake at meals and snacks, appropriate fat modifications, and consistent timing of meals and snacks instead of specific calorie levels.

**3** Meal plans that are labeled "no concentrated sweets," "no sugar added," "low sugar," and "liberal diabetic diets" are no longer appropriate. These diets do not reflect the current diabetes nutrition recommendations and unnecessarily restrict sucrose.

**4** Patients requiring clear-liquid or full-liquid diets should receive approximately 200 g of carbohydrate per day spread evenly throughout the day at meal and snack times to prevent starvation ketosis. Liquids included should not be sugar-free.

**5** Providing adequate nutrition is the primary concern for residents of long-term care facilities. It is appropriate to use the regular menu for residents with fairly consistent day-to-day amounts of carbohydrate at meals and snacks. Low-calorie meal plans are not generally needed.

## Methods for Teaching Food/Meal Planning

**1** No single meal planning approach works for every patient. For each phase of education, different educational resources may be needed. Basic nutrition interventions are needed for beginning education, and more complex tools may be needed as the counseling process continues. Preplanned printed diet sheets are ineffective and should not be used.

**2** Several meal planning approaches are available to teach basic nutrition and diabetes nutrition guidelines as well as more in-depth nutrition interventions.[121] The person with diabetes and the educator may begin with one meal planning approach and try other resources as the counseling process continues.

**3** Carbohydrate counting has become the preferred approach for food and meal planning.[122] This approach, which is appropriate for persons with all types of diabetes, is described in the next section.

**4** The following resources are some of the materials available from different organizations that can be used in teaching food/meal planning for diabetes.

   **A** *Dietary Guidelines for Americans*[4] and *The Food Guide Pyramid*[123] can be used as an introduction to basic nutrition and to begin the process of changing eating behaviors; these resources do not address issues specific to diabetes.

   **B** *The First Step in Diabetes Meal Planning*[24] is a basic, self-contained nutrition pamphlet based on the Food Guide Pyramid. It is designed to be given to patients to use until an individualized meal plan can be developed by a dietitian; this pamphlet also can be used in individualizing the meal plan.

   **C** *Healthy Food Choices*[124] is a pamphlet that illustrates the basics of good nutrition and the exchange lists. It opens into a mini-poster that provides a general overview of what to eat and when.

   **D** *Healthy Eating for People with Diabetes* (English and Spanish)[125] is a low-literacy booklet in which drawings are used to visually present nutrition concepts. The plate method for determining portion sizes is introduced.

   **E** *Exchange Lists for Meal Planning*[116,117] lists groups of measured foods of approximately the same nutritional value; foods in each list can be substituted or exchanged for other foods in the same list. The exchange lists are used with an individualized meal plan that specifies when and how many exchanges from each group are to be eaten for meals and/or snacks.

   **F** *Carbohydrate Counting: Getting Started*[126] is a booklet that introduces carbohydrate counting. It focuses on what foods contain carbohydrate, how to count carbohydrate, keeping simple food records, and how to eat consistent amounts of carbohydrate at meals and snacks.

   **G** *Carbohydrate Counting: Moving On*[127] is a booklet that focuses on identifying patterns in blood glucose levels related to food intake, diabetes medication (if used), and physical activity. It includes how to interpret records and take action based on blood glucose patterns.

   **H** *Carbohydrate Counting: Using Carbohydrate/Insulin Ratios*[128] is a booklet designed for people who take insulin and have chosen intensive diabetes management using multiple daily insulin injections or an insulin pump. Food and blood glucose records are used to fine-tune diabetes management by adjusting rapid-acting or short-acting insulin according to anticipated carbohydrate intake and physical activity. The relationship between food eaten and insulin injected is referred to as a *carbohydrate-to-insulin ratio*.

   **I** *My Food Plan*[129] is a booklet that provides a simplified approach to carbohydrate counting and meal planning. Common foods are grouped by approximate portion sizes. A personalized food plan provides for individualization; general guidelines for making healthful food choices are included. The booklet is also available in Spanish, *Mi Plan de Comidas*.[129]

**J** *My Food Plan for Kids & Teens*[130] teaches carbohydrate counting and good nutrition for youth with diabetes and includes fast foods, snack foods, and other favorites. *My Food Plan for Early Kidney Disease*[131] provides simple information about protein, phosphorous, and sodium. *My Food Plan Made Easy*[132] is a simplified, large-print version of *My Food Plan.*

**K** *Single-Topic Diabetes Resources*[133] is a set of 21 single-topic handouts that contain basic information about popular diabetes education topics as diverse as to how to treat hypoglycemia, nutrition and diabetes complications, and counseling parents of toddlers about food and diabetes.

**5** *Facilitating Lifestyle Change: A Resource Manual*[134] is designed to aid educators in working with patients who want to make changes in eating habits for blood glucose and/or weight control.

## Carbohydrate Counting

**1** Carbohydrate counting is useful for all persons with diabetes. Some individuals will benefit from simply knowing which foods are carbohydrates and how many servings or choices of carbohydrate to select for meals and/or snacks. Other individuals, usually those using intensive insulin therapy, will move on and use carbohydrate-to-insulin ratios to determine their premeal insulin doses.

**2** Emphasis is placed on the total amount of carbohydrate rather than the source or type. Sucrose and other sugars may be substituted for other carbohydrates as part of the food/meal plan. Healthy eating remains the bottom line.

**3** Foods are divided into 3 food groups: carbohydrates, meat and meat substitutes, and fat.
   **A** One carbohydrate serving or choice contains 15 g of carbohydrate.
   - Foods that contain carbohydrate are starches, fruits, milk, and desserts. Table 1.8 lists examples of common carbohydrate choices.
   - Vegetables also contain carbohydrate but generally in smaller amounts. The green and leafy vegetables only count as a carbohydrate if large amounts are eaten, such as a lunch that consists primarily of a large salad or a plate of cooked vegetables. However, starchy vegetables such as potatoes, corn, peas, or winter squash are considered carbohydrate choices.
   - A *free food* is defined as any food or drink that contains less than 5 g of carbohydrate or 20 calories per serving.
   **B** An average serving of meat, fish, or poultry is 3 oz or about the size of a deck of cards. An average serving of a meat substitute is 1 oz cheese, ¼ cup cottage cheese, 1 egg, or 2 Tb peanut butter.
   **C** Each fat serving has approximately 5 g of fat. Examples are 1 tsp of butter, margarine, mayonnaise, or oil; 1 Tb of reduced-fat mayonnaise or regular salad dressings; and 2 Tb of reduced-fat salad dressings, cream cheese, or sour cream.

**4** Individuals need to know how many carbohydrate choices are allowed for meals or snacks. A typical food/meal plan for adults with type 2 diabetes may start with 3 to 4 carbohydrate choices (45 to 60 g) per meal for women, 4 to 5 carbohydrate choices

(60 to 75 g) per meal for men, and 1 to 2 choices (15 to 30 g) for each snack. Food records and blood glucose monitoring data can then be used to determine if this amount is appropriate for the individual to consume.

## Table 1.8. Examples of Carbohydrate Choices or Servings

**Carbohydrate Choice = 15 g of carbohydrate**

*Starch*
- 1 slice bread
- ½ cup pasta
- ¾ cup dry cereal
- 4-6 crackers
- ⅓ cup rice
- 1 small potato

*Fruit*
- 1 small piece
- ½ cup juice

*Milk*
- 1 cup skim/low-fat
- ¾ cup yogurt

*Desserts/Others*
- 2 small cookies
- 1 Tb jam, honey, syrup
- ½ cup ice cream or frozen yogurt
- 2-in-square cake or brownie

**A** Education for the basics of carbohydrate counting (Level 1) covers the following information:
- Why carbohydrate is important in relation to blood glucose levels
- Which foods contain carbohydrate
- What portion sizes are equal to 1 carbohydrate choice or 1 serving of carbohydrate
- How to find and use carbohydrate information
- What portion tools are needed, such as measuring cups and spoons or visual estimations

**B** Identifying usual food intake and portion sizes through the use of food records or food recall enables individuals to determine usual carbohydrate intake at meals and snacks.

**C** Carbohydrate target ranges for meals and snacks are determined by the individual and dietitian based on usual carbohydrate intake and distribution, food/nutrition goals set mutually, medication, and level of physical activity.

**D** Self-monitoring of blood glucose provides the information needed by the individual and the healthcare team to determine the plan's effectiveness in reaching target blood glucose goals.

**E** In most cases, consistency of carbohydrate intake will reduce fluctuations in postprandial glucose levels. When variation in carbohydrate intake is desired, individuals can be taught to adjust medication and physical activity to maintain target blood glucose levels.

**F** As individuals gain more experience with the basics of carbohydrate counting, they become more skilled at estimating and recording carbohydrate intake using either the choice or gram method. Level 2 carbohydrate counting is designed to teach individuals about the relationship between food, activity, and glucose levels so that they can effectively manage their diabetes. The following skills enable individuals to use and benefit from this level of carbohydrate counting:

- How to subtract, multiply, and divide (a calculator is helpful)
- How to use a variety of resources such as reference books, carbohydrate lists, and nutrition labels to calculate the carbohydrate content of more complex foods (eg, combination food items, restaurant foods)
- How to determine the role of meats and fats in the carbohydrate counting system
- How to identify patterns related to glucose, food, medication, and activity
- How to perform pattern management (Figure 1.4 shows an example of pattern management).

**5** Persons with diabetes are taught to prioritize information on the food label.

**A** The serving size should be considered first. All of the information on the food label is based on the portion size.

**B** The next information that should be reviewed is total carbohydrate. This number shows the total grams of carbohydrate in 1 serving. Total carbohydrate includes all starches, sugars, and fiber; 15 g of carbohydrate equals 1 carbohydrate choice or serving.

**C** Grams of sugar can be ignored because they are included in the total grams of carbohydrate.

**D** If a food has 5 or more g of fiber, subtract the total grams of fiber from the total carbohydrate before converting the total grams of carbohydrate into choices.

**6** When using carbohydrate counting, the protein and fat content of foods must be considered because of the calories they contribute and, therefore, the potential for weight gain. In usual amounts, however, protein and fat have minimal effects on blood glucose levels.

## Carbohydrate-to-Insulin Ratios

**1** Carbohydrate-to-insulin ratios (Level 3 carbohydrate counting) are useful for intensive insulin therapy or for insulin pump therapy. The goal is to provide accurate rapid-acting or short-acting premeal insulin doses to cover the amount of carbohydrate that will be eaten for the meal.

**2** Individuals need to eat a consistent amount of carbohydrate at meals and determine the amount of premeal insulin needed to cover that amount of carbohydrate. After this amount has been determined, the premeal insulin dose is divided into the usual carbohydrate intake. For example, if 60 g of carbohydrate are eaten at breakfast and 4 units of rapid-acting insulin are used before breakfast to cover the carbohydrate consumed, the carbohydrate-to-insulin ratio is 15:1. To make insulin adjustments for consuming more or less carbohydrate, the premeal insulin dose can be adjusted accordingly. For more information on carbohydrate-to-insulin ratios, see Chapter 6, Insulin Pump Therapy and Carbohydrate Counting for Pump Therapy: Carbohydrate-to-Insulin Ratios in Diabetes Management Therapies.

# Figure 1.4. Example of Diabetes Daily Record

Name: JD
BG Goal: 80 to 150 mg/dL

| Day/Date | Time | Med/Insulin Type/Dose | BG, mg/dL Premeal | BG, mg/dL Postmeal | Food Intake Amt. | Food Intake Type (food/drink) | Carbohydrate Info Choices | Carbohydrate Info Grams | Exercise Type/Amount |
|---|---|---|---|---|---|---|---|---|---|
| Tues. 4/15 | 5:30 PM | Glucotrol/2.5 mg | 160 | | 4 oz | Ground beef | | 0 | Watch TV |
| | | | | | 8 oz | Baked potato | | 43 g | |
| | | | | | 1 c | Corn | | 30 g | |
| | | | | | | | | 73 g Total | |
| | 9:00 PM | | | 212 | | | | | |
| Wed. 4/16 | 5:30 PM | Glucotrol/2.5 mg | 141 | | 2 c | Macaroni and cheese | | 60 g | Shop, walk in mall 1 hour |
| | | | | | 1 c | Green peas | | 30 g | |
| | | | | | 1 pc | Bread | | 12 g | |
| | | | | | | | | 102 g Total | |
| | 9:00 PM | | | 183 | | | | | |
| Thurs. 4/17 | 5:45 PM | Glucotrol/2.5 mg | 170 | | 3 pc | Fried chicken | | 27 g | Walk 15 minutes |
| | | | | | 1 c | Mashed potatoes | | 30 g | |
| | | | | | 1/2 c | Gravy | | 6 g | |
| | | | | | 3 oz | Biscuit | | 34 g | |
| | | | | | | | | 97 g Total | |
| | 9:00 PM | | | 192 | | | | | |

## Essential Food Label Information for Food and Meal Planning[135,136]

**1** The Nutrition Labeling and Education Act (NLEA) of 1995 mandated nutrition labeling on almost all food products and provided a standard format for food labels. The Nutrition Facts label includes the following required information:

**A** Serving size and servings per container (similar food products have similar serving sizes); all of the nutrition information on the Nutrition Facts panel is based on the serving size

**B** Total calories per serving and calories from fat per serving

**C** Total fat (g), saturated fat (g), cholesterol (mg), sodium (mg), total carbohydrate (g), dietary fiber (g), sugars (g), and protein (g)

**D** Percentage of Recommended Dietary Allowances (RDA) for vitamin A, vitamin C, calcium, and iron

**E** Percent Daily Values for total fat, saturated fat, cholesterol, sodium, total carbohydrate, and dietary fiber based on a 2000-calorie diet; these values can be used to quickly compare foods and to see how the amount of a nutrient in a serving of food fits in 2000-calorie reference diet

**F** Calories per gram of fat, carbohydrate, and protein

**2** Descriptive terms that food manufacturers are allowed to put on a food package or label are also regulated. Common food label terms and their meanings are shown in Table 1.9.

## Table 1.9. Common Food Labels and Their Meaning

| | |
|---|---|
| **Free** | |
| *Fat-free* | ½ g or less fat per serving |
| *Sugar-free* | ½ g or less sugar per serving |
| *Calorie-free* | 5 calories or less per serving |
| **Low** | |
| *Low-fat* | 3 g or less fat per serving |
| *Low-calorie* | 40 calories or less per serving |
| *No sugar added* | No sugar added during processing, including ingredients that contain sugar, such as fruit juice |
| **Reduced** | |
| *Reduced or less fat* | At least 25% less fat than the regular food |
| *Reduced or less sugar* | At least 25% less sugar than the regular food |
| *Reduced or fewer calories* | At least 25% fewer calories than the regular food |
| *Light or lite* | ⅓ fewer calories or 50% less fat than the regular product |

**3** A *health claim* is a statement on the label that establishes a relationship between a nutrient and a disease or health-related condition. A food must meet certain nutrient levels to make a health claim, and these claims must be approved by the Food and Drug Administration. The following are examples of health claims and the health condition to which each relates:

**A** High in fiber: cancer, heart disease

**B** Low in fat, saturated fat, and cholesterol: heart disease, cancer

**C** Low in sodium: high blood pressure

**D** High in calcium: osteoporosis

**4** A food package or label is also required to show the list of ingredients used to make the food. All ingredients are listed in descending order by weight.

**5** Label information can be helpful in various meal planning methods. For example, 1 carbohydrate serving is based on the amount of food (eg, starch, fruit, milk, or other carbohydrate) that contains approximately 15 g of carbohydrate. One fat serving is based on the amount of food that contains approximately 5 g of fat.

## Ethnic and Cultural Appropriateness

**1** Successful diabetes prevention and treatment in diverse ethnic populations requires sensitivity to cultural differences in health beliefs and eating habits.

**2** Food choices and eating habits must be understood within the context of culture. Eating is a personal matter that may carry great cultural significance.

**3** Health professionals can use a 4-step process to improve cross-cultural counseling: (1) self-evaluation of their own cultural heritage; (2) pre-interview research on the cultural background of each client; (3) in-depth, cross-cultural interview to establish client's personal preferences and cultural background and eating habit adaptations made in the United States; and unbiased analysis of the data[137] (See Chapter 4, Cultural Competence in Diabetes Education and Care, in Diabetes Education and Program Management).

**4** Information on selected ethnic groups is published by the American Dietetic Association and the American Diabetes Association (see resource list at the end of this chapter). Each series is being revised to include a 2-page client education sheet on diabetes meal planning. Nutrition recommendations have been developed for the following: Alaska Native, Cajun and Creole, Chinese American, Filipino American, Hmong American, Indian and Pakistani, Jewish, Mexican American, Navajo, Northern Plains Indian, and Soul and Traditional Southern.

## Travel Adaptations

**1** When traveling to places where the time change is only 1, 2, or 3 hours, each morning insulin injection time can be moved one-half hour ahead or behind (depending on the direction the person is traveling) until the person is back on schedule. Insulin adjustments will need to be made when traveling overseas.

**A** When overseas travel is eastbound, there may be a 6-hour to 8-hour time difference, resulting in a shorter day. Background insulins such as intermediate-acting insulins or Ultralente need to be reduced. Some health professionals recommend following the guideline of decreasing the insulin dose by whatever percentage of 24 hours is lost. Rapid-acting or short-acting insulins are taken before meals.

**B** When overseas travel is westbound, days will be longer. Injections of regular insulin can be added for every 4 to 6 hours (before meals) to cover the additional time. Different guidelines may be recommended. Individuals should be taught to talk with their healthcare team about how to adjust insulin before traveling.

**2** Remind individuals to carry their medications, blood glucose monitoring equipment, and urine ketone testing materials when traveling. They also need to wear medical identification showing that they have diabetes. Individuals should be taught to protect their testing strips and insulin from extremes in temperature.

**3** Individuals need to be prepared for delays, cancelled flights, or changes in travel plans. Many flights offer only beverages and peanuts or pretzels. Individuals should be taught to carry extra snacks with them to help prevent hypoglycemia.

**4** Airplane travel is not the only time that an eating schedule may be disrupted. In many countries, it is customary to eat very late evening meals. With planning and flexible insulin regimens, travel and mealtime changes can be handled safely.

**5** Giving individuals general guidelines for estimating carbohydrate servings of unfamiliar foods can be helpful. For example, one half of a fist is equivalent to 1 carbohydrate choice.

**6** Other precautions for traveling include carrying carbohydrate for extra activity and for treating hypoglycemia, teaching travel companions how to give glucagon, carrying guidelines on how to handle acute illnesses, and carrying spare prescriptions for medications.

---

## Key Educational Considerations

**1** Emphasize the goals of meal planning for persons with either type 1 or type 2 diabetes: improve blood glucose control, lipids, and blood pressure. To prevent hyperglycemia and maintain euglycemia, food intake is balanced with insulin(s) taken by injection or insulin still being produced by the pancreas and with exercise. Strategies for improving blood glucose control for persons with type 2 diabetes that can be helpful include

**A** Eating less calories, fat, and carbohydrate through food selection (eg, decreasing fat intake) and eating smaller portion sizes

**B** Achieving moderate weight loss; the biggest improvement in blood glucose levels occurs with a modest weight loss

**C** Distributing carbohydrate and food intake throughout the day by eating smaller meals and snacks

**D** Increasing activity (exercise) levels

**E** Improving eating behaviors (eg, eating breakfast and lunch instead of consuming all calories late in the day)

**F** Using blood glucose monitoring results to evaluate the relationships between food, exercise, medication, coping skills, and the effectiveness of food/meal and exercise changes.

**2** Emphasize to individuals that they have not failed if their meal planning strategies have not improved their blood glucose control. A change in therapy may be needed to meet blood glucose goals; changing medications is a natural progression in the management of diabetes.

**3** To encourage participation in nutrition education, show individuals a list of the nutrition-related topics that are offered and let them choose what they want to learn at each session. This technique also relieves the educator of the unrealistic burden of trying to teach everything in one visit.

**4** To elicit past experiences with dietitians or weight loss, ask individuals or use examples of former patients (without identifying source of information). For example, start the discussion with the following patient history: "I worked with a woman who resisted making the initial appointment because her previous experience with dieting was in a program where she had to weigh in at every visit, measure her food at all times, and eat foods that she did not like. She was amazed that meal planning for blood glucose control could be so flexible. What's been your experience?"

**5** Use the Nutrition Facts label on food packages to point out the grams of carbohydrate, protein, fat, and number of calories per serving. Help patients understand that carbohydrate servings are based on 15 g of carbohydrate and fat servings are based on 5 g of fat. Use an actual food label to illustrate that the serving size on the food label may differ from the exchange value. For example, a label for brown rice lists a serving size of 1 cup while the serving size from the starch list for brown rice is 1/3 cup.

**6** Invite patients to teach the educator(s) about the ingredients in and preparation of cultural/ethnic foods. Combining the patient's cultural expertise with the diabetes and nutrition knowledge of the educator allows for a true exchange of information that will benefit the patient.

**7** Use menus from local restaurants or fast-food chains to help patients plan a meal according to their meal plan. Using a menu allows for patient preferences and variety and often brings some humor and realism to the teaching session. Through role playing, patients can also practice their assertiveness skills by asking their "waiter" partner questions about ingredients, preparation, and presentation of food.

**8** Conduct a supermarket tour to teach flexibility and variety in meal planning. Participants can read the food labels, learn where to find the recommended foods in the supermarket, learn the aisles to avoid, and compare the nutritional content of different brands of foods.

**9** Display a chart or test tubes showing the amounts of sucrose or fat in common foods.
  **A** Compare small portions of common foods such as a cookie, frozen yogurt, or ice milk with the sucrose in a 12-oz can of regular soft drink, Jello®, fruited yogurt, etc.

**B** Point out that small portions of sucrose-containing foods can be used as a carbohydrate serving in the meal plan, but that the calorie and fat content of sucrose-containing foods also need to be considered.

**10** Offer samples of products or coupons to encourage patients to try some new foods. Helping a patient change from the usual egg-and-bacon-on-a-roll breakfast may be more successful if the patient has tried and liked a new whole-grain cereal.

**11** The terms *sugar-free*, *fat-free*, and *lite* on foods do not mean that these foods are "free" or contain less calories than regular foods. To teach this concept, use food labels to demonstrate the number of calories in and the fat and carbohydrate content of a common sugar-free or fat-free product, or use the American Diabetes Association's booklet *A Guide to Fitting Foods with Sugar Substitutes and Fat Replacers into Your Meal Plan*. This booklet includes examples of food labels containing these products and is a guide to help individuals incorporate these foods into their meal plans.

**12** To teach patients how to consider the total amount of carbohydrate when selecting a piece of cake, the educator can offer a rule of thumb that a 2-in square contains approximately 15 g of carbohydrate and 5 g of fat (1 carbohydrate choices and 1 fat serving). One piece (1/6) of a frosted, 2-layer cake, however, contains approximately 45 g of carbohydrate and 10 g fat (3 carbohydrate choices and 2 fat servings).

**13** Emphasize the importance of accurate portion skills. Encourage use of a food scale, measuring spoons, and measuring cups. Consider using food labs to improve your own skills as well as the patient's. Practice repeatedly. Teach patients that periodic measuring and weighing needs to be an ongoing activity for accurate carbohydrate counting.

**14** Use the patient's records to demonstrate patterns in food, medication, activity, and blood glucose levels. Ask the patient what they think is happening. Initially, the educator can interpret the results. The patient can assume increasing responsibility for this over time.

**15** After determining individual carbohydrate-to-insulin ratios, provide ample opportunities for the patient to complete paper-and-pencil exercises that simulate situations in which insulin adjustments would be needed for larger- or smaller-than-usual meals or snacks. Examples include weekend brunch, pizza parties, or a light lunch.

**16** Monitor the patient's weight. If weight gain is a problem, emphasize portion control, limiting protein and fat intake, and using weight-management behaviors.

---

## Self-Review Questions

**1** What are the major goals of medical nutrition therapy (MNT) for persons with diabetes?

**2** How many calories per gram do carbohydrate, protein, fat, and alcohol contribute to the energy content of the diet?

**3** What factors determine the postmeal glycemic response of foods?

**4**   What are 2 priorities related to the carbohydrate content of the food/meal plan?

**5**   How are foods containing sucrose used in a food/meal plan?

**6**   Name 4 types of nonnutritive sweeteners currently available on the market and 4 nutritive sweeteners that are frequently substituted for sucrose in food products.

**7**   What is the effect of protein on the postmeal blood glucose response?

**8**   List 3 types of fatty acids found in foods and list 3 examples of foods containing each type of fatty acid. What is the major effect of each type of fatty acid on blood lipid levels?

**9**   What are recommendations for the use of alcoholic beverages for persons with diabetes?

**10**   What information is needed prior to the first nutrition visit?

**11**   How is the nutrition prescription determined?

**12**   List the exchange lists. Each list is based on how many calories and grams of carbohydrate, protein, and fat? Why is it helpful to know these values?

**13**   List the 4 groups of foods that contain carbohydrate. What are average portion sizes for common foods in each group?

**14**   Distinguish between initial versus continuing nutrition education. How are food diaries used?

**15**   Determine the approximate range of caloric requirement per day for an inactive man weighing 195 lb (75 kg).

**16**   Determine the approximate range of caloric requirement per day for an inactive woman weighing 165 lb (75 kg).

**17**   List 2 meal-planning tools that can be used to teach basic diabetes nutrition.

**18**   How can the values on food labels be prioritized?

**19**   What is the definition of a "free food" for carbohydrate counting?

**20**   State 2 primary principles of carbohydrate-to-insulin ratios.

**21**   Calculate how much insulin would be needed to cover 90 g of carbohydrate for someone using a carbohydrate-to-insulin ratio of 15 g of carbohydrate per 1 unit of insulin.

**22**   Why do individuals using carbohydrate-to-insulin ratios also need to be concerned about intake of dietary fat and protein?

---

## Learning Assessment: Case Study 1

AJ is a 45-year-old woman who was diagnosed with type 2 diabetes 5 years ago. She has not been in for a medical checkup for 3 years. She decided to return at this time because of chronic fatigue and blurry vision. Her HbA$_{1c}$ value is 8.3% (normal = 4% to 6%), cholesterol is 214 mg/dL (5.5 mmol/L), and triglycerides are 275 mg/dL (3.1 mmol/L). Her current weight is 175 lb (79.5 kg) and height is 5 ft 4 in (162 cm); body mass index (BMI) = 30 kg/m$^2$. She states that she hasn't returned for any follow-up visits because the only advice she gets is to lose weight and not eat sugar, neither of which she is able to do.

---

## Questions for Discussion

**1**   How should you deal with AJ's negative feelings about diabetes meal planning?

**2**   What are possible initial educational topics for AJ?

**3**   What are short-term food/meal planning strategies for AJ?

**4** What information and educational tools might be helpful for AJ at this time?

**5** How can continued education and counseling be planned and provided for AJ?

## Discussion

**1** Start the session by asking AJ about her concerns about diabetes and the symptoms she is experiencing. Ask how she believes you can be most helpful to her.

**2** The initial educational approaches that can be discussed with AJ include reviewing lifestyle strategies besides weight loss she can implement to improve her diabetes control. Explain to her the changes in the understanding of diabetes and management that have occurred since she was diagnosed. Diabetes is a progressive disease and the symptoms she is experiencing may be the result of a failing pancreas. It is important to start with lifestyle changes, and then decide whether medication(s) also needs to be added. She needs to understand she is not to blame herself. Ask if she is willing to identify a strategy to implement, and then review blood glucose monitoring and blood glucose goals with her.

**3** Short-term meal planning options for AJ include learning to count carbohydrate servings at meals and snacks and beginning some type of regular physical activity.

**4** AJ was introduced to carbohydrate counting. A simplified educational tool was used to help her understand that foods are grouped into carbohydrate, meat, and fat choices. Average portion sizes for different types of food were discussed. She felt that 3 to 4 carbohydrate choices at meals (breakfast, lunch, dinner), 1 to 2 carbohydrate choices for snacks (morning, afternoon, evening), 1 oz to 2 oz of meat at lunch, 3 oz to 4 oz of meat at supper, and 1 to 2 fat servings per meal would be a reasonable food plan. She also stated she would like to begin a walking program.

**A** AJ agreed to keep food and blood glucose records and return in 2 weeks for a follow-up visit. At that visit she will have the opportunity to identify problems she is having with the strategies she chose. The dietitian and AJ can also evaluate the effect of the food and exercise changes on her blood glucose levels. Changes will be made as needed.

**B** As an educator you realize that, depending on her previous eating habits and with her 5-year duration of diabetes, the expected outcome from MNT is approximately a 1% decrease in $HbA_{1c}$. Therefore, you need to evaluate if lifestyle changes alone will be adequate for AJ or whether medications need to be combined with MNT.

**5** At 3 months AJ is to return for an $HbA_{1c}$ test. At that time, the decision can be made as to whether MNT and exercise alone are adequate or if there is a need to add an oral agent or other medications. Her lipids should be retested in 3 to 6 months. At each visit, the emphasis should be on reaching blood glucose goals and not on weight loss.

## Learning Assessment: Case Study 2

JD is a 52-year-old male diagnosed with type 2 diabetes 6 years ago. His $HbA_{1c}$ value is 9.6% (normal = 4.4% to 6.1%). He has hypertension and is on antihypertensive medication, has elevated triglycerides, and has low HDL cholesterol. He is currently taking glipizide 2.5 mg, tid. JD has been asked to test his blood glucose before breakfast and dinner and at bedtime. His readings are consistently above his target goal ranges. He reports that over the years his blood glucose levels have continued to go up even though he hasn't changed what he eats. Lately, he has stopped testing because he reports that no matter what he does and how hard he tries to follow his diet, his blood glucose levels do not improve.

JD is 5 ft 10 in (178 cm), weighs 195 lb (89 kg), and his BMI is 28. His weight has been stable over the past 5 years. The food/nutrition assessment shows that JD eats 3 meals daily, a midafternoon and evening snack. His current estimated daily caloric intake is 2300 to 2500 calories. He eats breakfast at home, brings a lunch to work, and has his evening meal at home. He used to drink 2 to 3 beers per day but has been avoiding alcohol the past year. He is physically active in his job as a school custodian and walks to and from work Monday through Friday (2 miles round trip).

JD's doctor wants him to begin taking insulin and has recommended he start with 2 injections a day, taking rapid-acting insulin and NPH insulin before breakfast and before his evening meal. JD states that he attended diabetes classes when he was first diagnosed with diabetes. Three months ago he had a consult with a dietitian who introduced him to carbohydrate counting. He has been keeping a record of his food intake, blood glucose levels, and physical activity, but has been frustrated because they have not improved, so he is willing to try insulin.

## Questions for Discussion

**1** Why have JD's blood glucose levels increased even though his lifestyle has not changed and his food habits and physical activity level are better than a year ago?

**2** What food/meal planning skills will be important for JD as he starts taking insulin?

**3** What resources or tools can you recommend to JD to help him be more successful with carbohydrate counting?

**4** How can you determine JD's interest in his wife's involvement and her willingness to assist JD?

## Discussion

**1** Explain to JD about the progressive nature of type 2 diabetes and why at this time it is important for him to begin taking insulin. He appears to have mastered the basics of carbohydrate counting. He is willing to keep records of his food intake, blood glucose levels, and insulin so that his insulin dose can be adjusted to cover his preferred lifestyle. He plans to highlight blood glucose levels outside the target range and will focus on the influence of carbohydrate foods.

**2** It will be beneficial for JD to purchase a carbohydrate reference book and measuring cups so he can better determine portion sizes. He also needs to be alerted to the possibility of weight gain as his blood glucose levels improve and, therefore, to watch his meat and fat portions. He feels that he can eat a smaller midafternoon snack. On weekends he will also test his blood glucose levels before lunch. By using his food and testing information, JD hopes to determine what type of insulin regimen would be best for him.

**3** JD states that his wife is willing to alter her cooking and he needs her help and support. He is also willing to help with some of the cooking and grocery buying. How to read food labels, prevention and treatment of hypoglycemia, and how to deal with sick days should be reviewed with JD and his wife.

**4** JD and his wife plan to develop a list of dinner menus and bedtime snacks. He is also anxious to learn about carbohydrate-to-insulin ratios so eventually he can do more adjusting of his insulin doses. JD and his wife agreed to a follow-up visit in 3 weeks, at which time JD will bring his food and glucose data. Eventually JD will probably need a more intensive insulin regimen to give him the flexibility he wants.

## References

**1** American Diabetes Association. Nutrition recommendations for people with diabetes mellitus (position statement). Diabetes Care. 2001. In press.

**2** Franz MJ, Bantle JP, Beebe CA, et al. Evidence-based nutrition recommendations for diabetes and complications (technical review). Diabetes Care. 2001. In press.

**3** Franz MJ, Bantle JP, eds. The American Diabetes Association's Guide to Medical Nutrition Therapy for Diabetes. Alexandria, Va: American Diabetes Association; 1999.

**4** US Department of Agriculture and US Department of Health and Human Services. Nutrition and Your Health: Dietary Guidelines for Americans 2000. 5th ed. Hyattsville, Md: USDA Human Nutrition Information Service; 2000. Home and Garden Bulletin No. 232.

**5** Krauss RM, Eckel RH, Howard B, et al. AHA dietary guidelines. Revision 2000: a statement for healthcare professionals from the Nutrition Committee of the American Heart Association. Circulation. 2000;102:2284-2299.

**6** de Chavez M, Chavez A. Diet that prevents cancer: recommendations from the American Institute for Cancer Research. Int J Cancer. 1998;11(suppl):85-89.

**7** Kant AK, Schatzkin A, Graubard BI, Schairer C. A prospective study of diet quality and mortality in women. JAMA. 2000;283:2109-2115.

**8** Huijbregts P, Feskens E, Rasanen L, et al. Dietary patterns and 20 year mortality in elderly men in Finland, Italy, and The Netherlands: longitudinal cohort study. BMJ. 1997; 315:13-17.

**9** Appel LJ, Moore TJ, Obarzanek E, et al. A clinical trial of the effects of dietary patterns on blood pressure. N Engl J Med. 1997;336:1117-1124.

**10** Anderson JW, Hanna TJ, Peng X, Kryscio RJ. Whole grain foods and heart disease risk. J Am Coll Nutr. 2000;19:291S-299S.

**11** Liu S, Manson JE, Lee I-M, et al. Fruit and vegetable intake and risk of cardiovascular disease: the Women's Health Study. Am J Clin Nutr. 2000;72:922-928.

**12** Hu FB, Rimm EB, Stampfer MJ, Ascherio A, Spiegelman D, Willett WC. Prospective study of major dietary patterns and risk of coronary heart disease in men. Am J Clin Nutr. 2000;72:912-921.

**13** Lockwood D, Frey ML, Gladish NA, Hiss R. The biggest problem in diabetes. Diabetes Educ. 1986;12:30-33.

**14** Ary DV, Toobert D, Wilson W, Glasgow RE. Patient perspective factors contributing to nonadherence to diabetes regimen. Diabetes Care. 1986;9:168-172.

**15** Delahanty LM, Halford BN. The role of diet behaviors in achieving improved glycemic control in intensively treated patients in the Diabetes Control and Complications Trial. Diabetes Care. 1993;16:1453-1458.

**16** UK Prospective Diabetes Study (UKPDS) Group: UK Prospective Diabetes Study 7: response of fasting plasma glucose to diet therapy in newly presenting type II diabetic patients. Metabolism. 1990;39:905-912.

**17** Kulkarni K, Castle G, Gregory R, et al. Nutrition practice guidelines for type 1 diabetes mellitus positively affect dietitian practices and patient outcomes. J Am Diet Assoc. 1998;98:62-70.

**18** Franz MJ, Monk A, Barry B, et al. Effectiveness of medical nutrition therapy provided by dietitians in the management of non-insulin-dependent diabetes mellitus: a randomized, controlled clinical trial. J Am Diet Assoc. 1995;95:1009-1017.

**19** Diabetes Control and Complications Trial Research Group. The effect of intensive treatment of diabetes on the development and progression of long-term complications in insulin-dependent diabetes mellitus. N Engl J Med. 1993;329:977-986.

**20** UK Prospective Diabetes Study (UKPDS) Group. Intensive blood-glucose control with sulphonylureas or insulin compared with conventional treatment and risk of complications in patients with type 2 diabetes (UKPDS 33). Lancet. 1998;352:837-853.

**21** American Diabetes Association. Management of dyslipidemia in adults with diabetes (position statement). Diabetes Care. 2001;24(suppl 1): S58-S61.

**22** The Expert Panel on Blood Cholesterol Levels in Children and Adolescents. Report of the Expert Panel on Blood Cholesterol Levels in Children and Adolescents. Pediatrics. 1992;89(suppl):525-584.

**23** American Diabetes Association. Standards of medical care for patients with diabetes mellitus (position statement). Diabetes Care. 2001;24(suppl 1):S33-S43.

**24** The First Step in Diabetes Meal Planning. Alexandria, Va and Chicago: American Diabetes Association and American Dietetic Association; 1995.

**25** American Diabetes Association. Type 2 diabetes in children and adolescents (consensus statement). Diabetes Care. 2000;23:381-389.

**26** Helmrich SP, Ragland DR, Leung RW, Paffenbarger RS. Physical activity and reduced occurrence of non-insulin dependent diabetes mellitus. N Eng J Med. 1991;325:147-152.

**27** Manson JE, Rimm EB, Stampfer MJ, et al. Physical activity and incidence of non-insulin dependent diabetes mellitus in women. Lancet. 1991;338:774-778.

**28** Manson JE, Nathan DM, Krolewski AS, Stampfer MJ, Willett WC, Hennekens CH. A prospective study of exercise and incidence of diabetes among US male physicians. JAMA. 1992;268:63-67.

**29** Hu FB, Sigal RJ, Rich-Edwards JW, et al. Walking compared with vigorous physical activity and risk of type 2 diabetes in women. JAMA. 1999;282:1433-1439.

**30** Moore LL, Visioni AJ, Wilson PWF, D'Agostino RB, Finkle WD, Ellison RC. Can sustained weight loss in overweight individuals reduce the risk of diabetes mellitus? Epidemiology. 2000;11:269-273.

**31** Kulkarni K, Franz MJ. A dietitian's perspective on medical nutrition therapy for diabetes. In: Franz MJ, Bantle JP, eds. American Diabetes Association Guide to Medical Nutrition Therapy for Diabetes. Alexandria, Va: American Diabetes Association; 1999:3-17.

**32** Rabasa-Lhoret R, Garon J, Langlier H, Poisson D, Chiasson J-L. Effects of meal carbohydrate on insulin requirements in type 1 diabetic patients treated intensively with the basal-bolus (Ultralente-regular) insulin regimen. Diabetes Care. 1999;22:667-673.

**33** Lafrance L, Rabasa-Lhoret R, Poisson D, Ducros F, Chiasson J-L. The effects of different glycaemic index foods and dietary fibre intake on glycaemic control in type 1 diabetic patients on intensive insulin therapy. Diabetic Med. 1998;15:972-978.

**34** Wolever TMS, Hamad S, Chiasson J-L, et al. Day-to-day consistency in amount and source of carbohydrate intake associated with improved glucose control in type 1 diabetes. J Am Coll Nutr. 1999;18:242-247.

35 Chaturvedi N, Stevens LK, Fuller JH. The WHO Multinational Study of Vascular Disease in Diabetes. Mortality and morbidity associated with body weight in people with IDDM. Diabetes Care. 1995;18:761-765.

36 Purnell JQ, Hokanson JE, Marcovina SM, Steffes MW, Cleary PA, Brunzell JD. Effect of excessive weight gain with intensive therapy of type 1 diabetes on lipid levels and blood pressure. JAMA. 1998;280:140-146.

37 Williams KV, Erbey JR, Becker D, Orchard TJ. Improved glycemic control reduces the impact of weight gain on cardiovascular risk factors in type 1 diabetes. Diabetes Care. 1999;22:1084-1091.

38 Beebe CA. Nutrition therapy for type 2 diabetes. In: Franz MJ, Bantle JP, eds. American Diabetes Association Guide to Medical Nutrition Therapy for Diabetes. Alexandria, Va: American Diabetes Association; 1999:46-68.

39 Brownell KD, Wadden TA. Etiology and treatment of obesity: understanding a serious, prevalent, and refractory disorder. J Consult Clin Psychol. 1992;60:505-517.

40 Maggio CA, Pi-Sunyer FX. The prevention and treatment of obesity. Application to type 2 diabetes (technical review). Diabetes Care. 1997;20:1744-1766.

41 Foreyt JP, Goodrick GK. Evidence for success of behavior modification in weight loss and control. Ann Intern Med. 1993;119:698-701.

42 Wing RR, Venditti E, Jakicic JM, Polley BA, Lang W. Lifestyle intervention in overweight individuals with a family history of diabetes. Diabetes Care. 1998;21:350-359.

43 Markovic TP, Jenkins AB, Campbell LV, Furler SM, Kraegen EW, Chisholm DJ. The determinants of glycemic responses to diet restriction and weight loss in obesity and NIDDM. Diabetes Care. 1998;21:687-694.

44 Wing RR, Blair EH, Bononi P, et al. Caloric restriction per se is a significant factor in improvements in glycemic control and insulin sensitivity during weight loss in obese NIDDM patients. Diabetes Care. 1994;17:30-36.

45 Kelley DE, Wing R, Buonocore C, Sturis J, Polonsky K, Fitzsimmons M. Relative effects of calorie restriction and weight loss in non-insulin-dependent diabetes mellitus. J Clin Endocrinol Metab. 1993;77:1287-1293.

46 Wing RR, Koeske R, Epstein LH, et al. Long-term effects of modest weight loss in type II diabetic patients. Arch Intern Med. 1987;147:1749-1753.

47 Watts NB, Spanheimer RG, DiGirolamo M, et al. Prediction of glucose response to weight loss in patients with non-insulin-dependent diabetes mellitus. Arch Intern Med. 1990;150:803-806.

48 Markovic TP, Campbell LV, Balasubramanian S, et al. Beneficial effect on average lipid levels from energy restriction and fat loss in obese individuals with or without type 2 diabetes. Diabetes Care. 1998;21:695-700.

49 National Institutes of Health, National Heart, Lung, and Blood Institute. Clinical guidelines on the identification, evaluation, and treatment of overweight and obesity in adults—the evidence report. Obes Res. 1998;6:51S-209S.

50 Campbell PJ, Gerich JE. Impact of obesity on insulin action in volunteers with normal glucose tolerance: demonstration of a threshold for adverse effect of obesity. J Clin Endocrinol Metab. 1990;1114-1118.

51 Yamashita S, Nakamura T, Shimonura I, et al. Insulin resistance and body fat distribution. Diabetes Care.1996;19:287-291.

52 Fujimoto WY, Bergstrom RW, Boyko EJ, et al. Visceral adiposity and incident coronary heart disease in Japanese-American men. Diabetes Care. 1999;22:1808-1812.

53 Boden G, Chen X. Effects of fat on glucose uptake and utilization in patients with non-insulin dependent diabetes. J Clin Invest. 1995;96:1261-1267.

54 Mayer-Davis EJ, Monacao JH, Hoen HM, et al. Dietary fat and insulin sensitivity in a triethnic population: the role of obesity. The Insulin Resistance Atherosclerosis Study (IRAS). Am J Clin Nutr. 1997;65:79-87.

55 Mayer-Davis EJ, Levin S, Marshall JA. Heterogeneity in associations between macronutrient intake and lipoprotein profile in individuals with type 2 diabetes. Diabetes Care. 1999;22:1632-1639.

56 Lissner L, Levitsky DA, Strupp BJ, Kalkwarf HJ, Roe DA. Dietary fat and the regulation of energy intake in human subjects. Am J Clin Nutr. 1987;46:886-892.

57 Schaefer EJ, Lichtenstein AH, Lamon-Fava S, et al. Body weight and low-density lipoprotein cholesterol changes after consumption of a low-fat ad libitum diet. JAMA. 1995;274:1450-1455.

58 Hegstad DM, Ausman LM, Johnson JA, Dallal GE. Dietary fat and serum lipids: an evaluation of the experimental data [published erratum appears in Am J Clin Nutr 1993;58:245]. Am J Clin Nutr. 1993;57:875-883.

59 Garg A, Bantle JP, Henry RR, et al. Effects of varying carbohydrate content of diet in patients with non-insulin dependent diabetes mellitus. JAMA. 1994;271:1421-1428.

60 Mayer-Davis EJ, D'Agostino RJ, Karter AJ, et al. Intensity and amount of physical activity in relation to insulin sensitivity. The Insulin Resistance and Atherosclerosis Study (IRAS). JAMA 1998;270:669-674.

61 Schneider SH, Khachadurian AK, Amorosa LF, et al. Ten-year experience with exercise-based outpatient life-style modification program in the treatment of diabetes mellitus. Diabetes Care. 1992;15:1800-1810.

62 Yamanouchi K, Shinozaki T, Chikada K, et al. Daily walking combined with diet therapy is a useful means for obese NIDDM patients not only to reduce body weight but also to improve insulin sensitivity. Diabetes Care. 1995;18:775-778.

63 Albright A, Franz M, Hornsby G, et al. American College of Sports Medicine position stand. Exercise and type 2 diabetes. Med Sci Sports Exerc. 2000;32:1345-1350.

64 Arnold L, Mann J, Ball M. Metabolic effects of alterations in meal frequency in type 2 diabetes. Diabetes Care. 1997;20:1651-1654.

65 Jenkins DJ, Ocana A, Jenkins AL, et al. Metabolic advantages of spreading the nutrient load: effects of increased meal frequency in non-insulin-dependent diabetes. Am J Clin Nutr. 1992;55:461-467.

66 Bertelsen J, Christiansen C, Thomsen C, et al. Effect of meal frequency on blood glucose, insulin, and free fatty acids in NIDDM subjects. Diabetes Care. 1993;16:4-7.

67 Ruggiero L, Prochaska JO. Readiness for change, application of the transtheoretical model to diabetes. Diabetes Spectrum. 1993;6:21-60.

68 Monk A, Barry B, McClain K, et al. Practice guidelines for medical nutrition therapy provided by dietitians for persons with non-insulin-dependent diabetes mellitus. J Am Diet Assoc. 1995;95:999-1006.

69 Report of a Joint FAO/WHO Expert Consultation. Carbohydrates in Human Nutrition. Rome, Italy: Food and Agriculture Organization of the United Nations and World Health Organization; 1998.

70 Nuttall FQ, Gannon MC. Carbohydrates and diabetes. In: Franz MJ, Bantle JP, eds. American Diabetes Association Guide to Medical Nutrition Therapy for Diabetes. Alexandria, Va: American Diabetes Association; 1999:85-106.

71 Gannon MC, Nuttall FQ. Protein and diabetes. In: Franz MJ, Bantle JP, eds. American Diabetes Association Guide to Medical Nutrition Therapy for Diabetes. Alexandria, Va: American Diabetes Association; 1999:107-125.

72 Fraser RJ, Horowitz M, Maddox AF, Harding PE, Chatterton BE, Dent J. Hyperglycemia slows gastric emptying rate in type I (insulin-dependent) diabetes mellitus. Diabetologia. 1990;33;675-680.

73 Schvarcz E, Palmer M, Aman J, Lindkvist B, Beckman K-W. Hypoglycemia increases gastric emptying rate in patients with type I diabetes mellitus. Diabetic Med. 1993;10:660-663.

74 Jarvi A, Karlstrom B, Grandfeldt Y, Bjorck I, Vesby B. The influence of food structure on postprandial metabolism in patients with NIDDM. Am J Clin Nutr. 1995; 61:837-842.

75 Parillo M, Giacco R, Ciardullo AV, Rivellese AA, Riccardi G. Does a high-carbohydrate diet have different effects in NIDDM patients treated with diet alone or hypoglycemic drugs. Diabetes Care. 1996; 19:498-500.

76 Bantle JP, Swanson JE, Thomas W, Laine DC. Metabolic effects of dietary sucrose in type II diabetic subjects. Diabetes Care. 1993;16:1301-1305.

77 Peterson DB, Lambert J, Gerring S, et al. Sucrose in the diet of diabetic patients - just another carbohydrate? Diabetologia. 1986;29:216-220.

78 Rickard KA, Loghmani E, Cleveland JL, Fineberg NS, Greidenberg GR. Lower glycemic response to sucrose in the diets of children with type 1 diabetes. J Pediatr. 1998;133:429-432.

79 Malerbi DA, Paiva ES, Duarte AL, Wajchenberg BL. Metabolic effects of dietary sucrose and fructose in type II diabetic subjects. Diabetes Care. 1996;19:1249-1256.

80 Chandalia M, Garg A, Luthohann D, vonBergmann K, Grundy SM, Brinkley LJ. Beneficial effects of a high dietary fiber intake in patients with type 2 diabetes. N Engl J Med. 2000;342:1392-1398.

81 Nuttall FQ. Dietary fiber in the management of diabetes. Diabetes. 1993;42:503-508.

82 Hollenbeck CG, Coulston AM, Reaven GM. To what extent does increased dietary fiber improve glucose and lipid metabolism in patients with noninsulin-dependent diabetes mellitus (NIDDM)? Am J Clin Nutr. 1986;43:16-24.

83 Toeller M, Buyken AE, Heitkamp G, et al. Fiber intake, serum cholesterol levels, and cardiovascular disease in European individuals with type 1 diabetes. Diabetes Care. 1999;22(suppl 2):B21-B28.

84 Bantle JP, Swanson JE, Thomas W, Laine DC. Metabolic effects of dietary fructose in diabetic subjects. Diabetes Care. 1992;15:1468-1476.

85 Bantle JP, Raatz SK, Thomas W, Georgopoulos A. Effects of dietary fructose on plasma lipids in healthy subjects. Am J Clin Nutr. 2000;72:1128-1134.

86 Akgum S, Ertel NH. A comparison of carbohydrate metabolism after sucrose, sorbitol, and fructose meals in normal and diabetic subjects. Diabetes Care. 1980; 3:582-585.

87 Butchko HH, Kotsonis FN. Acceptable daily intake vs actual intake: the aspartame example. J Am Coll Nutr. 1991;10:258-266.

88 Powers M. Sugar alternatives and fat replacers. In: Franz MJ, Bantle JP, eds. American Diabetes Association Guide to Medical Nutrition Therapy for Diabetes. Alexandria, Va: American Diabetes Association; 1999:148-164.

89 London R. Saccharin and aspartame. Are they safe to consume during pregnancy? J Reprod Med. 1988;33:17-21.

90 World Health Organization Expert Committee on Food Additives. Toxicological Evaluation of Certain Food Additives and Food Contaminants. Geneva, Switzerland: World Health Organization. 1981;16:11-27 and 1983;18:12-14.

91 Franz MJ. Protein controversies in diabetes. Diabetes Spectrum. 2000;13: 132-141.

92 Henry RR. Protein content of the diabetic diet. Diabetes Care. 1994;17:1502-1513.

93 Nuttall FQ, Mooradian AD, Giannon MC, Billington C, Krezowski P. Effect of protein ingestion on the glucose and insulin response to a standardized oral glucose load. Diabetes Care. 1984;7:465-470.

94 Peters AL, Davidson MB. Protein and fat effects on glucose responses and insulin requirements in subjects with insulin-dependent diabetes mellitus. Am J Clin Nutr. 1993;58:555-560.

**95** Gray RO, Butler PC, Beers TR, Kryshak EJ, Rizza RA. Comparison of the ability of bread versus bread plus meat to treat and prevent subsequent hypoglycemia in patients with insulin-dependent diabetes mellitus. J Clin Endocrinol Metab. 1996;81:1508-1511.

**96** American Diabetes Association. Diabetic nephropathy (position statement). Diabetes Care. 2001;24(suppl 1):S70-S73.

**97** Hu FB, Stampfer MJ, Rimm EB, et al. A prospective study of egg consumption and risk of cardiovascular disease in men and women. JAMA. 1999;281:1387-1394.

**98** Madigan C, Ryan M, Owens D, Collins P, Tomkin GH. Dietary unsaturated fatty acids in type 2 diabetes. Diabetes Care. 2000;23:1472-1477.

**99** Heilbronn L, Noakes M, Clifton P. Effect of energy restriction, weight loss, and diet composition on plasma lipids and glucose in patients with type 2 diabetes. Diabetes Care. 1999; 22:889-895.

**100** Montori VM, Farmer A, Wollan PC, Dinneen SF. Fish oil supplementation in type 2 diabetes: a quantitative systematic review. Diabetes Care. 2000;23:1407-1415.

**101** Warshaw H, Franz M, Powers MA, Wheeler M. Fat replacers: their use in foods and role in diabetes medical nutrition therapy (technical review). Diabetes Care. 1996;19:1294-1301.

**102** Kelly SM, Shorthouse M, Cotterell JC, et al. A 3-month, double-blind, controlled trial of feeding with sucrose polyester in human volunteers. Br J Nutr. 1998;80:41-49.

**103** Tuck M, Corry D, Trujillo A. Salt-sensitive blood pressure and exaggerated vascular reactivity in the hypertension of diabetes mellitus. Am J Med. 1990;88:210-216.

**104** The sixth report of the Joint National Committee on Prevention, Detection, Evaluation, and Treatment of High Blood Pressure. Arch Intern Med. 1997;2413-2446.

**105** Sacks FM, Svetkey LP, Vollmer WM, et al. Effects on blood pressure of reduced dietary sodium and the Dietary Approaches to Stop Hypertension (DASH) diet. N Engl J Med. 2001;344:3-10.

**106** Mooradian AD, Failla M, Hoogwerf B, Maryniuk M, Wylie-Rosett J. Selected vitamins and minerals in diabetes mellitus: a technical review. Diabetes Care. 1994;17:464-479.

**107** Kanis JA. The use of calcium in the management of osteoporosis. Bone. 1999;24:279-290.

**108** Koehler KM, Pareo-Tubbeh SL, Romero LJ, Baumgartner RN, Garry PJ. Folate nutrition and older adults: challenges and opportunities. J Am Diet Assoc. 1997;97:167-173.

**109** Yusuf S, Dagenais G, Pogue J, Bosch J, Sleight P. Vitamin E supplementation and cardiovascular events in high-risk patients. The Heart Outcomes Prevention Evaluation Study Investigators. N Engl J Med. 2000;342:154-160.

**110** Franz MJ. Alcohol and diabetes. In: Franz MJ, Bantle JP, eds. American Diabetes Association Guide to Medical Nutrition Therapy for Diabetes. Alexandria, Va: American Diabetes Association; 1999:192-210.

**111** Koivisto VA, Tulokas S, Toivonen M, et al. Alcohol with the meal has no adverse effects on postprandial glucose homeostasis in diabetic patients. Diabetes Care. 1993;16:1612-1614.

**112** Valmadrid CT, Klein R, Moss SE, Klein BK, Cruickshanks KJ. Alcohol intake and the risk of coronary heart disease mortality in persons with older-onset diabetes mellitus. JAMA. 1999;282:239-246.

**113** Solomon CG, Hu FB, Stampfer MJ, et al. Moderate alcohol consumption and risk of coronary heart disease among women with type 2 diabetes. Circulation. 2000;102:494-499.

**114** Ajani UA, Gaziano M, Lotufo PA, et al. Alcohol consumption and risk of coronary heart disease by diabetes status. Circulation. 2000;102:500-505.

**115** Kulkarni K, Castle G, Gregory R, et al, and the Diabetes Care and Education Practice Group of the American Dietetic Association. Nutrition practice guidelines for type 1 diabetes: an overview of the content and application. Diabetes Spectrum. 1997;10:248-256.

**116** Exchange Lists for Meal Planning. Alexandria, Va and Chicago: American Diabetes Association and American Dietetic Association; 1995.

**117** Wheeler ML, Franz M, Barrier P, Holler H, Cronmiller N, Delahanty LM. Macronutrient and energy database for the 1995 exchange lists for meal planning: a rationale for clinical practice decisions. J Am Diet Assoc. 1996; 96:1167-1171.

**118** Maryniuk MD. Counseling and education strategies for improved adherence to nutrition therapy. In: Franz MJ, Bantle JP, eds. American Diabetes Association Guide to Medical Nutrition Therapy for Diabetes. Alexandria, Va: American Diabetes Association; 1999:369-386.

**119** Schafer RG, Bohannon B, Franz M, et al. Translation of the diabetes nutrition recommendations for health care institutions (technical review). Diabetes Care. 1997; 20:96-105.

**120** American Diabetes Association. Translation of the diabetes nutrition recommendations for health care institutions (position statement). Diabetes Care. 2000;23(suppl 1):S47-S49.

**121** Holler HJ, Pastors JG. Diabetes Medical Nutrition Therapy: A Professional Guide to Management and Nutrition Education Resources. Chicago: American Dietetic Association; 1997.

**122** Gillespie S, Kulkarni K, Daly A. Using carbohydrate counting in diabetes clinical practice. J Am Diet Assoc. 1998;98:897-899.

**123** US Department of Agriculture. The Food Guide Pyramid. Hyattsville, Md: USDA Human Nutrition Information Service; 1992.

**124** Healthy Food Choices. Alexandria, Va and Chicago: American Diabetes Association and American Dietetic Association; 1986.

**125** Healthy Eating for People With Diabetes and Comida Saludable para Personas con Diabetes. Minneapolis: IDC Publishing; 1997.

**126** Carbohydrate Counting: Getting Started (Level 1). Alexandria, Va and Chicago: American Diabetes Association and American Dietetic Association; 1996.

**127** Carbohydrate Counting: Moving On (Level 2). Alexandria, Va and Chicago: American Diabetes Association and American Dietetic Association; 1996.

**128** Carbohydrate Counting: Using Carbohydrate/Insulin Ratios (Level 3). Alexandria, Va and Chicago: American Diabetes Association and American Dietetic Association; 1996.

**129** My Food Plan and Mi Plan de Comidas. Minneapolis: IDC Publishing; 2000.

**130** My Food Plan for Kids and Teens. Minneapolis: IDC Publishing; 1998.

**131** My Food Plan for Early Kidney Disease. Minneapolis: IDC Publishing; 2000.

**132** My Food Plan Made Easy. Minneapolis: IDC Publishing; 2000.

**133** Single-Topic Diabetes Resources. Alexandria, Va and Chicago: American Diabetes Association and American Dietetic Association; 1996.

**134** Facilitating Lifestyle Change: A Resource Manual. Alexandria, Va and Chicago: American Diabetes Association and American Dietetic Association; 1996.

**135** American Diabetes Association. Food labeling (position statement). Diabetes Care. 2001,24 (suppl): 5102-5103.

**136** Wheeler ML, Franz MJ, Heins J, et al. Food labeling (technical review). Diabetes Care. 1994;17:480-487.

**137** Kittler PG, Sucher KP. Diet counseling in multicultural society. Diabetes Educ. 1990;16:127-134.

## Resources

### Annual Listing of Publications

American Diabetes Association. Diabetes Resource Catalog. Alexandria, Va: American Diabetes Association. Updated annually.

American Dietetic Association and Diabetes Association. Ethnic and Regional Food Practices: Alaska Native, Chinese American, Filipino American, Hmong, Jewish, Mexican American, Navajo, Northern Plain Indian. Chicago: American Dietetic Association.

Diabetes Care and Education Dietetic Practice Group, American Dietetic Association. Selected Diabetes and Nutrition Education Resources: For the Diabetes Professional. Chicago: American Dietetic Association. Updated annually.

IDC Publishing. Making a Difference in Diabetes Education. Minneapolis: International Diabetes Center. Updated annually.

### Other Resources

References 119 to 128 are valuable patient education tools.

Franz MJ, Bantle JP, eds. American Diabetes Association Guide to Medical Nutrition Therapy for Diabetes. Alexandria, Va: American Diabetes Association; 1999.

The new shape of medical nutrition therapy. Diabetes Spectrum. 2000;13.

The art of nutrition: multiple aspects of diabetes medical nutrition therapy. Diabetes Spectrum. 1996;9.

Compu-Cal handheld computers. Olympia, Wash: Compu-Cal, Inc.

Foster-Powell K, Miller JB. International tables of glycemic index. Am J Clin Nutr. 1995;62:871S-893S.

Powers MA, ed. Handbook of Diabetes Nutritional Management. Rockville, Md: Aspen Publishers Inc; 1996.

Tinker LF, Heins JM, Holler HJ. Commentary and translation: 1994 nutrition recommendations for diabetes. J Am Diet Assoc. 1994;94:507-511.

Wasserman DH, Zinman B. Exercise in individuals with IDDM (technical review). Diabetes Care. 1994;17:924-937.

**Carbohydrate Counting Resource Books**
(Chapter 6, part 2, entitled Carbohydrate Counting for Pump Therapy: Carbohydrate-to-Insulin Ratios, in Diabetes Management Therapies, also includes a list of resources for carbohydrate counting.)

Exchange Lists for Meal Planning. Alexandria, Va and Chicago: American Diabetes Association and American Dietetic Association; 1995.

Franz M. Exchanges for All Occasions. 4th ed. Minneapolis: IDC Publishing; 1997.

Holzmeister LA. The Diabetes Carbohydrate and Fat Gram Guide. Alexandria, Va and Chicago: American Diabetes Association and American Dietetic Association; 1997.

Pennington J. Food Values of Portions Commonly Used. New York: JB Lippincott Company; 1994.

**Eating Out, Convenience, and Fast Food Guides**
Franz M. Fast Food Facts. 5th ed. Minneapolis: IDC Publishing; 1998.

Monk A. Convenience Food Facts. Minneapolis: IDC Publishing; 1996.

Month of Meals: Classic Cooking, Meals in Minutes, Ethnic Delights, Old-Time Favorites, Vegetarian Pleasures. Alexandria, Va: American Diabetes Association.

Warshaw H. American Diabetes Association's Guide to Healthy Restaurant Eating. Alexandria, Va: American Diabetes Association; 2000.

# Learning Assessment: Post-Test Questions

## Medical Nutrition Therapy for Diabetes

**1**

**1** Which of the following persons with type 2 diabetes would most benefit from medical nutrition therapy (MNT)?
  **A** 42-year-old female with a cholesterol of 205 mg/dL
  **B** 51-year-old male with low-density lipoproteins (LDL) of 134 mg/dL
  **C** 36-year-old female with triglycerides of 150 mg/dL
  **D** 60-year-old male with high-density lipoproteins (HDL) of 50 mg/dL

**2** An effective strategy for achieving blood glucose goals in a person with type 1 diabetes is
  **A** Moderate caloric restriction
  **B** Eating meals and snacks at specific times
  **C** Increasing NPH insulin if carbohydrate intake exceeds usual consumption
  **D** Integrating insulin regimen into usual eating habits

**3** The macronutrient that exerts the greatest influence on postprandial blood glucose levels is
  **A** Protein
  **B** Carbohydrate
  **C** Fat
  **D** Fiber

**4** Insulin affects the use and storage of nutrients in each of the following ways except
  **A** Facilitates cellular transport
  **B** Promotes lipogenesis by inactivating lipoprotein lipase
  **C** Stimulates glycogen synthesis
  **D** Suppresses gluconeogenesis (glucose production by the liver)

**5** Which of the following intakes of the sugar substitute aspartame on a daily basis exceeds the acceptable daily intake (ADI) for a female who weighs 130 lb?
  **A** 14 cans (12 oz) of diet soft drinks
  **B** 18 cans (12 oz) of diet soft drinks
  **C** 45 packets of a tabletop sweetener
  **D** 75 packets of a tabletop sweetener

**6** ML is a 39-year-old person with type 1 diabetes who weighs 121 lb (55 kg) and has overt nephropathy. Her protein requirement is
  **A** 35 g
  **B** 44 g
  **C** 50 g
  **D** 55 g

**7** If ML eats a meal that includes 1 serving from the starch group, 1 serving of meat (1 oz), 1 serving of fruit (1/2 c), and 1 serving of milk (8 oz), what will be her intake of protein?
  **A** 10 g
  **B** 14 g
  **C** 18 g
  **D** 20 g

**8** Which of the following MNT strategies is consistent with the goal of attaining optimal lipid levels?
  **A** Limit fat consumption to 20% of daily calories in a person with normal lipid levels
  **B** Restrict dietary cholesterol to less than 200 mg/day if triglycerides are elevated
  **C** Limit saturated fatty acids to less than 10% of daily calories if LDL cholesterol is the primary concern
  **D** Increase polyunsaturated fat to 15% of total fat calories if VLDL levels are a primary concern

**9** Assuming that blood glucose goals are being met, the guidelines for the use of alcohol in persons with diabetes include all of the following except:
  **A** Teach adult men with diabetes to limit consumption to 2 drinks with their regular meal plan
  **B** Eliminate 1 or more carbohydrate servings for each alcoholic beverage consumed
  **C** A 12-oz beer, 5-oz wine, or 1½-oz of hard liquor (spirits) is considered 1 drink
  **D** Avoid consumption of alcoholic beverages if triglycerides are elevated

**10** Persons with type 2 diabetes who are sodium sensitive and taking medications for hypertension should

   **A** Limit their intake of sodium to 3000 mg daily

   **B** Use no more than 2 tsp (5 g) of table salt as part of their total daily intake

   **C** Be encouraged to consume entrees with 800 mg sodium or less per serving

   **D** Limit their intake to low-sodium foods having 140 mg of sodium or less

**11** Guidelines for the role of carbohydrate in meal planning include

   **A** The amount of carbohydrate to be included in the meal plan is determined before the protein and fat

   **B** The amount of carbohydrate included will depend on the individual's current eating patterns and nutrition goals

   **C** It is more important to count the carbohydrate from simple sugars than the total daily intake of carbohydrate

   **D** The amount of fiber in the diet can be ignored since it is not digested (available to the body)

**12** Which of the following statements accurately describes the carbohydrate counting approach to meal planning?

   **A** Individuals are ready to learn pattern management once they learn carbohydrate-to-insulin ratios

   **B** Use of the basic diet planning guidelines is integral to a carbohydrate counting approach

   **C** Individuals who are familiar with the exchange system for meal planning may more easily grasp the carbohydrate counting approach

   **D** The carbohydrate counting approach restricts carbohydrate choices to starches and fruits

**13** PS is a marketing director with type 1 diabetes who learned about carbohydrate-to-insulin ratios a month ago and has managed to reach her glucose goals since she implemented this approach. She now wants to adjust her insulin for a corporate dinner she will be attending and asks your assistance. Her usual carbohydrate-to-insulin unit ratio is 2 (for each 1 carbohydrate choice she takes 2 units of lispro), and she usually takes 8 units of lispro with her evening meal. She anticipates that she will select 6 carbohydrate choices at this dinner, which is more than her usual. How many additional units of insulin will she need to take?

   **A** 1 unit

   **B** 2 units

   **C** 4 units

   **D** 6 units

**14** With her new flexibility in meal planning, she has also started to exercise. You advise her that

   **A** Her carbohydrate-to-insulin ratio will probably not change

   **B** She'll need to recheck her carbohydrate-to-insulin ratios if she continues to exercise regularly

   **C** She will need to add additional protein to her exercise snack

   **D** She should eat higher calorie snacks with sufficient fat content to adjust for the increase in flexibility in carbohydrate intake and to cover for exercise

**15** GH is an assembly line worker with type 2 diabetes and the equivalent of a fifth grade education. She was referred to you by her employer for nutrition counseling because she has had to take more than the usual number of bathroom breaks while working. Which approach to meal planning is more likely to be appropriate for her?

   **A** Carbohydrate counting

   **B** Exchange system

   **C** Diabetes nutrition guidelines

   **D** Booklets featuring monthly menus

*See next page for answer key.*

# Post-Test Answer Key

## Medical Nutrition Therapy for Diabetes

**1**

| | | | | |
|---|---|---|---|---|
| **1** | B | | **9** | B |
| **2** | D | | **10** | C |
| **3** | B | | **11** | B |
| **4** | B | | **12** | C |
| **5** | B | | **13** | C |
| **6** | B | | **14** | B |
| **7** | C | | **15** | C |
| **8** | C | | | |

# A Core Curriculum for Diabetes Education
Diabetes Management Therapies

## Exercise 2

*Catherine A. Mullooly, MS, RCEP*SM*, CDE*
*Joslin Clinic*
*Boston, MA*

## Introduction

**1** The beneficial effects of exercise in treating diabetes were recognized as early as the ancient times.[1] Centuries later in the 1920s, exercise was first recommended as a therapeutic tool for lowering blood glucose levels.[2,3]

**2** Today, exercise continues to be regarded as a primary component of diabetes management.

**3** Much of the morbidity and mortality among persons with diabetes is attributed to cardiovascular disease. Epidemiological evidence suggests that regular exercise and physical fitness are associated with decreased cardiovascular disease in the general population as well as a decreased occurrence of type 2 diabetes.[4]

**4** Because individuals, including people with diabetes, are living longer, the prevalence of diabetes in the elderly and the total number of people with diabetic complications are increasing. Consequently, the role of exercise becomes even more significant.

**5** This chapter focuses on the benefits, effects, risks, and precautions of exercise for persons with diabetes. Also discussed are exercise options for special populations, strategies for enhancing exercise, guidelines for developing exercise prescriptions and strategies for self-directed exercise programs.

## Objectives

Upon completion of this chapter, the learner will be able to

**1** State the benefits of exercise.

**2** Describe the physiologic response to exercise in individuals with and without diabetes.

**3** Identify the risks associated with exercise and ways to minimize risks.

**4** Explain the principles of an exercise program for people with diabetes.

**5** Identify appropriate exercise therapies for special populations.

**6** Describe strategies for self-directed exercise programs.

## Benefits of Exercise

**1** Exercise generally is regarded as having a salutary effect for everyone. The benefits are many and may be even more favorable for the person with diabetes.

**2** Most of the benefits result from chronic (regular, long-term), aerobic (cardiovascular) exercise.

**3** Resistance exercise to increase muscle strength is an important means of preserving and increasing muscular strength and endurance and of preventing falls and increasing mobility among the elderly.[5]

**4** Because persons with diabetes have an increased risk of cardiovascular disease, the role of exercise in reducing modifiable risks has primary importance. The potential benefits of exercise for persons with diabetes include the following:[6,7]

**A** Improved functioning of the cardiovascular system

**B** Improved strength and physical work capacity

**C** Decreased risk factors for coronary artery disease (CAD)
  - Reduction in plasma cholesterol, triglycerides, and low-density lipoproteins (LDL)
  - Increase in high-density lipoproteins (HDL), particularly in the presence of weight loss

**D** Increased insulin sensitivity[7,8]

**E** Reduced hyperinsulinemia, a proposed risk factor for atherosclerosis[9-11]

**F** Enhanced fibrinolysis
  - Hypercoagulability frequently is present in persons with diabetes
  - Chronic exercise can enhance fibrinolysis and affect other mechanisms responsible for this hypothesized risk factor for atherosclerosis[12,13]

**G** Favorable changes in body composition (reduction of body fat and weight; increase in muscle mass)

**H** Adjunct therapy for controlling hypertension

**I** Improved quality of life and self-esteem; reduced psychological stress[14]

**5** The chronic effects of exercise appear to benefit the person with type 2 diabetes by reducing HbA1c, improving insulin sensitivity, assisting in attainment and maintenance of desirable body weight, and decreasing CAD risk factors.[15]

  **A** Several long-term studies[16-19] demonstrate a sustained improvement in glucose control while a regular exercise program is maintained.

  **B** Thus, exercise is an essential component of diabetes self-management education for all individuals with type 2 diabetes.

**6** Exercise is also a critical part of the overall diabetes self-management education for type 1 diabetes, especially in light of the increased risk for macrovascular disease in this patient population.

  **A** Regular exercise in type 1 has not been shown consistently to result in improved diabetes control as evidenced by HbA1c.[20-22] This finding may be due to the difficulty of balancing insulin adjustments with food in concordance with physical activity.

  **B** It may be possible, however, for select patients to obtain a sustained decrease in HbA1c.[23-26]

  **C** Recommendations for the prevention of exercise-induced hypoglycemia must be included in the exercise plan and educational program.

**7** Because of its effects on self-esteem and stress reduction, the addition of a regular exercise program can serve as the first step in self-directed behavior change for many individuals with diabetes.

## Physiology of Exercise in Individuals Without Diabetes

**1** Plasma glucose levels in individuals without diabetes who exercise remain relatively stable due to an intricate regulation between the increase in glucose uptake by exercising muscles and increased hepatic glucose production.[27]

**2** The contribution of carbohydrate (stored as glycogen in the liver and muscles) and fat (stored as triglyceride in adipose tissue) depends on exercise intensity, duration, fitness level, and time and content of the last meal.[6,28] This regulation involves a hormonal balance between decreased insulin secretion and increased action of catecholamines, glucagon, growth hormone, and cortisol (counterregulatory hormones).

**A** At the onset of exercise, fuel utilization by muscles progresses from fat (extracted from the bloodstream as free fatty acids [FFA] at rest) to high-energy phosphate compounds, such as adenosine triphosphate (ATP) and phosphocreatine (CP), to glucose utilization from intramuscular stores of glucose, and triglycerides.

- The immediate fuel sources available for muscle contraction are ATP and CP. The breakdown of these high-energy phosphate compounds contributes to the immediate resynthesis of ATP (the primary fuel source for muscle contraction).
- ATP and CP stores are limited and can only supply the energy needs of quick, powerful movements, such as sprinting for time periods of 8 to 12 seconds.
- As exercise moves from the quick, initial muscle action to an extended exercise session, the fuel supply for the contracting muscles shifts from the immediate high energy phosphate groups to the second system from which ATP is produced (glycolysis).[29]

**B** During the first few minutes of exercise, intramuscular glucose is broken down *anaerobically* (without oxygen present). Although this pathway does not provide an abundant quantity of ATP, this pathway is important at the onset of exercise when oxygen availability is limited. As exercise continues, an adequate supply of oxygen becomes available for the breakdown of carbohydrates, fats, and proteins, if necessary, for the resynthesis of ATP.

- During sustained exercise, carbohydrate, protein, and fat continually recharge the phosphate pool.
- After the first 5 to 10 minutes, glycogen breakdown decreases, as circulating glucose from the liver becomes a major fuel source (*hepatic glycogenolysis*).[30]

**C** As exercise continues beyond 20 to 30 minutes, the muscle glycogen stores are depleted. Plasma glucose is maintained as glucose is broken down from the liver (hepatic glycogenolysis) and free fatty acids (FFA) (triglycerides mobilized from adipose tissue) are utilized.

- At the beginning of exercise, hepatic glucose production is mainly derived from glycogenolysis.
- As exercise continues, gluconeogenesis becomes increasingly important in providing glucose. The main substrates for hepatic gluconeogenesis during exercise are lactate, amino acids, and glycerol.

**D** As exercise duration increases, the contribution of FFA as a fuel increases relative to glucose, from about 35% at 40 minutes of exercise to nearly 70% at 4 hours of exercise.[6,30]

- Exercise of low-to-moderate intensity relies primarily on FFA as the oxidative fuel for muscle.[6]
- The oxidation of fat-derived fuels cannot replace the utilization of glucose. When carbohydrate is limited, fat is not completely oxidized and ketone bodies are formed.

**E** Hormonal response to exercise determines substrate utilization during exercise (Table 2.1).

- Secretion of counterregulatory hormones increases and helps maintain glucose homeostasis.[26,31]
- Insulin secretion is decreased during exercise as a result of increased activity of the sympathetic nervous system.[31,32]

## Table 2.1. Hormonal Response and Metabolic Effects During Exercise in Individuals Without Diabetes

| Hormone | Response During Exercise | Metabolic Effect |
|---|---|---|
| *Insulin* | ⬇ | • Facilitates hepatic glucose and FFA production |
| *Glucagon* | ⬆ | • Increases hepatic glucose production, increases blood glucose |
| *Epinephrine* | ⬆ | • Stimulates FFA production, which provides glycerol as a substrate for glucogenesis |
| *Norepinephrine* | ⬆ | • Stimulates hepatic and muscle glycolysis, stimulates lipolysis |
| *Growth hormone/Cortisol* | ⬆ | • Increases lipolysis, decreases insulin-stimulated glucose uptake, increases gluconeogenetic substrates |

- The suppression of insulin secretion facilitates hepatic glucose production and lipolysis, which allows blood glucose to be maintained.[28,30,33]

**F** An ongoing increased uptake of glucose by muscle occurs during the postexercise period as one means of replenishing glycogen stores.
- Replenishment of glycogen stores may take 24 to 48 hours.[6,34]
- The postexercise recovery, particularly after exhaustive work, is characterized by enhanced insulin sensitivity.[35,36]

**G** Trained athletes demonstrate the following responses:
- A reduction in fasting insulin secretion in response to a glucose load
- An increase in muscle sensitivity to insulin despite reduced insulin secretion[28,37]
- Less of a generalized secretion of counterregulatory hormones than sedentary individuals[32]
- Less glucose utilization than sedentary individuals during exercise that is of similar intensity and duration and, as a result, a slower rate and duration of glycogen usage as well as a greater reliance on fats for fuel, which are associated with greater endurance.[31,32]

## Physiology of Exercise in Individuals With Diabetes

**1** A person with diabetes who exercises may have a decreased need for, or better utilization of, insulin; the result may be a decrease in diabetes medications needed to reach glucose goals.

  **A** Acute effects of exercise generally cause a reduction in plasma glucose.

  **B** Chronic exercise results in improved insulin sensitivity and glucose tolerance because of changes in body composition and the additive effects of daily exercise.

**C** The hormonal response to exercise depends on the degree of diabetes control, medication, time and content of the last meal, fitness level, and type of exercise.
  - Because the person with type 1 diabetes does not have a normal compensatory decrease in insulin secretion with exercise, metabolic abnormalities may occur.[9,27,32,33,38]

**2** Hypoglycemia is the most commonly encountered problem in individuals with diabetes who exercise and are treated with insulin or insulin secretagogues.
  - **A** Normally, plasma insulin decreases with exercise in individuals without diabetes. This decrease, along with increases in plasma counterregulatory hormones, allows hepatic glucose production and lipolysis to match glucose utilization.
  - **B** In persons with diabetes taking insulin, the plasma insulin concentration does not decrease. Because the insulin is exogenous in origin, the plasma insulin concentration actually may increase due to increased sensitivity or mobilization from subcutaneous depots (Table 2.2).

---

## Table 2.2. Factors That Contribute to Hypoglycemia in Type 1 Diabetes

- Accelerated absorption of insulin
- Nonsuppressible plasma insulin levels
- Increased insulin sensitivity
- Possible impaired counterregulatory hormonal response

*autonomic neuropathy*

---

  - A high plasma insulin level during exercise may enhance glucose uptake and further stimulate glucose oxidation in the exercising muscle.[7]
  - A high plasma insulin level inhibits hepatic glucose production and FFA mobilization.[33] As a result, hepatic glucose production does not keep pace with peripheral glucose utilization and the blood glucose concentration falls.
  - Hypoglycemia also can result from exercise in patients with type 2 diabetes treated with insulin secretagogues (sulfonylureas, meglitinide, and nateglinide) or insulin.[38] These individuals are less prone to exercise-induced hypoglycemia, although it still can occur, and very rarely develop hyperglycemia with ketosis. Improvements in insulin sensitivity, insulin secretion, and glucose disposal rates have been well documented in type 2 diabetes as a result of regular exercise, although the mechanisms underlying these improvements have not been clearly explained.[7,40] Changes in body composition (decrease in fat weight and increase in muscle mass) contribute to increasing sensitivity to endogenous and exogenous insulin. The potential result is a reduction in exogenous insulin and/or anti-hyperglycemic agents.

**3** Another major concern for persons with diabetes who are taking insulin, or sulfonylureas or meglitinides, particularly those with type 1 diabetes, is *post-exercise, late-onset hypoglycemia* (PEL) (that is, hypoglycemia occurring 4 or more hours following exercise). This is more frequently encountered in those individuals with type 1 diabetes.

**A** PEL generally occurs following exercise of moderate to high intensity with a duration greater than 30 minutes.

**B** PEL results from increased insulin sensitivity, ongoing glucose utilization, and repletion of glycogen stores.[41]

**4** In type 1 individuals with hyperglycemia and/or ketosis, acute exercise may result in a worsening of metabolic control.[7,42] A certain amount of insulin is required for glucose uptake. In the absence of adequate insulin, exercise raises plasma glucose, FFA, and ketones (Table 2.3).

**5** Exercise of a high intensity can also cause blood glucose levels to be higher after exercise than before, even though blood glucose levels are in the normal range before beginning exercise. This hyperglycemia can also extend into the postexercise state and is mediated by the counterregulatory hormones. Hepatic glucose production no longer matches, but, in fact, exceeds the rise in glucose use.[43-45]

## Table 2.3. Consequences of Insufficient Insulin

- Impaired peripheral glucose utilization
- Excessive counterregulatory hormones
- Enhanced hepatic glucose production, lipolysis, and ketogenesis
- Rapid rise in already elevated blood glucose level and increased ketosis

## Special Considerations and Precautions of Exercise

**1** The primary side effect of acute exercise is hypoglycemia. Occasionally, hyperglycemia and ketosis also occur in individuals with type 1 diabetes (Table 2.4).

**A** Blood glucose response to exercise is affected by the type, amount, and intensity of exercise; the timing and type of previous meal and medication; the preexercise blood glucose level; and the fitness level.[8,29,30]

**B** Hypoglycemia is a significant threat to persons who exercise while taking insulin, or sulfonylureas or meglitinide; nateglinide, however, has a low potential for hypoglycemia. Persons who use biguanides, thiazolidinediones, alpha-glucosidases, or meal planning and exercise alone to control type 2 diabetes are not at risk of hypoglycemia when exercising.

**C** General guidelines to either increase carbohydrate consumption or decrease medication(s) are based on planned versus unplanned exercise. Initial guidelines should be provided and then adjusted based on the individual's response to the exercise program.

**2** Exercise-induced hypoglycemia can be largely prevented by implementing certain guidelines.

**A** During planned exercise/activity, the following self-management tasks can reduce the risk of hypoglycemia.

## Table 2.4. Exercise Considerations for People With Diabetes

*Hypoglycemia (if diabetes is treated with insulin, or sulfonylureas or meglitinides)*
- Exercise-induced hypoglycemia
- Postexercise, late-onset hypoglycemia (PEL)

*Hyperglycemia after very strenuous (high-intensity) exercise*

*Hyperglycemia and ketosis in insulin-deficient type 1 patients*

*Precipitation or exacerbation of cardiovascular disease*
- Presence of silent heart disease: arrhythmia, cardiac dysfunction
- Excessive increases in blood pressure with exercise
- Angina pectoris
- Myocardial infarction
- Sudden death

*Worsening of long-term complications with inappropriately prescribed exercise program*
- Proliferative retinopathy: vitreous hemorrhage, retinal detachment
- Nephropathy: increased proteinuria
- Peripheral neuropathy: soft tissue and joint injury, foot ulcers, orthopedic injury
- Autonomic neuropathy: decreased cardiovascular response to exercise, decreased maximum aerobic capacity, impaired response to dehydration, orthostatic hypotension, impaired counterregulatory response

*Source:* Adapted from Horton ES. Prescription for exercise. Diabetes Spectrum 1991;4:250-257.

- Adjustments are needed to prevent hypoglycemia in the insulin-treated individual because hepatic glucose production is blocked or partially inhibited by exogenous insulin.[29,33] The physiological decrease in circulating insulin levels that occurs with exercise cannot take place in patients treated with insulin.
- A reduction of the rapid-acting or short-acting insulin of 30% to 50% has been demonstrated to decrease the risk of hypoglycemia.[38,46]
- Also effective would be to decrease the insulin acting during the time of exercise by 10% of the total daily insulin.
- The recommendation to change the injection site to a part of the body not involved in the activity to prevent hypoglycemia was based on published reports in the 1970s.[47] These studies demonstrated an increase in serum insulin levels in patients who exercised shortly after an insulin injection. The recommendation to inject in the arm or abdomen instead of the leg if the activity was jogging or cycling emerged from these studies. Despite the increased absorption rate, subsequent research[48] demonstrated that simply changing the insulin injection site was not effective for preventing hypoglycemia. If the level of circulating insulin is elevated for any reason, hypoglycemia is likely to occur. Dose reductions should accompany any exercise that is performed during the peak action of the insulin.[49]
- Proper administration of insulin requires injecting into the subcutaneous fat layer. Teach patients to avoid intramuscular injection of insulin prior to exercise because muscle contractions accelerate the absorption of insulin into the circulation.[49]

- Blood glucose monitoring before and after exercise provides needed feedback for the individual who is learning to adjust insulin and/or carbohydrate (CHO) with exercise.
- Tailor adjustments to the specific exercise response of each individual (Table 2.5). The choice between decreasing medication or increasing carbohydrate will depend on the individual's goals.

## Table 2.5. Exercise Adjustments

|  | Individual's Goals |
| --- | --- |
| *Insulin Adjustment* | • Weight loss<br>• Improved control<br>• Planned, regularly scheduled exercise |
| *Carbohydrate Replacement* | • Long duration of exercise<br>• Unplanned exercise |

B During unplanned exercise/activity, carbohydrate replacement may be necessary to prevent hypoglycemia when insulin adjustments are not made or when exercise occurs several hours after a meal or when exercise is of a long duration.

- The amount of additional carbohydrate needed depends on the time of exercise in relation to medication and previous meal; the type, intensity, and duration of exercise (Table 2.6); and the preexercise blood glucose level.
- Exercise performed 1 to 3 hours after a meal may not require any additional carbohydrate supplement.

## Table 2.6. Carbohydrate Replacement During Exercise[51]

| Intensity | Duration (minutes) | Carbohydrate Replacement | Frequency |
| --- | --- | --- | --- |
| *Mild-to-moderate* | <30 | May not be needed | — |
| *Moderate* | 30 to 60 | 15 g | Each hour |
| *High* | 60+ | 30 to 50 g | Each hour |

- Moderate intensity exercise increases glucose uptake by the muscle 2 to 3 mg/kg/body weight/min above resting levels.[38] For example, a 154 lb (70 kg) individual would require an additional 140 to 210 mg of glucose for every minute of moderate exercise. This would mean an additional 8.4 to 12.6 g of glucose is required for every hour of exercise.
- For high-intensity exercise, the rate of glucose utilization by the muscle may increase to as much as 5 to 6 mL/kg/body weight/min or an additional 350 to 420 mg of

glucose for every minute of exercise. Even though the rate of glucose utilization increases, the demand on glucose stores and risk of hypoglycemia is less because exercise of this intensity cannot be sustained for long periods of time.[38]

- A snack is needed when the preexercise blood glucose level places the person at risk for hypoglycemia during or at the end of the exercise session.
- Unfortunately, the starting blood glucose level that places an individual at risk for hypoglycemia is sometimes only defined after a period of trial and error. Blood glucose monitoring can help to determine the minimum level at which a carbohydrate snack is required.
- Preexercise snacks have been demonstrated to prevent post-exercise hypoglycemia when taken 15 to 30 minutes before exercise of short duration (less than 45 minutes).[50]

**C** For individuals participating in extended periods of exercise (longer than 2 hours), reducing insulin may be easier than continually supplementing with carbohydrate. It may be necessary to reduce the dose of both rapid-acting or short-acting, and intermediate-acting or long-acting insulins depending on the time and type of exercise.

**D** Hypoglycemia remains a risk with exercise for persons using insulin pump therapy.
- The chances of developing hypoglycemia may be less for insulin pump users due to the steady infusion of insulin. Also, basal rates and boluses can be adjusted based on the timing, duration, and type of exercise performed.
- The amount of insulin decrease or the amount of carbohydrate supplement depends on a person's fitness level and the duration and intensity of the exercise.[46,52]
- Options for insulin pump users to maintain euglycemia with exercise include reducing the basal infusion rate, consuming additional carbohydrates, or temporarily suspending pump use.[46,50,52,53]

**E** A link between the time of day when exercise is performed and the risk of exercise-induced hypoglycemia has not been confirmed with research.
- The risk for hypoglycemia with exercise may be lower when the level of circulating insulin is low. For example, exercise performed prior to the morning insulin injection presents a low risk of hypoglycemia.
- The risk for nocturnal hypoglycemia is increased when exercise is performed during the evening hours. However, decreasing the evening insulin dose can reduce this risk.

**F** The likelihood of exercise-induced hypoglycemia can be decreased by avoiding exercise when the injected insulin is reaching the peak level. However, an insulin adjustment usually is required because it may be difficult to avoid exercise when medication is peaking.

**3** Postexercise, late-onset hypoglycemia (PEL) occurs several hours following an exercise session and is a significant concern to persons treated with insulin; it also can occur in persons treated with insulin secretogogues.

**A** PEL can be the result of acutely increased insulin mobilization and sensitivity, increased glucose utilization, replenishment of glycogen stores, and defective counterregulatory mechanisms.[27,41]

**B** Options to minimize the occurrence of PEL include
- Providing patient education to increase awareness
- Reducing the insulin that peaks during the postexercise period

- Supplementing carbohydrate during the postexercise phase
- Avoiding exercise prior to bedtime
- Monitoring blood glucose frequently during the postexercise period[41]

**4** Exercise-induced hyperglycemia can occur in individuals with type 1 diabetes.

  **A** Hyperglycemia and worsening of ketosis can result if exercise is initiated when fasting blood glucose levels are greater than 250 mg/dL (13.9 mmol/L) and ketones are present.[42]

- Teach patients to delay exercise until blood glucose levels improve and ketones are negative.
- If a type 1 patient has a postmeal blood glucose level greater than 250 to 300 mg/dL (13.9 to 16.7 mmol/L) due to a dietary indiscretion, an insulin deficiency may not be indicated. Exercise under this condition generally will cause a drop in blood glucose levels.
- Negative urine ketones confirm the absence of insulin deficiency.
- A patient with type 1 diabetes should use caution if exercise is going to be performed with a blood glucose level that is greater than 300 mg/dL (16.7 mmol/dL) even in the absence of ketones.

  **B** Occasionally, high-intensity, short-term, exhaustive exercise causes an acute rise in blood glucose levels in persons with well-controlled diabetes.[43-45]

- Participation in highly competitive sports can sometimes result in postexercise hyperglycemia. This phenomenon may be due to excess sympathetic stimulation as a result of high-intensity exercise; catecholamines are released that act on the liver to produce glucose. This has been observed to cause initial increases, followed by declines, in blood glucose levels. However, the existence of an undetected hypoglycemic reaction during exercise should not be overlooked as this sometimes can cause the same sympathetic response.
- An extra injection of insulin should not be administered in response to the hyperglycemia. The insulin action will coincide with the postexercise increase in insulin sensitivity and potentially result in severe hypoglycemia.

## Other Safety Precautions

**1** Teach all persons with diabetes who are treated with insulin, sulfonylureas, or meglitinides to carry some type of carbohydrate with them while exercising.

**2** Blood glucose monitoring, both pre- and postexercise, is the key to safety and understanding of how exercise affects blood glucose.

**3** Advise persons with diabetes to wear some form of diabetes and personal identification.

**4** Avoid vigorous exercise if the environment is extremely hot, humid, smoggy, or cold.

**5** Proper equipment and exercise shoes appropriate for the activity will reduce the likelihood of injury.

**6** Include a warm-up and cool-down sessions with each workout. Stretching exercises performed following the cool-down enhance flexibility and prevent injury.

**7** Certain medications can impair exercise tolerance. Beta-blockers alter the heart-rate response to exercise as well as mask hypoglycemia and the body's counterregulatory response.

**8** Adequate hydration should be maintained while exercising.

**9** Stop exercise if pain, light-headedness, or shortness of breath occurs.

**10** The American Diabetes Association recognizes that an exercise tolerance test may be helpful if a patient is going to participate in a moderate- to high-intensity exercise program or for anyone at high risk for underlying cardiovascular disease.[42] Direct special attention during assessments toward identifying a history of cardiac disease (including silent heart disease), the presence of complications, medications, medical and family history, and degree of diabetes control. Physical activity assessments are useful for patients and educators when planning exercise.

## Exercise Programs

**1** There are two types of exercise: aerobic and anaerobic.

**A** *Aerobic exercise* is defined as exercise that involves repetitive, submaximal contraction of major muscle groups (eg, swimming, cycling, jogging) and requires oxygen to sustain muscular effort.[40,54] Aerobic exercise provides the greatest benefits for people with diabetes in terms of blood glucose control and cardiovascular status. The health-related benefits of exercise do not appear to be dependent on the type of aerobic exercise.

**B** *Anaerobic exercise* is defined as exercise that does not require sustained oxygen to meet the energy demands and generally does not induce the same health benefits as an aerobic program.

• Anaerobic exercise and certain types and intensity levels of aerobic exercise may cause excessive rises in blood pressure, cardiac workload, and intraocular pressure. These reactions could be potential problems in persons with diabetes and vascular disease or complications.

• Studies[55,56] suggest that properly designed resistance programs may improve indices of cardiovascular function, glucose tolerance, strength, and body composition provided the person with diabetes does not have contraindications to weight training.

**2** The duration of exercise is inversely related to the intensity of the exercise: lower intensity exercise needs to be conducted over a longer period of time than higher intensity exercise for maximum benefit. The duration of exercise to meet the required weekly energy expenditure is 20 to 60 minutes per session.[15]

**A** All workouts should include a 5- to 10-minute warm-up and cool-down.

• The warm-up increases core body temperature and prevents muscle injury; the cool-down prevents blood pooling in the extremities and facilitates removal of metabolic by-products.

• Initiate exercise in the warm-up and conclude in the cool-down phase.[57]

**B** New studies have shown similar cardiorespiratory gains to occur when physical activity is done in shorter bouts (~10 minutes) accumulated throughout the day, as when activity of similar duration and intensity occurs for one prolonged session (~30 minutes).[5,57] However, 30 minutes of continuous exercise seems to have a greater impact on weight loss.[58]

- These findings, although beneficial in terms of cardiorespiratory gains, have not been studied in the diabetes population.
- It may be necessary for severely deconditioned individuals to exercise in multiple sessions of short duration (~10 minutes).[57]

**3** To achieve the desired fitness level, exercise needs to be done 5 times per week or 3 to 4 times per week for maintenance.[40]

**A** The duration of glycemic improvement after the last exercise session usually is greater than 12 hours but less than 72 hours.[18]

**B** To improve glycemic control, exercise needs to be done at least every other day, on at least 3 nonconsecutive days, and ideally 5 days per week.

**C** Obese individuals may need to exercise more frequently (5 to 7 days per week) to optimize weight loss or maintenance.

**D** Exercise that is limited to 2 days per week generally does not produce a meaningful change in maximal uptake.

**E** The minimum physical conditioning for health benefits requires expending at least 700 calories per week.

**F** For maximum health benefits, 2000 calories per week are required; there is limited substantial health benefit to expending greater than 2000 calories per week.[57]

**4** The intensity of exercise should be 60% to 85% of the maximal age-adjusted heart rate (comparable to 50% to 70% of maximal oxygen uptake or $VO_{2\,max}$).

**A** Training intensity can be calculated accurately using the results of an exercise stress test.

**B** Based on the individual's maximum heart-rate response to the exercise stress test, the following heart-rate (HR) reserve formula is commonly used to calculate target heart-rate zone: target heart-rate range = [($HR_{max}$ - $HR_{rest}$) × 0.50 and 0.85] + $HR_{rest}$.

- Select a range between 50% to 85% based on the individual's fitness level, duration of diabetes, degree of complications, and patient's goals.

**C** The following equation can be used to estimate the true maximal heart rate when the actual maximal exercise heart rate is unknown: $HR_{max}$ = 220 – patient's age.

- This procedure may overestimate the maximal heart rate of some type 2 patients, particularly those with autonomic neuropathy.[40,57]
- Due to the high prevalence of occult cardiovascular disease, caution is required when applying standard heart-rate formulas to the diabetes population.

**D** Exercise performed at low levels (<50% $HR_{max}$) has less effect on glucose disposal than exercise performed at higher intensities. The effect on glucose disposal during high-intensity exercise is roughly proportional to the total work performed (time × intensity). However, high-intensity exercise may result in transient hyperglycemia and cause an excessive rise in blood pressure.

**E** When initiating an exercise program, it may be necessary to begin at low levels (50%) with brief rest intervals and progress weekly to higher intensity, continual exercise.[57]

**5** Exercise components of duration, frequency, and intensity will help achieve aerobic training effects.

**A** Individual factors such as fitness level, age, and health status can affect the attainment of these goals.

**B** Medications (eg, ß-blockers) and the presence of secondary complications may affect the exercise plan and individual tolerance (Table 2.7).

## Table 2.7. Summary of Exercise Recommendations

| | |
|---|---|
| *Screening* | • Presence of vascular and neurological complications, silent heart disease, stress ECG (GXT*) in patients >35, type 2 diabetes >10 years' duration, type 1 diabetes >15 years' duration, microvascular disease (proliferative retinopathy or nephropathy), peripheral vascular disease, autonomic neuropathy. [42] |
| *Exercise Prescription* | *Type 2 Diabetes*[40]<br>• Aerobic preferred; anaerobic allowed if no secondary limitations (2 times/wk)<br>*Intensity*<br>• 50% to 85% of heart rate reserve or 60% to 90% of maximal heart rate (40% to 70% of maximum aerobic capacity)<br>*Duration*<br>• 30 to 60 min (can be divided into three 10-min sessions)<br>*Frequency*<br>• 3 nonconsecutive days up to 5 times per week; schedule every other day |
| *Exercise Prescription* | *Type 1 Diabetes*[42]<br>• All levels of exercise can be performed by those who do not have complications and are in good blood glucose control. |
| *Safety Precautions* | • Warm up/cool down<br>• Careful selection and progression of exercise program<br>• Patient education<br>• Monitor blood glucose pre-/postexercise<br>• Adjust guidelines to prevent hypoglycemia<br>• Management by healthcare personnel |

*GXT = graded exercise test.
*Source:* Adapted from the American Diabetes Association. Exercise and NIDDM: a technical review.[41]

**6** It has been recommended that strength-developing exercises be included with cardiorespiratory endurance activities in order to improve musculoskeletal health, maintain independence in performing daily activities, and reduce the possibility of injury.[5,59] The acute components of a resistance-training program include the following:

**A** The choice of which exercises to perform is based upon what the individual wants to achieve with the strengthening program.

- If an individual wants to achieve specific strength gains, then the resistance program is planned to target the particular action and muscular components that are essential in the desired activity.
- Individuals who are interested in basic fitness can select exercises that use each of the major muscle groups of the body (shoulders, back, chest, abdomen, and legs).[60]

**B** Advise patients to exercise in a specific order to use the larger muscle groups first and then move to the smaller muscle groups.

- By working the larger muscle groups and then proceeding to the smaller groups, the demanding exercises are performed early in the workout while the energy supply is the greatest and the individual has an abundance of energy.
- If one chooses to perform the exercises in an alternative manner, the exercises which have a small energy demand will start to deplete energy stores, leaving the individual with a reduced energy supply to complete more debilitative exercises (exercises including the larger muscle groups).[61]

**C** For individuals with diabetes and no known cardiac disease, it is important to find out what physical attributes are necessary to attain their goal before determining the appropriate resistance. Once these parameters have been identified, the resistance and repetition load can be determined.

- The resistance used is determined though the individual's *repetition maximum* (RM), which is defined as the amount of weight that allows for successful completion of a specified number of repetitions (no more, no less).[61]
- Studies have shown repetitions of 8 RM or less to produce the greatest strength gains, and muscular endurance is maximized through the use of resistance that allows for the performance of more than 12 repetitions.
- For an individual who wants to achieve both muscular strength and endurance, 8 to 12 repetitions would be the most appropriate range.
- When working with individuals with cardiac disease, particular attention must be focused on blood pressure and heart-rate response to the resistance training. It is recommended that these individuals start at lighter resistance loads and perform exercises that utilize a smaller amount of muscle mass, which in turn will decrease the myocardial oxygen demand on the heart.[61] The heart rate and blood pressure need to remain within the limits established by the exercise tolerance test and, therefore, should be monitored throughout the training session.

**D** Performing 1 to 2 sets of each exercise has been proven to be beneficial to increase general muscle strength and endurance.

- Instruct individuals with a low fitness level or little training experience to complete just 1 set of each exercise for the first 4 to 6 weeks. Once they are comfortable with the exercise and have demonstrated good technique, the number of sets can be increased.

**E** Rest for an adequate amount of time between sets to allow for successful completion of the next set.

- For individuals training at lower intensities, rest periods are short (15 seconds to 1 minute).
- Individuals training at higher intensities will take longer to recover and may take up 2 minutes to regain enough energy to successfully complete the next set.[60]

**7** Special precautions need to be taken by patients with diabetes prior to starting a resistance-training program.

**A** Before starting the exercise sessions, teach the individual proper weight lifting technique:

- Keep the body properly aligned.
- Breathe properly, exhaling during the phase in which the muscle is exerting its force against the apparatus and inhaling while lowering the weight.
- Control the lifting movement.
- Obtain the adequate range of motion.
- Make sure the equipment is adjusted to fit the body frame.

**B** Individuals with long-term microvascular or macrovascular complications will require program modifications to decrease the strain on their cardiovascular systems due to the resistive exercises.

- Teach patients with proliferative retinopathy or nephropathy to avoid resistive training. Resistive exercises may be harmful due to the excessive systolic pressure responses experienced.[61]
- Individuals with diabetes who also have cardiovascular disease should possess an ejection fraction of = 45% and a cardiorespiratory fitness level of = 7 metabolic equivalents (METs), without ischemic ST segment depression on their electrocardiogram, hypo- or hypertensive responses, serious ventricular arrhythmias, or symptoms of cardiovascular disease, prior to beginning a resistance training program.[62]
- Patients with any complications that may be exacerbated by resistance training should always receive approval from their physician before starting a program.

---

## Exercise Considerations for the Elderly

**1** Age-associated changes in body composition in the elderly account for decreases in basal metabolic rate, muscle strength, activity levels, and a decreased energy expenditure.

**A** Reductions in lean body mass occur primarily as a result of loss of skeletal muscle mass and increase in body fat. This decrease in muscle mass is a direct cause of the decrease in muscle strength seen in older adults.

**B** Research has provided evidence that muscle mass, not muscular function, is the major determinate of age- and gender-related differences in strength.[63] As physical activity levels decline with advancing age, muscle power and strength become critical elements in walking ability.

**C** The capacity of the elderly to respond to an exercise program is often underrated. Individuals over the age of 60 years have demonstrated greater benefits from aerobic and strength training in fitness capacity, strength, functional capacity, and glucose tolerance than comparable younger groups.

**D** Special attention needs to be directed toward potential hazards for the elderly population.[64,65]

- A thorough physical exam is required prior to initiation of an exercise program. Emphasis is placed on detecting occult heart disease, cardiovascular and/or peripheral vascular disease, joint/bone disease, and secondary complications.
- Strength training improves performance activities of daily living and counteracts muscle weakness. Teach patients to train each major muscle group 2 to 3 times per week. Muscular toning can be accomplished via free weights, strap-on

ankle/wrist weights, and traditional strengthening machines (eg, Nautilus®). The appropriate intensity is in the range of 1 set of 8 to 12 repetitions "somewhat hard" on the perceived exertion rating (12 to 13).[57]

- Aerobic fitness is beneficial for older persons (Table 2.8). Because of the progressive decline in oxygen transport and functional capacity, an effective training stimulus for this age group may be much less than is needed in a younger person.[64]

**E** Teach individuals with degenerative joint disease or osteoarthritis to avoid orthopedic or musculoskeletal stress. Vary exercise so that it is primarily weight-bearing one day and nonweightbearing on alternate days.[57]

**F** Sedentary individuals have an increased risk for cardiac arrest and cerebral vascular accidents if exercise is too vigorous. Teach these patients to initiate exercise at lower levels, progress slower, and gradually increase in duration and frequency to reach their desired fitness level.

## Table 2.8. Guidelines for Aerobic Exercise in the Elderly

*Beneficial aerobic activities include cycling, brisk walking, swimming, dancing, rowing.*

*Intersperse initial exercise with brief rest periods; continuous exercise is achieved over time.*

*Adding 2 to 5 minutes per week to the workout usually is appropriate for achieving the following desired goals[64]:*
- Duration of 30 to 40 minutes
- Frequency of 5 to 6 times per week
- Intensity based on graded exercise test (GXT), risk factors, medical history (typical training heart rate in the elderly is 60% to 75% of maximal heart rate)

*Assess progress and reevaluate the exercise plan in about 4 to 6 weeks.*

## Exercise Considerations for Obese Persons

**1** Combined programs of exercise, meal planning, and behavior change are effective for obese persons.

**A** The therapeutic approach that emphasizes increased levels of physical activity offers the advantage of enhancing caloric expenditure and providing the benefits of exercise in terms of influencing blood lipids, blood glucose control, blood pressure, mood, and attitude.[54]

**B** Often, the initial fitness goal of the obese person is to simply increase the amount of physical activity from an inactive state.

**C** A combination of meal planning plus exercise has been shown to be more effective at long-term weight control than either meal planning or exercise alone. The addition of exercise to a weight-control program may facilitate more permanent weight loss than total reliance on caloric restriction.[8]

**D** Regular exercise during a weight-control program helps to maintain muscle mass while promoting fat loss. Weight loss achieved by caloric restriction alone may lead to loss of lean muscle mass and less loss of fat.

**E** Continuous aerobic exercise has the greatest impact on weight loss because of enhanced caloric expenditure.

- Walking is an effective choice for continuous aerobic exercise. Alternative types of exercise include cycling and water exercise.
- Less effective options are swimming (less likely to induce weight loss or provide aerobic effects) and running (too much knee stress for obese individuals).

**F** As the duration of exercise increases, so does the utilization of fat as a fuel. A longer duration (eg, greater than 45 minutes) has been shown to have a greater calorie-burning and fat-mobilization effect than shorter exercise periods.[6,57]

**G** Intensity should be at the low end of the target heart-rate range.

- The duration of exercise should be sufficient to expend 200 to 300 kcal per session.
- This calorie expenditure may be accomplished with low-intensity exercise of long duration (40 to 60 minutes) such as walking.[57]

**H** Frequency of exercise should be a minimum of 3 times per week. An exercise frequency of 5 times per week is recommended for increased weight loss and facilitation of blood glucose goal attainment.

## Exercise Considerations for Persons With Diabetes Complications

**1** Persons with chronic complications of diabetes often do not take part in physical activity programs. Yet, it is useful for this group to undertake an exercise program to improve or maintain their functional capacity, strength, and flexibility.[66] Since persons with diabetes have an increased risk of cardiovascular disease, comprehensive assessments may be necessary to determine the most appropriate exercises.

**2** Patients with established cardiovascular disease usually require supervision in a cardiac rehabilitation program.

**A** Hypertension and a hypertensive response to exercise (systolic blood pressure >260 mm Hg, diastolic blood pressure >125 mm Hg) frequently are seen in persons with diabetes.[57]

- Exercise should be performed at an intensity that avoids a hypertensive response.
- If the patient is hypertensive, advise them to avoid exercises that involve heavy lifting, straining, and Valsalva-like maneuvers.
- Exercise that involves the upper body and arms generally induces larger increases in systolic blood pressure than similar workloads performed by the legs alone.

**B** Rhythmic exercises using the lower extremities are recommended, such as walking, light jogging, and cycling. Weight training should involve low resistance with high repetitions.[57]

**3** Patients with peripheral vascular disease will experience ischemic pain during physical activity as a result of insufficient oxygen supply and demand for the active muscles.

**A** A walking program for intermittent claudication may improve collateral circulation and muscle metabolism and, in turn, decrease pain.[67]

**B** An interval training program of walk/rest periods results in greater exercise tolerance of pain-limited work capacity.

- The distance and duration of the walk is determined by a pain-limited threshold.
- Advise patients to keep the intensity low because higher intensity demands a greater blood supply and induces claudication pain.[65]
- Teach patients that conversation, music, etc. can divert attention from the discomfort and pain.
- Discontinue exercise when the discomfort or pain accelerates from moderate to intense discomfort and the individual's attention cannot be diverted.[57]

**C** Weight-bearing activities are preferred, although non weight-bearing activities may allow for longer duration and higher intensity exercise.

**D** Pain at rest and during the night are indications of severe peripheral vascular disease, which is an absolute contraindication for a walking exercise program.[68]

**E** Daily exercise will maximize tolerable pain.[57]

**4** Patients with advanced retinopathy have significant restrictions on exercise participation.

**A** Provide exercise recommendations based on the severity and stage of diabetic retinopathy. In general, exercise has not been shown to accelerate retinopathy.

**B** In the early stages of retinopathy, there are limited restrictions on exercise.
- Exercise may actually reduce the risk of developing proliferative diabetic retinopathy (PDR) and diabetic macular edema by its positive effects on blood pressure and HDL, which are associated with retinopathy.
- For patients with active PDR, strenuous activity may precipitate vitreous hemorrhage or traction retinal detachment; clearance for exercise must be provided by the patient's ophthalmologist.

**C** The level of retinopathy determines which activities are appropriate and which activities are to be avoided (Table 2.9).[69]

**5** For persons with recent visual impairment, and for some with long-standing visual loss, aerobic capacity may be reduced due to loss of independent mobility.

**A** Suitable options for exercise include swimming (using lane guides), stationary cycling, treadmill walking, tandem cycling, and folk dancing (using the sighted person as an anchor).

**B** Various teaching adaptations and organizations have broadened sports participation (snow skiing, track-and-field competition) for visually impaired individuals.[66]

**6** Nearly all known risk factors for coronary artery disease are found in persons with end-stage renal disease, thus underscoring the need for a properly planned exercise program.

**A** Although aerobic activities are preferred, the ability to perform this type of exercise depends on the degree of kidney impairment. These individuals usually have low functional and aerobic capacity.

**B** Recommend beginning any aerobic activity at a low level, perhaps using interval work, followed by a gradual, progressive exercise plan.[70] Brisk walking, swimming, and cycling are beneficial choices.

**7** Peripheral neuropathy can result in sensory losses of pain, touch, and balance. For example, neuroarthropathy (Charcot's foot) can lead to disarticulations and injury in sensory-impaired individuals.

## Table 2.9. Exercise Guidelines for Persons With Diabetic Retinopathy

| Level of Retinopathy | Exercise Recommendation(s) |
| --- | --- |
| *No diabetic retinopathy* | • No exercise limitations. |
| *Mild nonproliferative* | • No exercise limitations. |
| *Moderate nonproliferative* | • Avoid activities that dramatically elevate blood pressure (eg, power lifting). |
| *Severe to very severe nonproliferative* | • Limit increase in systolic blood pressure (eg, Valsalva maneuvers), and avoid activities that jar the head. Heart rate should not exceed that which elicits a systolic blood pressure response greater than 180 mm Hg (eg, boxing and intense competitive sports).[66] |
| *Proliferative* | • Avoid strenuous activity, high-impact activities, Valsalva maneuvers, and activities that jar the head (eg, weight lifting, jogging, high-impact aerobic dance, racquet sports, strenuous trumpet playing, and competitive sports). <br> • Encourage activities that are low-impact and aerobic and stress cardiovascular conditioning (eg, swimming without diving, walking, low-impact aerobic dance, stationary cycling, and endurance exercising).[69] |

**A** Exercise cannot reverse the symptoms of neuropathy, but it can prevent further loss of muscle strength and flexibility that commonly is seen in patients with sensory polyneuropathy. Adaptive shortening of connective tissue can occur due to immobilization or limited proprioception. Thus, daily range-of-motion exercises are recommended.

**B** Extra care is needed to avoid injury and overstretching by sensory-impaired individuals.[66]

　• Weight-bearing activities usually are not recommended because of the increased likelihood of soft tissue and joint injury.

　• Because avoiding orthopedic stress is important, exercises such as cycling and swimming are beneficial choices.

　• If balance is not impaired, brisk walking may be another alternative.[54]

　• Jogging is contraindicated because it places a threefold increase on the foot compared with walking.

**C** Proper footwear and inspection of the feet after exercise are strategies to prevent blisters and detect injuries. For persons with limited mobility, chair exercises may improve flexibility and strength.

**8** Exercise in people with autonomic neuropathy should be approached with caution because of the role of the autonomic nervous system in hormonal and cardiovascular regulation during exercise.

**A** Symptoms of angina are not reliable indicators of coronary artery disease due to the higher frequency of silent ischemia and myocardial infarction among people with diabetes.[27]

**B** Physical working capacity is reduced.

**C** High-intensity exercise should be avoided.

**D** Because dehydration may be a risk in individuals who have difficulty with thermoregulation, exercise in hot or cold environments should be avoided. Hypotension and hypertension following vigorous exercise are possibilities.

**E** Recumbent cycling and water aerobics are options for persons with orthostatic hypotension.

**F** Frequent blood glucose monitoring also is recommended during exercise for people with defective counterregulatory mechanisms.[66]

## Exercise Participation

**1** Little is known about how to increase and maintain participation in exercise programs.

**A** Only 22% of American adults participate in an exercise program that has been recommended for health benefits (light-to-moderate physical activity sustained for at least 30 minutes). About 54% are somewhat active but do not meet this objective, and 24% or more are completely sedentary.[71-73]

**B** More is known about exercise relapse than effective interventions. Approximately 50% of people who join an exercise program drop out during the first 3 to 6 months.

**2** The transtheoretical model for change has been applied to exercise participation, weight loss, smoking cessation, and mammography screening.[74,75]

**A** A perception of the pros (benefits) versus the cons (demands) of exercising determine the transition from consideration to participation to maintenance of an exercise program.

**B** The stages of change can be used to tailor intervention strategies and exercise outcomes to include both readiness and behavioral changes (see Chapter 3, Behavior Change, in Diabetes Education and Program Management, for more information).

**3** Stage-matched interventions are the most effective. These interventions provide strategies for overcoming barriers to participation at each stage.

**A** In the precontemplation stage, exercise is not even a consideration. People in this stage lack confidence in their ability to begin or continue an exercise program and avoid reading, talking, and thinking about it.
  - Asking that they begin to exercise will have a negative effect.
  - Building a trusting relationship and providing information are needed at this stage.

**B** Individuals in the contemplation stage think about exercise and perceive the advantages and disadvantages to be equal, but they do not exercise.
  - Be supportive of these patients; they are looking for assistance and validation.
  - It is important not to criticize any ambivalence about exercise but rather to encourage discussion of concerns, questions, and personal reasons to exercise.

**C** In the preparation stage, the individuals have thought about exercise and are ready to begin.
  - The patient is ready to set goals and develops a self-exercise plan.
  - This stage is probably the most rewarding time for patients.

**D** In the action stage, the individuals are exercising. They have achieved a regular level of exercise at least 20 minutes 3 times per week. There is a high risk of relapse because the behavior is new.

**E** In the maintenance stage, the rewards of exercise are more subtle after 6 months. However, as the potential for relapse still exists, the educator's role is to keep activities interesting and assist the individuals in progressing with their program.

**F** Most people are not successful with their first try; they may need 3 or 4 attempts before exercise becomes a long-term habit. When relapse does occur, feelings of failure, embarrassment, guilt, or shame may surface. Fifteen percent of people become demoralized and resist trying again, so support is important in all stages.

- Eighty-five percent will try again.
- Sixty percent of all New Year's resolutions are repledged the following year.
- People progress through the stages as they learn from their mistakes and try something different the next time.
- The more action taken, the better chance of progressing forward.

## Self-Directed Exercise Programs

**1** Anecdotal reports suggest that personally designed programs enhance enjoyment and are more likely to be sustained. Patients who choose an activity that they enjoy are more likely to participate in it on a regular basis. Exercise is more likely to occur when it is convenient (eg, close to home or work).

**2** Asking patients if they are thinking about exercising and their feelings about it provides cues for how to provide information.

**3** It is important for patients to establish realistic and practical goals at the beginning of an exercise program. Goals that are too vague, too ambitious, or too distant do not provide enough self-motivation to maintain long-term interest.

**A** This is probably the most rewarding time for patients.

**B** Ask patients to identify barriers and develop strategies to overcome possible interruptions in their regular exercise schedule (eg, inclement weather, seasonal change, vacations, and holidays).

**C** Teach patients strategies to optimize social support from the family, exercise class members, or a buddy system.

**D** Suggest to patients that they develop stimulus control strategies to initiate and continue exercise participation (eg, write exercise in appointment books, set watch alarms for exercise time).

**E** Suggest patients compare the time it takes to walk 2 miles at the beginning of their exercise program with the time required to walk this distance after they have been exercising for a period of time.

**F** One method of feedback for people with diabetes is to keep a log of pre- and postexercise blood glucose levels or to chart HbA1c for the duration of the training program.

## Key Educational Considerations

**1** Assist individuals in designing an exercise plan that will help them to safely achieve their goals. Reevaluate the exercise goals and plan between 5 and 7 weeks to establish new goals, as necessary, that reinforce the effects, benefits, and principles of the exercise program.

**2** Assist individuals to identify barriers to the exercise program and determine options for overcoming the barriers. For example, to overcome fear of hypoglycemia, discuss ways to make adjustments to prevent hypoglycemia.

**3** Ask the individuals to check blood glucose levels pre- and postexercise and record the results along with information about medication, food/carbohydrate intake, and the type and time of any symptoms that develop during or after exercise. By reviewing these records with the individuals, the educator can discuss the effects of exercise and offer ideas about needed adjustments in management. Furthermore, record keeping may provide reinforcement for the exercise program.

**4** Ask individuals to perform self-assessments to evaluate exercise results. Compare current level of physical activity to the amount of exercise performed at the beginning of the exercise program. Other parameters that can be monitored that reflect progress with the exercise program include weight, blood glucose, and lipid levels.

**5** Assist individuals who may be self-conscious because of their weight or fitness level to find a group or class of similar status and with comparable goals. A significant deterrent for many overweight people is joining an exercise class that consists of people who are lean and relatively fit.

## Self-Review Questions

**1** List the benefits of regular exercise for individuals with diabetes.
**2** Discuss the mechanisms for exercise-induced hypoglycemia.
**3** Describe precautions that can be taken to help prevent exercise-induced hypoglycemia, including postexercise, late-onset hypoglycemia.
**4** For persons with type 1 diabetes, describe when and why exercise can result in a worsening of hyperglycemia and ketosis.
**5** Describe components and give examples of aerobic exercise.
**6** Discuss strategies to improve adherence to an exercise program.
**7** State the potential risks of exercise for persons with type 1 and type 2 diabetes.
**8** Briefly discuss and identify exercise that would be appropriate or contraindicated for persons with retinopathy and neuropathy.
**9** Describe the importance of self-directed goals for exercise.

## Learning Assessment: Case Study

AB is a 41-year-old female with a 26-year history of type 1 diabetes. She has come to the diabetes center because she wants to start an exercise program. She is very enthusiastic about using some new exercise equipment, but she wants to know where to begin.

During the assessment she tells you, "I have nonproliferative retinopathy and my feet are a little numb, but otherwise my diabetes is well controlled." AB is 5 ft 4 in tall, weighs 170 lb (76.5 kg), and her HbA1c is >11% (normal = < 6.2%). She is on a split dose of regular and NPH insulins at breakfast and dinner. She checks her blood glucose levels in the morning, and her results are around 180 mg/dL (10.8 mmol/L). She states that she hasn't seen her doctor in awhile.

## Questions for Discussion

**1** What questions would you ask AB about her diabetes management?

**2** What does AB need to know before beginning her exercise program?

**3** What kind of program is safe for AB (eg, exercise type, intensity, duration, restrictions)?

## Discussion

**1** Although AB states that her diabetes is fine, she has an elevated HbA1c level. This finding, together with her comments about her eyes and feet, indicate to the diabetes educator certain key facts about AB's diabetes.

  **A** Her diabetes is not adequately controlled.

  **B** Complications could be well established.

  **C** AB may not be adequately informed regarding diabetes and its management.

**2** Since AB has not seen her physician for some time, she is encouraged to do so prior to initiating an exercise program.

**3** Based on the American College of Sports Medicine guidelines for her age and duration of diabetes, a graded exercise stress electrocardiogram test (GXT) is warranted prior to initiating an exercise program. The results of the GXT allow accurate and safe determinations of exercise tolerances and limitations.

**4** A medical exam also is necessary and should include a plasma lipid profile and blood chemistries, kidney function tests, and a comprehensive eye exam. These assessments are important in view of AB's history and are necessary before she can safely exercise.

**5** Results of the GXT show no cardiac dysfunction during exercise but reveal a poor tolerance for exercise, indicating a deconditioned state. When AB walked on the treadmill, her exercise systolic blood pressure was >200 mm Hg when her heart rate was 145 beats per minute. Maximal exercise heart rate was 165 beats per minute.

**6** Further assessments showed elevated lipids and a low HDL:LDL ratio (risk factors for CAD), slight proteinuria, and stable nonproliferative retinopathy.

**7** AB and her doctor decide that she will continue with the same insulin regimen, perform more frequent blood glucose monitoring, reevaluate her meal plan with the assistance of a dietitian, and begin an exercise program. AB is referred to an exercise specialist.

**8** The goals of an exercise program AB identifies are a weight loss of about 10 to 15 lb (4.5 to 6.8 kg) (combined with a meal plan), improved lipid profile, improved aerobic capacity, improved overall diabetes control (combined with an education program), and increased feelings of control and self-worth.

**9** An aerobic exercise program is established with AB.
  **A** Because treadmill walking at a heart rate of 145 beats per minute resulted in an elevated systolic blood pressure, AB's recommended intensity will be based on blood pressure response to exercise.
  **B** Due to the correlation of elevated blood pressure to increased proteinuria and retinopathy, the exercise will be performed at an intensity that does not induce large systolic changes.
   • AB's training intensity is 165 ($HR_{max}$) × 0.60 to 0.85 = 99 to 140 beats per minute.
   • At 132 beats per minute, her systolic blood pressure was 160 mm Hg, which is an appropriate training intensity.
   • Because AB has been inactive and is obese, she will need to initiate her exercise program at a lower training intensity (eg, 110 beats per minute).
   • Initially, she may need some brief rest periods during the workout, performing only 15 minutes of exercise at a time.
   • Alternating weekly additions of time and intensity to the workout will help accomplish the ultimate goal (within 6 to 8 weeks) of continual exercise for 45 to 60 minutes at a heart rate of 130 beats per minute.
  **C** AB decides to exercise 5 times per week. Focusing on increasing duration instead of only intensity will aid in fat mobilization and favorably alter the lipid profile.
  **D** Prior to initiating the exercise prescription, her blood glucose profile showed late-afternoon hyperglycemia.
   • While a consistent exercise program will eventually result in better blood glucose control 24 hours a day, an optimal time for AB to exercise now is between 2 PM and 4 PM, when her blood glucose levels are high. This is also AB's preferred time because her work is finished and her children are not yet home from school.
   • Exercising at this time will control her late-afternoon hyperglycemia.
   • Her NPH insulin may be peaking at this point or even waning if she takes human insulin. Therefore, AB will monitor pre- and postexercise blood glucose levels at this time of day to determine her blood glucose response to exercise. Her late afternoon blood glucose level may improve, in which case she can adjust her insulin to prevent hypoglycemia. If her blood glucose levels do not improve and remain elevated, this may be suggestive of underinsulinization and an increase in insulin may be needed.

**10** AB's feet are a little numb; therefore, jogging, stair climbing, or heavy weight-bearing exercises are not appropriate exercise choices. Cycling, walking, or water walking could be suggested as alternatives.

# References

1 Sushruta SCS. Vaidya Jadavaji Trikamji Acharia. Bombay, India: Sagar, 1938.

2 Allen FM, Stillman E, Fitz R. Total Dietary Regulation in the Treatment of Diabetes. Exercise 1919; Monograph 11.

3 Lawrence RH. The effects of exercise on insulin action in diabetes. Br Med J. 1926;1:648-652.

4 Helmrich SP, Ragland DR, Leung RW, Paffenbarger RS Jr. Physical activity and reduced occurrence of non-insulin-dependent diabetes mellitus. N Engl J Med. 1991;325:147-152.

5 US Department of Health and Human Services. Physical Activity and Health: A Report of the Surgeon General. Atlanta: US Department of Health and Human Services, Centers for Disease Control and Prevention, National Center for Chronic Disease Prevention and Health Promotion; 1996.

6 McArdle WD, Katch FI, Katch VL. Essentials of Exercise Physiology. Philadelphia: Lippincott, Williams & Wilkins; 2000.

7 Horton ES. Role and management of exercise in diabetes mellitus. Diabetes Care. 1988;11:201-211.

8 Bogardus C, Ravussin E, Robbins DC, Wolfe RR, Horton ES, Sims EAH. Effects of physical training with diet therapy on carbohydrate metabolism in patients with glucose intolerance and non-insulin-dependent diabetes mellitus. Diabetes. 1984;33:311-318.

9 Stout RW. Insulin and atheroma: 20 year perspective. Diabetes Care. 1990;13:631-654.

10 Fontbonne AM, Eschwege EM. Insulin and cardiovascular disease: Paris prospective study. Diabetes Care. 1991;14:461-469.

11 Schneider SH, Ruderman NB. Exercise and physical training in the treatment of diabetes mellitus. Compr Ther. 1986;12:49-56.

12 Colwell JA. Effects of exercise on platelet function, coagulation and fibrinolysis. Diabetes Metab Rev. 1986;1:501-512.

13 Hornsby WG, Boggess KA, Lyons TJ, Barnwell WH, Lazarchick J, Colwell JA. Hemostatic alterations with exercise conditioning in NIDDM. Diabetes Care. 1990;13:87-92.

14 Rodin J. Physiological effects of exercise. In: William RS, Wallace AG, eds. Biological Effects of Physical Activity. Champaign, Ill: Human Kinetics; 1990.

15 Schneider SH, Amorosa LF, Khachadurian AK, Ruderman NB. Studies on the mechanism of improved glycemic control during regular exercise in type II diabetes. Diabetologia. 1984;26:355-360.

16 Eriksson KF, Lindgarde F. Prevention of type II diabetes mellitus by diet and physical exercise. The 6-year Malmo Feasibility Study. Diabetologia. 1991;34:891-898.

17 Heath GW, Wilson RH, Smith J, Leonard BE. Community-based exercise and weight control: diabetes risk reduction and glycemic control in Zuni Indians. Am J Clin Nutr. 1991;53:S1642-S1646.

18 Schneider SH, Khachadurian AK, Amorosa LF, Clemow L, Ruderman NB. Ten-year experience with an exercise-based outpatient lifestyle modification program in the treatment of diabetes mellitus. Diabetes Care. 1992; 15(suppl 4):1800-1810.

19 Vanninen E, Uusitupa M, Siitonen O, Laitinen J, Lansimies E. Habitual physical activity, aerobic capacity, and metabolic control in patients with newly diagnosed type II diabetes mellitus: effect of a 1-year diet and exercise intervention. Diabetologia. 1992;35:340-346.

20 Stratton R, Wilson DP, Endres RK, Goldstein DE. Improved glycemic control after supervised 8-wk exercise program in insulin-dependent diabetic adolescents. Diabetes Care. 1987;10:589-593.

**21** Landt KW, Campaigne BN, James FW, Sperling MA. Effects of exercise training on insulin sensitivity in adolescents with type 1 diabetes. Diabetes Care. 1985;8:461-465.

**22** Wallberg-Henrikssonn H, Gunnarsson R, Henriksson J, et al. Increased peripheral insulin sensitivity and muscle mitochondrial enzymes but unchanged blood glucose control in type 2 diabetics after physical training. Diabetes. 1982;31:1044-1050.

**23** Peterson CM, Jones RL, Dupuis A, Levine BS, Bernstein R, O'Shea M. Feasibility of improved blood glucose control in patients with insulin-dependent diabetes mellitus. Diabetes Care. 1979;2:329-335.

**24** Wallberg-Henriksson H, Gunnarsson R, Henriksson J, Ostman J, Wahren J. Influence of training on formation of muscle capillaries in type 1 diabetes. Diabetes. 1984;33:851-857.

**25** Zinman B, Zuniga-Guajardo S, Kelly D. Comparison of the acute and long-term effects of exercise on glucose control in type 1 diabetics. Diabetes Care. 1984;7:515-519.

**26** Stratton R, Wilson DP, Endres RK. Acute glycemic effects of exercise in adolescents with insulin-dependent diabetes mellitus. Physician Sport Med. 1988;16:150-157.

**27** Vitug A, Schneider SH, Ruderman NB. Exercise in type 1 diabetes. In: Terjung RL, ed. Exercise and Sport Sciences Reviews. New York: Macmillan; 1988:285-304.

**28** Vranic M, Berger M. Exercise and diabetes. Diabetes. 1979;28:147-163.

**29** Tzankoff SP, Norris AH. Longitudinal changes in basal metabolism in man. J Appl Physiol. 1978;45:536-593.

**30** Franz MJ. Exercise and diabetes: fuel metabolism, benefits, risks and guidelines. Clin Diabetes. 1988;6:58-60.

**31** Winder WW. Regulation of hepatic glucose regulation during exercise. In: Terjung RL, ed. Exercise and Sport Sciences Reviews. New York: Macmillan; 1985:1-32.

**32** Hartley LH, Mason JW, Hogan RP, et al. Multiple hormonal responses to graded exercise in relation to physical training. J Appl Physiol. 1972;33:602-606.

**33** Zinman B, Vranic M, Albisser AM, Leibel BS, Marliss ED. The role of insulin in the metabolic response to exercise in the diabetic man. Diabetes. 1979;28(suppl 1):76-81.

**34** Wahren J. Glucose turnover during exercise in healthy men and in patients with diabetes mellitus. Diabetes. 1979;29(suppl 1):82-88.

**35** Ahlborg G, Felig P. Lactate and glucose exchange across the forearm, legs and splanchnic bed during and after prolonged leg exercise. J Clin Invest. 1982;69:45-54.

**36** Richter EA, Garetto LP, Goodman M, Ruderman N. Muscle glucose metabolism following exercise in the rat: increased sensitivity to insulin. J Clin Invest. 1982;69:785-793.

**37** Mondon CE, Dolkas CB, Reaven GM. Site of enhanced insulin sensitivity in exercise-trained rats at rest. Am J Physiol 1980;239(Endocrinol Metab 2):E169-177.

**38** Wasserman DH, Zinman B. Exercise in individuals with IDDM (technical review). Diabetes Care. 1994;17:924-937.

**39** Kemmer FW, Tacken M, Berger M. Mechanism of exercise-induced hypoglycemia during sulfonylurea treatment. Diabetes. 1987;36:1178-1182.

**40** Albright A, Franz M, Hornsby G, et al. for American College of Sports Medicine. Exercise and type 2 diabetes. Position stand. Med Sci Sports Exerc. 2000; 32:1345-1360.

**41** MacDonald MJ. Postexercise late-onset hypoglycemia in insulin dependent diabetic patients. Diabetes Care. 1987; 10:584-588.

**42** American Diabetes Association. Diabetes mellitus and exercise (position statement). Diabetes Care. 2001; 24(suppl 1): S51-S55.

**43** Mitchell TH, Abraham G, Schiffrin A, Leiter A, Marliss EB. Hyperglycemia after intense exercise in IDDM subjects during continuous subcutaneous insulin infusion. Diabetes Care. 1988;11:311-317.

**44** Calles J, Cunningham JJ, Nelson L, et al. Glucose turnover during recovery from intensive exercise. Diabetes. 1983;32:734-738.

**45** Purdon C, Brousson M, Nyveen SL, et al. The roles of insulin and catecholamines in the glucoregulatory response during intense exercise and early recovery in insulin-dependent diabetic and control subjects. J Clin Endocrinol Metab. 1993;76:566-573.

**46** Schiffrin A, Parikh S. Accommodating planned exercise in type I diabetic patients on intensive treatment. Diabetes Care. 1985;8:337-342.

**47** Koivisto VA, Felig P. Effects of leg exercise on insulin absorption in diabetic patients. N Engl J Med. 1978;298:79-83.

**48** Kemmer FW, Berchtold P, Berger M, et al. Exercise-induced fall of blood glucose in insulin-treated diabetics unrelated to alteration in insulin mobilization. Diabetes. 1979;28:1131-1137.

**49** Frid A, Ostman J, Linde B. Hypoglycemia risk during exercise after intramuscular injection of insulin in thigh in IDDM. Diabetes Care. 1990;13:473-477.

**50** Nathan D, Madnek SF, Delahanty L. Programming preexercise snacks to prevent postexercise hypoglycemia in intensively treated insulin dependent diabetics. Ann Intern Med. 1985;102:483-486.

**51** Franz MJ. Nutrition: can it give athletes with diabetes a boost? Diabetes Educ. 1991;17:163-172.

**52** Sonnenberg GE, Kemmer FW, Berger M. Exercise in type I diabetic patients treated with continuous subcutaneous insulin infusion. Diabetologia. 1990;33:696-703.

**53** Beaser RS. Outsmarting Diabetes. Minneapolis: Chronimed; 1994.

**54** Roitman JL, Kelsey M, LaFontaine TP, Southard DR, Williams MA, York T, eds. American College of Sports Medicine. Resource Manual for Guidelines for Exercise Testing and Prescription. 3rd ed. Philadelphia: Lea & Febiger; 1998.

**55** Durak EP, Jovanovic-Peterson L, Peterson CM. Randomized crossover study of effect of resistance training on glycemic control, muscular strength and cholesterol in type I diabetic men. Diabetes Care. 1990;13:1039-1043.

**56** Goldberg AP. Aerobic and resistive exercise modify risk factors for coronary heart disease. Med Sci Sports Exer. 1989;21:669-674.

**57** Franklin BA, Whaley MH, Howley ET, eds. American College of Sports Medicine. Guidelines for Exercise Testing and Prescription. 6th ed. Baltimore: Williams & Wilkins; 2000.

**58** Fulton JE, Mâsse LC, Tortolero SR, et al. Field evaluation of energy expenditure from continuous and intermittent walking in women. Med Sci Sports Exerc. 2001; 33:163-170.

**59** National Institutes of Health. NIH Consensus Statement: Physical Activity and Cardiovascular Health. Bethesda, Md: Department of Health and Human Services, Public Health Service; 1995:13(3).

**60** Kraemer WJ, Fleck SJ. Resistance training: exercise prescription. Physician Sport Med. 1988;16:69-81.

**61** Soukup JT, Maynard TS, Kovaleski JE. Resistance training guidelines for individuals with diabetes mellitus. Diabetes Educ. 1994;20:129-137.

**62** Franklin B, Bonzheim K, Gordon S, Timmis G. Resistance training in cardiac rehabilitation. J Cardiopulmonary Rehabil. 1991;11:99-107.

**63** Frontera WR, Hughes VA, Lutz KJ, Evans WJ. A cross-sectional study of upper and lower extremity muscle strength in 45- to 78-year-old men and women. J Appl Physiol. 1991;71:644-650.

**64** Graham C. Exercise and aging: implications for persons with diabetes. Diabetes Educ. 1991;17:189-195.

**65** Schwartz RS. Exercise training in treatment of diabetes mellitus in elderly patients. Diabetes Care. 1990;13(suppl 2):77-85.

**66** Graham C, Lasko-McCarthey P. Exercise options for persons with diabetic complications. Diabetes Educ. 1990;16:212-220.

**67** Hiatt WR, Regensteiner JG, Hargarten ME, Wolfel EE, Brass EP. Benefit of exercise conditioning for patients with peripheral arterial disease. Circulation. 1990;81:602-609.

**68** Levin, ME. The diabetic foot. In: Ruderman NB, Devlin JT, eds. The Health Professional's Guide to Diabetes and Exercise. Alexandria, Va: American Diabetes Association; 1995.

**69** Aiello LM, Cavallerano J, Aiello LP, Bursell SE. Retinopathy. In: Ruderman NB, Devlin JT, eds. The Health Professional's Guide to Diabetes and Exercise. Alexandria, Va: American Diabetes Association; 1995.

**70** Painter P. Exercise in end-stage renal disease. In: Terjung RL, ed. Exercise and Sport Sciences Reviews. New York: Macmillan; 1988:305-340.

**71** Pate RR, Pratt M, Blair SN, et al. Physical activity and public health: a recommendation from the Centers for Disease Control and Prevention and the American College of Sports Medicine. JAMA. 1995;273:402-407.

**72** Marcus BH, Rakowski W, Rossi JS. Assessing motivational readiness and decision making for exercise. Health Psychol. 1992;11:257-261.

**73** Dishman RK, Sallis JF, Orenstein DR. The determinants of physical activity and exercise. Public Health Rep. 1985;100:158-171.

**74** Marcus BH, Simkin LR. The transtheoretical model: applications to exercise behavior. Med Sci Sports Exerc. 1994;26:1400-1404.

**75** Marcus BH, Selby VC, Niaura RS, Rossi JS. Self-efficacy and the stages of exercise behavior change. Res Q Exerc Sport. 1992;63:60-66.

## Suggested Readings

*General Exercise Physiology*

Durstine JL, Bloomquist LE, Figoi SF, et al. eds. American College of Sports Medicine. Exercise Management for Persons With Chronic Diseases and Disabilities: Diabetes. Champaign, Ill: Human Kinetics; 1997:94-100.

McArdle WD, Katch FI, Katch VL. Essentials of Exercise Physiology: Diabetes Mellitus. Philadephia: Lippincott, Williams & Wilkins; 2000.

*Exercise and Diabetes*

Albright A, Franz M, Hornsby G, et al. for American College of Sports Medicine. Exercise and type 2 diabetes. Position stand. Med Sci Sports Exerc. 2000;32:1345-1370.

American Diabetes Association. Diabetes mellitus and exercise (position statement). Diabetes Care. 2001; 23(suppl 1):S51-S55.

Franz M. Exercise and diabetes. In: Haire-Joshu D, ed. Management of Diabetes Mellitus: Perspectives of Care Across the Life Span. 2nd ed. St. Louis: Mosby Year Book; 1996:162-201.

Goodyear, LJ. Exercise, glucose transport, and insulin sensitivity. Annu Rev Med. 1998;49:235-261.

Hornsby WG, ed. The Fitness Book for People with Diabetes. Alexandria, Va: American Diabetes Association; 1994.

Ivy, JL. Role of exercise training in the prevention and treatment of insulin resistance and NIDDM. Sport Med. 1997; 24: 321-326.

Ivy JL, Aderic TW, Donovan FL. American College of Sports Medicine. Prevention and treatment of non-insulin-dependent diabetes mellitus. In: Exercise and Sport Sciences Reviews. Philadelphia: Lippincott, Williams & Wilkins; 1999:(27):1-35.

Ruderman NB, Devlin JT, eds. The Health Professional's Guide to Diabetes and Exercise. Alexandria, Va: American Diabetes Association; 1995.

Wallberg-Henriksson, H, Rincon J, Zierath JR. Exercise in the management of non-insulin-dependent diabetes mellitus. Sports Med. 1998;25:25-35.

Zinker, BA. Nutrition and exercise in individuals with diabetes. Clin Sports Med. 1999;18:585-606, vii-viii.

# Learning Assessment: Post-Test Questions

## Exercise                                                    2

**1**  Which of the following are benefits of exercise?
  **A** Reduced plasma cholesterol and triglycerides and enhanced fibrinolysis
  **B** Reduced body fat, muscle mass, and weight
  **C** Improved glucose tolerance and hypercoagulability
  **D** Increased insulin sensitivity and decreased high-density lipoproteins

**2**  In persons without diabetes, during the first 5 to 10 minutes of exercise, the major fuel for energy is:
  **A** Free fatty acids from adipose tissue
  **B** Intramuscular glucose from glycogen
  **C** Hepatic glucose from glycogenolysis
  **D** Hepatic glucose from gluconeogenesis

**3**  In persons without diabetes, during the post-exercise recovery period, there is:
  **A** Replenishment of glycogen stores for 12 hours
  **B** Lessened insulin sensitivity
  **C** Increased uptake of glucose by muscle
  **D** Suppression of glucogenesis by the liver

**4**  After exercise, which factor contributes to hypoglycemia in type 1 diabetes?
  **A** Mobilization of free fatty acids
  **B** Depletion of muscle glycogen stores
  **C** Normal counterregulatory hormonal response
  **D** Accelerated absorption of insulin

**5**  BD has type 1 diabetes and is on the high school track team. He runs the 4th leg of the 200-meter relay which is a short, very intense workout. Ten minutes after the race, BD's blood glucose is 350 mg/dL. He should:
  **A** Inject himself with some regular insulin to cover the high blood glucose.
  **B** Test his urine for ketones.
  **C** Eat a snack of 1 bread exchange and 1 meat exchange.
  **D** Run for about 40 more minutes to decrease his blood glucose.

**6**  CN is age 55 years and has had type 2 diabetes for 10 years. He is 6 ft 1 in and weighs 300 lb. His fasting blood glucose is 145 mg/dL, and he is on metformin. He wants to start an exercise program. Which of the following would be the least important to teach him?
  **A** See his provider and have a stress test before beginning to exercise
  **B** Wear properly fitting exercise shoes
  **C** Carry glucose tablets for hypoglycemia
  **D** Have an eye examination prior to his exercise program

**7**  What frequency of exercise is optimal for weight loss for CN?
  **A** 2 to 3 days/week
  **B** 3 to 4 days/week
  **C** 4 to 5 days/week
  **D** 5 to 7 days/week

**8**  What maximum age-adjusted heart rate would provide an optimum aerobic workout for CN?
  **A** 50% to 70%
  **B** 55% to 75%
  **C** 60% to 85%
  **D** 65% to 90%

**9**  Which exercise routine is most appropriate for an elderly patient with a degenerative joint disease?
  **A** No exercise at all
  **B** Aerobic exercise only
  **C** Anaerobic exercise only
  **D** Alternating aerobic and strength training exercise

**10**  Patients with moderate nonproliferative retinopathy should:
  **A** Avoid all strenuous activity.
  **B** Avoid exercise that dramatically increases their blood pressure.
  **C** Limit exercise to 2 days a week.
  **D** Gradually incorporate resistance training into their normal exercise routine.

*See next page for answer key.*

# Post-Test Answer Key

## Exercise 2

| | | | | |
|---|---|---|---|---|
| 1 | A | | 6 | C |
| 2 | B | | 7 | D |
| 3 | C | | 8 | C |
| 4 | B | | 9 | D |
| 5 | B | | 10 | B |

## Pharmacologic Therapies

*John R. White, Jr., RPh, PharmD, PA-C*
*Washington State University*
*Spokane, Washington*

*R. Keith Campbell, RPh, MBA, CDE*
*Washington State University*
*Spokane, Washington*

*Peggy C. Yarborough, RPh, MS, BC-ADM, CDE*
*Campbell University and*
*Wilson Community Health Center*
*Wilson, North Carolina*

## Introduction

**1** For some people with diabetes, nonpharmacologic interventions will suffice to attain an optimal level of blood glucose control:

**A** Medical nutrition therapy

**B** Regular physical activity

**C** Blood glucose monitoring

**D** Attention to relevant clinical educational and psychosocial needs

**2** For the majority of people with diabetes, however, treatment will also require pharmacologic intervention. Approximately 90% of persons with diabetes require oral antidiabetes medications, insulin injections, or both, to reach glucose goals.[1]

**3** In addition to antidiabetes drugs, the pharmacologic therapies for a person with diabetes often include other agents to treat the myriad of associated comorbid conditions or complications of diabetes. These pharmacologic therapies are considered part of standard diabetes care even though they are not used for the purpose of altering blood glucose levels.

**4** Diabetes educators must be cognizant of the total range of therapies that are available for comprehensive diabetes care, not just the therapies that are used for glycemic control. They also need to be able to advise patients about the effects of other drugs on blood glucose levels, diabetes complications, and other aspects of self-management.

**5** This chapter will provide an update of the pharmacologic therapies for glycemic control and an overview of the impact of other drugs on diabetes management. The goal is for the educator to understand and be able to teach patients some of the intricacies of the pharmacologic interventions that are necessary for comprehensive diabetes self-management.

## Objectives

Upon completion of this chapter, the learner will be able to

**1** Explain the physiologic effects of insulin.

**2** Differentiate insulin preparations based upon species/source, type, purity, and concentration.

**3** Describe proper administration and storage guidelines for insulin.

**4** Explain the limitations for insulin mixing.

**5** Explain the similarities and differences of potential insulin therapy regimens, including the use of insulin pumps, and indications for specific insulin products.

**6** Explain the mechanism(s) of action of sulfonylureas, meglitinides, biguanides, alpha-glucosidase inhibitors, and thiazolidinediones.

**7** Describe the clinical use of alpha-glucosidase inhibitors, metformin, sulfonylureas, repaglinide, nateglinide, and the thiazolidinediones.

**8** Explain the use of combination therapy in patients with type 2 diabetes.

**9** Explain the clinical use of glucagon.

**10** Identify 3 categories of drug-related effects on diabetes.

**11** List 2 or more classes of medications that commonly are prescribed for patients with diabetes, and describe potential drug-disease, drug-drug or drug-food interactions.

**12** List suggestions the diabetes educator may offer to help patients prevent, minimize, or be prepared for a drug-related problem.

## Physiologic Effects of Insulin and Indications for Its Use

**1** The following describes the physiologic actions and release of endogenous insulin:

**A** *Insulin* is a hormone produced in the beta cells of the Islets of Langerhans in the pancreas; it is formed from a substance called *proinsulin* (Figure 3.1).

- When the pancreas is stimulated, primarily by an elevated blood glucose level, the proinsulin is cleaved at 2 sections of the molecule—at the glycine position identified as the #1 amino acid of the "A" chain and at the alanine position identified as the #30 amino acid of the "B" chain (see Figure 3.1). When the proinsulin molecule is then broken apart, insulin and the connecting peptide (C-peptide) are both secreted and enter the bloodstream in equimolar amounts. Some uncleaved proinsulin also enters the blood.

- Once in the blood stream, the half-life of free insulin has been reported to be in the order of 5.2 +/-0.7 minutes and may be increased in persons with diabetes who have high insulin antibody titers.

- Normal daily insulin secretion in a healthy, nonpregnant, nonobese adult is approximately 0.5 to 0.7 unit insulin per kg per day.

- Since insulin and C-peptide are jointly secreted, a measurement of C-peptide level can be used as a clinical monitor of endogenous insulin production and to determine type of diabetes. Direct measurement of insulin secretion is difficult, except under controlled or research conditions, because insulin is rapidly removed from the blood as it exerts its pharmacologic action.

- Demonstration of measurable levels of C-peptide (normal fasting [0.78 to 1.89 ng/mL]) may also be used to rule out fictitious insulin administration as a cause of unexplained hypoglycemia in a person without insulin-requiring diabetes.

- Because insulin and C-peptide have different biologic durations, a measurement of C-peptide level may not accurately reflect the endogenous insulin level at that period of time.

**B** Insulin exerts varied effects on body tissues.

- Stimulates entry of amino acids into cells, enhancing protein synthesis.
- Enhances fat storage (*lipogenesis*) and prevents the mobilization of fat for energy (*lipolysis* and *ketogenesis*).
- Stimulates the entry of glucose into cells for utilization as an energy source and promotes the resultant storage of glucose as glycogen (*glycogenesis*) in muscle and liver cells.
- Inhibits production of glucose from liver or muscle glycogen (*glycogenolysis*).
- Inhibits formation of glucose from noncarbohydrates, such as amino acids (*gluconeogenesis*).

**C** The major untoward effect of insulin therapy is hypoglycemia. Virtually all persons who inject insulin will experience hypoglycemia at some time.

- Frequent causes of hypoglycemia include too much (excessive dosage of) insulin; delayed, missed, or insufficient food intake; or too much (unplanned) exercise.

## Figure 3.1. Biochemical Formation of Human Insulin from Proinsulin

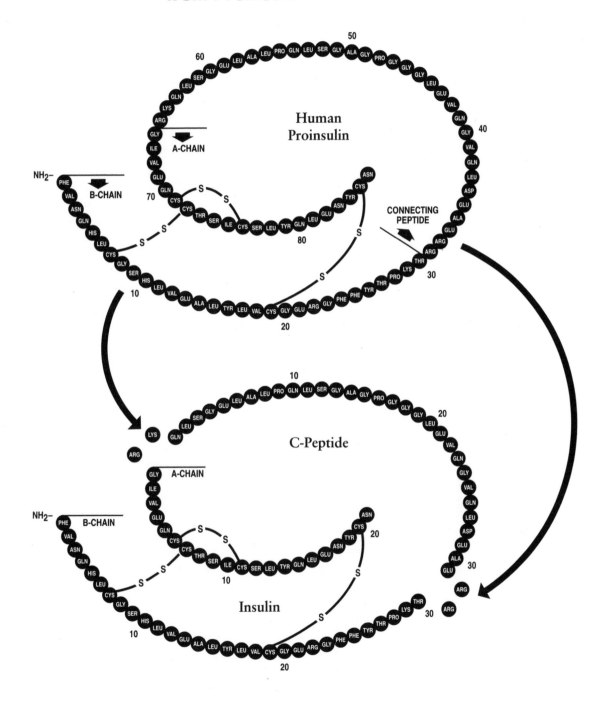

- Strategies to reduce the risk of hypoglycemia include routine self-monitoring of blood glucose levels; observing for and responding quickly to early symptoms of hypoglycemia; ingesting appropriate quantities and choices of a pre-exercise carbohydrate supplement; and using a consistent food/meal plan and pattern. (See Chapter 7, Hypoglycemia, in Diabetes Management Therapies, for additional information.)
- Instruct all insulin-using patients concerning the symptoms, prevention, and treatment of hypoglycemia. In addition, teaching patients to routinely carry a source of carbohydrate can help to prevent mild reactions from becoming severe.

**D** *Endogenous insulin* is defined as insulin that is supplied from the pancreas, while *exogenous insulin* is defined as injected pharmaceutical insulin.

**2** There are several hormones in the body that exert antagonistic effects to the hypoglycemic actions of insulin. These hormones are collectively referred to as *counterregulatory hormones*. Blood glucose management in diabetes needs to take into account, and make compensation for, the release of one or more of these hormones throughout the day in response to a variety of stimuli. The primary counterregulatory hormones include

**A** Glucagon (produced in the alpha cells of the pancreas)

**B** Epinephrine

**C** Norepinephrine

**D** Growth hormone

**E** Cortisol

**3** Insulin is indicated for specific patients with diabetes or in certain medical conditions.

**A** All individuals with type 1 diabetes require exogenous insulin to sustain life. In type 1 diabetes, production of insulin by beta cells is completely or largely lost.

**B** Individuals with type 2 diabetes may need insulin if other forms of therapy do not adequately control blood glucose levels or during periods of physiological stress such as surgery or infection.

**C** Women with gestational diabetes may need insulin if medical nutrition therapy alone does not adequately control blood glucose levels.

**D** Diabetic or nondiabetic patients receiving parenteral nutrition or high-caloric supplements to meet an increased energy need may require exogenous insulin to maintain normal glucose levels during periods of insulin resistance or increased insulin demand.

**E** Insulin is necessary in the treatment of diabetic ketoacidosis (DKA).

**F** Insulin is often needed in the treatment of hyperosmolar hyperglycemic state (HHS).

**G** Individuals with secondary diabetes, such as diabetes secondary to pancreatitis or other disease that severely diminishes beta cell production of insulin, may require insulin.

## Insulin Species/Source, Type, Purity, and Concentration

**1** Insulin preparations are differentiated by specific product characteristics (Table 3.1).

## Table 3.1.  Insulins Available in the US

| | Product | Manufacturer | Strength |
|---|---|---|---|
| *Rapid-Acting* | **Human Insulin Analogue** | | |
| | Humalog® lispro | Lilly | U-100 |
| | Novolog® aspart | Novo Nordisk | U-100 |
| *Short-Acting* | **Human** | | |
| | Humulin® R (regular) | Lilly | U-100, U-500 |
| | Novolin® R (regular) | Novo Nordisk | U-100 |
| | Velosulin® BR (regular) | Novo Nordisk | U-100 |
| | **Pork** | | |
| | Iletin® II regular | Lilly | U-100 |
| | Purified Pork regular | Novo Nordisk | U-100 |
| *Intermediate-Acting* | **Human** | | |
| | Humulin® L (Lente) | Lilly | U-100 |
| | Humulin® N (NPH) | Lilly | U-100 |
| | Novolin® L (Lente) | Novo Nordisk | U-100 |
| | Novolin® N (NPH) | Novo Nordisk | U-100 |
| | **Pork** | | |
| | Iletin® II Lente | Lilly | U-100 |
| | Iletin® II NPH | Lilly | U-100 |
| | Purified Pork Lente | Novo Nordisk | U-100 |
| | Purified Pork NPH | Novo Nordisk | U-100 |
| *Long-Acting* | **Human** | | |
| | Humulin® U (Ultralente) | Lilly | U-100 |
| | **Human Insulin Analogue** | | |
| | Lantus® (insulin glargine) | Aventis | U-100 |
| *Fixed Combination (all are U-100 insulins)* | | | |
| | **Human** | | **NPH/reg Ratio** |
| | Humulin® 70/30 | Lilly | 70/30 |
| | Novolin® 70/30 | Novo Nordisk | 70/30 |
| | Humulin® 50/50 | Lilly | 50/50 |
| | **Human Insulin Analogue** | | **NPL/lispro Ratio** |
| | Humalog® Mix 75/25 | Lilly | 75/25 (neutral protamine lispro/lispro) |

**2** The species/sources for insulin are beef, pork, and human.  The 5 product types include pork, which is isolated from animal pancreas glands; biosynthetic human insulin derived from bacteria (E coli), or fungal cells (Saccharomyces cerevisiae); and biosynthetic human insulin analogue.

**A** Beef insulin differs from human insulin at 3 amino acid sites, while pork insulin differs at only 1 amino acid site (Table 3.2).  Because of this difference, beef insulin induces more antigenic reactions than pork insulin.  Beef-pork combination products were generally thought to induce the most antigenic reactions and were discontinued for this reason.  Beef insulin is not available in the US.

## Table 3.2. Amino Acid Sequence Differences Between Various Insulin Species

| Species | A Chain | | | B Chain | | | |
|---------|-----|------|------|------|------|------|-----------|
| | A-8 | A-10 | A-21 | B-30 | B-29 | B-28 | B chain terminal |
| *Human* | Threonine | Isoleucine | Asparagine | Threonine | Lysine | Proline | |
| *Lispro* | Threonine | Isoleucine | Asparagine | Threonine | **Proline** | **Lysine** | |
| *Aspart* | Threonine | Isoleucine | Asparagine | Threonine | Lysine | **Aspartate** | |
| *Glargine* | Threonine | Isoleucine | **Glycine** | Threonine | Lysine | Proline | 2 Arginines added |
| *Bovine* | **Alanine** | **Valine** | Asparagine | **Alanine** | Lysine | Proline | |
| *Porcine* | Threonine | Isoleucine | Asparagine | **Alanine** | Lysine | Proline | |

**B** Human insulin, the human insulin analogue lispro, the human insulin analogue aspart, and the human insulin analogue glargine are manufactured by using recombinant-DNA technology (biosynthetic). Human insulin and rapid-acting insulins are less antigenic than beef insulin and slightly less antigenic than pork insulin.

**C** Human biosynthetic NPH, Lente, and Ultralente insulins appear to be absorbed faster and therefore act more quickly than animal-derived insulins, even though they have similar pharmacologic effects. Commercially prepared human insulins are effective and chemically identical to endogenous human insulin.

**D** There are virtually no contraindications to human insulin, although there are rare instances of hypersensitivity.

**E** Human insulin has provided an option for vegetarians, Moslems, Orthodox Jews, or Hindus who prefer not to use pork or beef insulins.

**F** Animal-derived insulins induced insulin antibody formation to a greater degree than human insulins or rapid-acting insulins. When insulin is bound to insulin antibodies the predictability of the insulin's peak effect and duration of action will be altered.

**3** Insulin is generally classified according to peak effect and duration of action (Table 3.3).[2] The currently available rapid-acting insulins are lispro and aspart, the short-acting insulin is regular, the intermediate-acting insulins are NPH and Lente, and the long-acting insulin is Ultralente. Additionally, a true "peakless" long-acting insulin analogue Lantus® (*insulin glargine*) is now available.

**A** Regular insulin, lispro and aspart, and glargine are the clear insulins or solution of insulin; all of the others are suspensions. Regular insulin is the only insulin product routinely used for intravenous administration, although lispro may be given intravenously.

## Table 3.3. Onset, Peak, and Duration of Human Insulin Preparations

| Insulin Preparation | Onset of Action, h | Peak Action, h | Duration | |
|---|---|---|---|---|
| | | | Effective Duration of Action, h | Maximum Duration of Action, h |
| *Rapid-acting* Lispro or aspart insulin | 0.2 to 0.5 min | 0.5 to 1.5 | 3 to 4 | 4 to 6 |
| *Short-acting* Regular | 0.5 to 1 | 2 to 3 | 3 to 6 | 6 to 8 |
| *Intermediate-acting* NPH | 2 to 4 | 6 to 10 | 10 to 16 | 14 to 18 |
| Lente | 3 to 4 | 6 to 12 | 12 to 18 | 16 to 20 |
| *Long-acting* Ultralente | 6 to 10 | 10 to 16 | 18 to 20 | 20 to 24 |
| Insulin glargine | 1.1 | - | 24 | 24+ |
| *Combinations* 70/30; 50/50; 75/25 | 0.5 to 1 | Dual | 10 to 16 | 14 to 18 |

*Source:* Adapted with permission from Skyler.[2]

**B** *Insulin lispro* is an insulin analogue identical to human insulin in its structure with the exception of the juxtaposition of lysine and proline in positions 28 and 29 on the B chain (see Figure 3.1). This molecular alteration yields insulin with a faster rate of absorption than regular human insulin.[3]

- A dose of lispro insulin peaks in half the time and in double the concentration of a comparable subcutaneous injection of regular insulin.[3]
- Lispro insulin can generally be used in place of regular insulin to provide better coverage of postprandial glycemic excursions.[4]
- Lispro insulin can be injected immediately prior to eating (generally less than 15 minutes preprandially); injecting lispro insulin 30 to 60 minutes prior to meals may result in profound hypoglycemia.
- Several studies show reduced hypoglycemia in patients with type 1 diabetes treated with lispro insulin compared with those treated with regular human insulin.[5-7]
- Insulin lispro has also been shown to be a suitable pump insulin.[8,9] Insulin lispro insulin pump therapy compared to regular insulin reduced HbA1c; however, both reduced the incidence of hypoglycemia compared to injected insulin.[9]
- Lispro insulin is available in the US only by prescription.

**C** *Insulin aspart* is an insulin analogue in which aspartic acid has been substituted for the amino acid proline at the B28 position (see Figure 3.1). In comparison to human short-acting insulin, insulin aspart can improve postprandial glycemic control by reducing hyperglycemic and hypoglycemic excursions.[10,11]

### Figure 3.2. Time Action Profiles of Glargine vs NPH Insulin in Type 1 Diabetes

*Source:* Reprinted with permission from Lepore.[15]

- Insulin aspart has a glucose-lowering response similar to insulin lispro and its duration of action is shortest after abdominal subcutaneous injection.[12]
- Compared to regular human insulin, insulin aspart is associated with a lower number of hypoglycemic episodes.[10]
- Insulin aspart is also reported to be effective when used in insulin pump therapy.[13]

**D** NPH contains protamine and some zinc to prolong the duration of action.
Lente and Ultralente insulins have high zinc levels to prolong the duration of action.

- Both protamine and zinc have occasionally been implicated as the causative agents of immunologic reactions such as urticaria at the injection site.

**E** *Insulin glargine* (Lantus) is a long-acting human insulin analogue which differs from human insulin in that asparagine at position A-21 is replaced by glycine and 2 arginines are added to the C terminus of the B chain.[14]

- Insulin glargine is a long-acting, "peakless" insulin which provides insulin in a basal pattern for 24 hours (see Figure 3.2).[15]
- Studies in persons with type 1 and type 2 diabetes have shown that insulin glargine when administered once daily provides similar control to NPH insulin administered once or twice daily.[16,17] In addition in individuals with type 2 diabetes treated with insulin glargine, there was a lower risk of nocturnal hypoglycemia and less weight gain compared with NPH.[17]
- Insulin glargine should be administered once daily at bedtime.[16]
- Insulin glargine should not be mixed in the same syringe with other insulins.
- The most common adverse event reported with glargine use is pain of mild intensity at the injection site.[16]
- Insulin glargine provides only basal insulin coverage and in many cases will be used in combination with other insulin preparations, with oral agents, or possibly in the future with inhaled insulin.

**F** *Insulin detemir* (NN304)) is a scluble basal insulin analog also being developed to cover basal insulin requirements. It has been shown to be as effective as NPH in maintaining glycemic control, with reduced risk of hypoglycemia, but has a higher mean dose requirement compared to NPH.[18]

**4** Purity of animal-source insulin is expressed as parts per million (ppm) of proinsulin, the primary contaminant after extraction from the pancreas. Concern about purity is a less significant issue in insulin therapy today than previously, as all insulins are now highly purified.

**5** The concentrations of insulin currently available in the US are U-100 and U-500, indicating 100 units/mL or 500 units/mL, respectively.[19] U-100 insulin is the insulin of choice for nearly all patients. U-100 insulin is not always available worldwide; instruct patients to take extra supplies when traveling to foreign countries.

   **A** Patients requiring large doses of insulin may benefit by using U-500 regular insulin. The onset and duration of action of U-500 is not the same as U-100 regular.

   **B** U-500 regular insulin (Humulin R, Eli Lilly) is available in the US only by prescription.

## Administration and Storage Guidelines

**1** Effective use of insulin requires the correct equipment, insulin preparation, and consistent use of proper technique.

**2** Teach patients to store insulin according to the manufacturer's recommendations.

   **A** Generally, insulin should be refrigerated at 36°F to 46°F (2C° to 8°C).
   - Unopened insulin products may be stored under refrigeration until the expiration date noted on the product label.

   **B** To reduce local irritation at the injection site that may occur when injecting cold insulin, advise patients to roll the prepared syringe between the palms, bring the bottle of insulin to room temperature before withdrawing the dose, or store the insulin at room temperature. Opened or unopened vials of insulin may be stored at a controlled room temperature of 59°F to 86°F (15°C to 30°C) for a period of 1 month; unused insulin should be discarded after that time.[19]

   **C** Storage guidelines differ for use and storage of used (punctured) or unused cartridge insulin (Penfill®) and disposable prefilled insulin pens.
   - Insulin cartridges or regular prefilled insulin pens may be kept unrefrigerated for 28 days (1.5-mL or 3.0-mL cartridges).
   - Humalog Mix 75/25 may be used for 10 days capped at room temperature (72°F) and out of direct sunlight; unused can be stored without refrigeration for 28 days, but should be stored in the refrigerator.
   - 70/30 insulin cartridges or prefilled insulin pens may be kept unrefrigerated for 10 days.
   - NPH insulin cartridges or prefilled insulin pens may be kept unrefrigerated for 14 days.

   **D** Keep extemporaneously prepared, prefilled syringes of either single formulations or mixtures of insulins refrigerated and use within 21 to 30 days.[19]

   **E** Availability of insulin and supplies may vary; teach patients to carry insulin and supplies when traveling. Due to variance of temperature, insulin should not be left in a car or checked through in airline baggage.

   **F** Instruct patients to examine vials of insulin for sediment or other visible changes before withdrawing the insulin into the syringe. Cloudiness or discoloration of clear insulin, clumping of insulin suspensions, or flocculation (frosting) of insulin suspensions indicates that the insulin has lost potency and should not be used but returned to the pharmacy for exchange. The incidence of frosting may be minimized if temperature is stabilized through refrigeration and if agitation or shaking of the vial is minimized.

**3** Insulin administration equipment includes the following and requires consistent use of proper technique.

**A** Disposable insulin syringes with attached needles for U-100 insulin are available in different syringe sizes, chosen according to the dose of insulin to be injected: 0.25 mL (for doses <25 units), 0.3 cc (for doses <30 units), 0.5 cc (for doses <50 units) or 1 cc (for doses 50 to 100 units). Needle length may be 5/16-inch or 1/2-inch. The "short needle" (5/16-inch length) is appropriate only for individuals with normal or near-normal body mass index (BMI <27 kg/m$^2$).

**B** In most circumstances, and with proper training, syringes and needles may be safely reused; however, reuse may carry an increased risk of infection for some individuals.[19] Advise patients who choose to reuse syringes that the markings on the syringe may rub off and that the needle becomes dull with repeated use. Instruct patients to safely recap the needle and store at room temperature.

**C** Alternative equipment to the traditional syringe-needle unit is available. The variety of injection devices includes automatic needle injectors, automatic needle and insulin injectors, pen injectors, and needle-free jet injectors. The needle-free jet injectors propel insulin through the skin by air pressure.

**D** *Insulin pumps*, also known as continuous subcutaneous insulin infusion (CSII) devices, are programmed to deliver a continuous infusion of insulin subcutaneously; before ingestion of food, the patient programs the device to administer a bolus (rapid release) of insulin.[20] This method can provide a more physiologic pattern of insulin delivery than attained by multiple injections of insulin (see Chapter 6, Insulin Pump Therapy, in Diabetes Management Therapies).

- Frequent blood glucose monitoring provides patients and professionals with the data needed for decision-making and flexibility.
- Because of the expense of pumps, patients need to consider pump therapy carefully in collaboration with their healthcare team.
- Insulin pumps currently available for daily use utilize an open-loop system. A continuous basal dose is programmed, and the patient then adjusts bolus doses of insulin based on blood glucose levels, food intake, and activity levels.

**4** Teach patients to follow a specific routine for insulin injections, including consistent technique, accurate dosage, and site rotation.

**A** Injections are given into the subcutaneous tissue. Most individuals are able to lightly grasp a fold of skin and inject at a 90° angle. Thin individuals or children may need to pinch the skin and inject at a 45° angle to avoid intramuscular injection.[19]

**B** Insulin may be injected into the subcutaneous tissue of the upper arm, the anterior and lateral aspects of the thigh, the buttocks, and the abdomen (with the exception of a circle with a 2-inch radius around the navel).[19] These sites are chosen because of the low potential for adverse reactions as well as general patient acceptability and accessibility (see Chapter 4, Monitoring, in Diabetes Management Therapies).

- Areas for injection must be determined individually, allowing for scar tissue, areas with less subcutaneous fat, and patient preference.

- Both the patient and the health professional need to examine injection areas at regular intervals to detect bruising, redness, infection, lipoatrophy, or lipohypertrophy.
- Teach patients to rotate injection sites to prevent local irritation. Rotating within one area is recommended (eg, rotating injections systematically within the abdomen) rather than rotating to a different area with each injection. This practice may decrease variability in absorption from day to day.[19]

**C** Insulin absorption may vary depending upon several parameters.

- Abdominal injection provides the most rapid absorption followed by the arms, thighs, and buttocks.[19] However, note that insulin glargine does not display this difference of absorption rates at different sites.[21] Deeper intramuscular injections induce faster absorption and shorter duration of action. High levels of insulin antibodies can also inhibit insulin action following injection.
- Exercise or massage of the injection site may induce more rapid absorption and action from a dose of insulin probably by increasing the rate of blood flow through the tissue around the site.[19]

**5** Various problems or complications may arise from insulin impurity, species/source, and improper injection technique.

**A** Insulin impurity can cause lipodystrophies (atrophy and hypertrophy).

- *Atrophy*, which is a concavity or pitting of the fatty tissue, is an immune phenomenon that occurs in a small number of patients and is related to species/source or purity. Use of highly purified insulins such as human insulin or purified pork reduces the occurrence of atrophy. Patients who develop this problem may benefit from injecting human or highly purified insulin around the periphery of the atrophied areas.[22]
- *Hypertrophy*, which is a fatty thickening of the lipid tissue, is best prevented by rotation of injection sites.

**B** Allergies to insulin are rare. Insulin allergy may occur as local reactions (rash, urticarial cutaneous reaction) or systemic reactions (serum sickness, anaphylaxis).

- Prior to insulin purification, local cutaneous reactions were more common.
- Zinc or protamine in the insulin, preservatives, and rubber or latex stoppers have all been implicated in inducing allergic reactions.
- Both local and systemic reactions appear to be immunologically mediated through induction of high titers of IgG and IgE antibodies.
- If systemic reaction occurs, desensitization to the insulin will be necessary.

## Mixing Insulins

**1** Organizing the necessary materials prior to insulin injection will limit errors.

**2** Guidelines for extemporaneous insulin mixtures are listed in Table 3.4. These standards are based on published data.[23]

**A** Varying the time delay for injecting after mixing may result in a different insulin action.

**B** As a general rule, the 2 insulins being mixed should be of the same brand.

**C** Rapid-acting or regular insulin is usually drawn up first, followed by the intermediate-acting insulin. This practice limits the potential for contamination, which may result in dose variance.

## Table 3.4. Guidelines for Mixing Insulin and/or Prefilling Syringes

| | |
|---|---|
| *Regular and NPH* | • Mixture stable in any ratio<br>• Mixture of choice, if regular and intermediate combination is needed<br>• Extemporaneously prepared syringes that are refrigerated are stable for at least 1 month<br>• Prefilling is acceptable |
| *Regular and Lente* | • Binding of regular begins immediately<br>• Binding continues for 24 hours<br>• Activity of regular is blunted<br>• Velosulin should not be mixed with Lente insulins<br>• If mixed or prefilled, the interval between mixing the insulins and administering the insulin should be standardized |
| *Commercially Prepared Premixed Insulins* | • Prefilling is acceptable |
| *Lente and Ultralente* | • Mixture stable in any ratio<br>• Mixture stable for 18 months<br>• Prefilling is acceptable |
| *Lispro Insulin with NPH or Ultralente* | • Mixture stable in any ratio<br>• Administer immediately after mixing |
| *Glargine* | • Should not be mixed with other insulins |

*Source:* From American Diabetes Association.[19]

**3** Commercially available premixed insulins (70/30, 50/50, 75/25) are manufactured and stabilized by altered buffering. These products may be advantageous for individuals unable to mix insulins accurately or reliably.

## Insulin Therapy Programs

**1** Insulin dosing schedules vary among individuals (see Chapter 5, Pattern Management of Blood Glucose, in Diabetes Management Therapies).

    **A** Physiologically, insulin is released throughout the day in frequent bursts in response to a variety of stimuli such as the glycemic rise from ingestion of food or the release of counterregulatory hormones. Insulin release in response to food intake is referred to as a *bolus secretion*; insulin release to counteract ongoing hormonal or other glycemic influences is referred to as *basal secretion*. Thus, the physiologic insulin profile is one of peaks (boluses) and valleys (basal) of insulin release throughout the day (Figure 3.3).

    **B** A goal of insulin therapy is to mimic, as nearly as possible, the physiologic profile of insulin secretion (eg, the peaks and valleys). Such a pattern is difficult to achieve with infrequent injections of insulin.

## Figure 3.3. Time Action of Physiologic (Endogenous) Insulin*

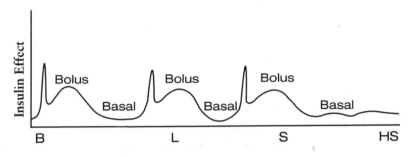

B = breakfast, L = lunch, S = supper, HS = bedtime.

"Bolus" secretion: The biphasic release of insulin in response to food intake.
"Basal" secretion: The release of insulin to counteract ongoing hormonal or other glycemic influences.

*Schematic representation only

    **C** To optimize glycemic control, the pharmacology and pharmacokinetics of insulin require that a person receive small amounts of insulin continuously (basal), with boluses of insulin before meals and snacks.

    **D** The evolution of insulin management in the US is clearly moving from single injection therapy with intermediate-acting insulin to multiple injection therapy with human insulins.

    **E** The kinetics of various insulin products is shown in Table 3.3.

**2** The starting dose and schedule of insulin administration is based on the clinical assessment of insulin deficiency and suspected insulin resistance and on the person's preferences for eating times and amounts of carbohydrate, exercise, and waking/sleep patterns.[24]

    **A** Insulin requirements for individuals with type 1 diabetes or who are within 20% of ideal body weight are usually 0.5 to 1.0 unit/kg body weight/day.

    • Insulin requirements will be higher (even double) in the presence of intercurrent illness or other metabolic instability.

    • Insulin requirements will be less (0.2 to 0.6 unit/kg body weight/day) during the *honeymoon phase*, the period of relative remission early in the course of the disease.

    **B** Insulin requirements for individuals with type 2 diabetes vary considerably and may range from as little as 5 to 10 units/day to as much as several hundred units per day.[25] This variability may be attributed to interpatient variability of insulin deficiency and insulin resistance.

    **C** Insulin requirements for women with preexisting diabetes during the second and third trimesters of pregnancy gradually increase and are usually 0.9 to 1.2 units/kg body weight/day (as much as twice the total daily dosage of insulin needed before pregnancy).[26] These increases in plasma insulin are opposed by diminished

*[handwritten: Type 1]*
*[handwritten: .5 – 1]*

responsiveness to insulin action due to placental production of contrainsulin hormones. Women should be treated with an intensive insulin regimen.

**D** Approaches to insulin therapy for gestational diabetes differ greatly. A total dose of 20 to 30 units given before breakfast, is commonly used to initiate therapy.[26] The total dose is usually divided into two-thirds intermediate-acting insulin and one-third rapid-acting or short-acting insulin. For obese women, a higher starting dosage of insulin is usually necessary. The total initial dosage may be as high as 0.8 to 1.0 units/kg body weight/day.[26]

**E** Target blood glucose levels for test times before meals, after meals, and during sleep should be established. Setting targets with the patient (rather than for the patient) enhances patient understanding and decision-making as the person observes changes in blood glucose levels in relation to changes in food, exercise, stress, or illness.

**F** Subsequent adjustments in dose or timing of the insulin are based on self-monitoring of blood glucose (SMBG) and clinical signs and symptoms of hypoglycemia or hyperglycemia.

**G** Other parameters used to refine the insulin dose and schedule include glycosylated hemoglobin levels, achievement of weight or lipid goals, and variability of lifestyle or activities from day to day.

**3** Regimens for insulin monotherapy vary as needed, to meet the needs of the individual's daily habits with regard to meals, exercise, medications, work or activity schedule, and emotional factors. Note: The following regimens assume that the patient's lifestyle includes a waking time in the morning, meals spaced consistently during the day and waking hours, with a late evening bedtime. Appropriate alterations can be made in the insulin program to accommodate a midnight or rotating work schedule or other lifestyle preferences. Combination therapy using insulin with antidiabetes oral agents is discussed later.

**A** In a single daily injection regimen, insulin is administered in the morning or at bedtime (Figure 3.4A).

- Is not indicated for type 1 diabetes.
- Usually utilizes an intermediate-acting or a long-acting insulin, but could include a combined dose of a rapid-acting or short-acting and intermediate-acting insulin product.
- Bedtime administration may offer the advantage of improved fasting blood glucose control by suppressing nocturnal hepatic glucose production or increasing the basal-metabolic clearance of glucose.[27]
- Single daily doses of intermediate-acting or long-acting insulins may be used when doses are <30 units/day; however, for larger daily insulin doses, 2 or more doses will likely be needed.

**B** In 2-injection regimens, insulin is administered in the morning before breakfast and before the evening meal or at bedtime.

- It can include only intermediate-acting insulin (Figure 3.4B), or doses of regular or rapid-acting insulins mixed with intermediate-acting insulin, or premixed formulations (ie, mixtures such as Humalog Mix 75/25)[28] at one or both injection times. Mixed doses in the morning and before the evening meal is often called a *split-mixed regimen* and is considered *conventional insulin therapy*.

## Figure 3.4. Time Action of Insulin*, One or Two Daily Injections

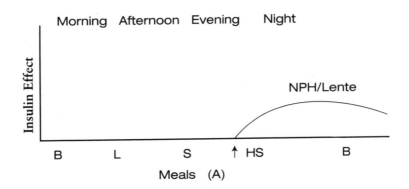

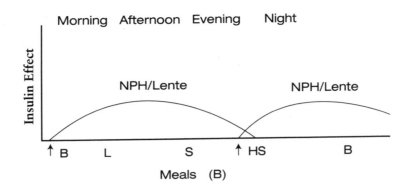

A: Idealized insulin effect provided by insulin regimen consisting of a bedtime (HS) injection of intermediate-acting insulin (NPH or Lente).
B: Idealized insulin effect provided by insulin regimen consisting of 2 daily injections of intermediate-acting insulin.

B = breakfast; L = lunch; S = supper; HS = bedtime snack; arrow = time of insulin injection, 30 minutes before meals
*Schematic representation only

*Source:* Reprinted with permission from Skyler.[2]

2/3    1/3
1:2    1:1

- Usually two thirds of the total daily dose of insulin is given before breakfast (using a ratio of 1 part rapid-acting or short-acting insulin to 2 parts intermediate-acting insulin) and one third is given before the evening meal (using a ratio of 1:1 or 1:2, rapid-acting or short-acting to intermediate insulin) (Figure 3.5A and B).
- **C** Multiple injections of insulin (3 or more) are components of the system called *intensive insulin therapy*. In 3-injection regimens, insulin is administered in the morning before breakfast, before the evening meal, and at bedtime, or before each meal.

## Figure 3.5. Time Action of Insulin*, Two Split-Mixed Daily Injections

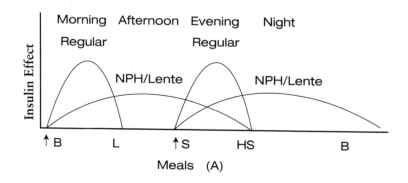

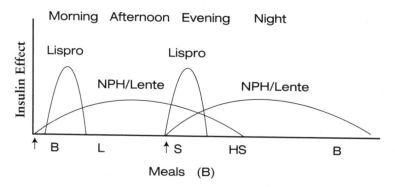

A: Idealized insulin effect provided by split-mixed insulin regimens consisting of 2 daily injections of short-acting insulin (regular) and intermediate-acting insulin (NPH or Lente).

B: Idealized insulin effect provided by insulin regimen consisting of rapid-acting insulin (lispro) and intermediate-acting insulin.

B = breakfast; L = lunch; S = supper; HS = bedtime snack; arrow = time of insulin injection, 30 minutes before meals
*Schematic representation only

*Source:* Reprinted with permission from Skyler.[2]

- Combination of rapid-acting or short-acting and intermediate-acting insulin before breakfast, rapid-acting or short-acting insulin alone before the evening meal, and intermediate-acting insulin at bedtime is illustrated in Figure 3.6A and B. This type of therapy reduces the risk of nocturnal (2 to 4 AM) hypoglycemia, allows better insulin coverage for early morning (5 to 10 AM) hyperglycemia from the release of cortisol and growth hormone (the dawn phenomenon), and, in some cases, may accommodate "sleeping in."

# Figure 3.6. Time Action of Insulin*, Three Multiple-Dose Daily Injections

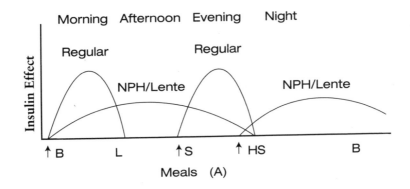

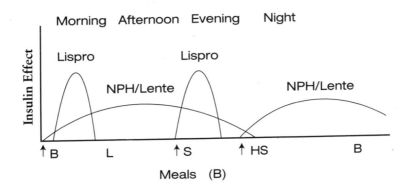

Idealized insulin effect provided by insulin regimen consisting of a morning injection of short-acting insulin and intermediate-acting insulin (NPH or Lente), a presupper injection of short-acting insulin, and a bedtime (HS) injection of intermediate-acting insulin.

A: Regular insulin
B: Rapid-acting insulin (lispro)

B = breakfast; L = lunch; S = supper; HS = bedtime snack; arrow = time of insulin injection, 30 minutes before meals
*Schematic representation only

*Source:* Reprinted with permission from Skyler.[2]

- • Ultralente insulin combined with rapid-acting or short-acting insulin before breakfast, before lunch, and before the evening meal is illustrated in Figure 3.7A and B. Individuals with unusual schedules may find this protocol particularly useful.
- ◘ In 4-injection regimens, insulin is administered in the morning before breakfast, before lunch, before the evening meal, and at bedtime and is illustrated in Figure 3.8 A and B.

## Figure 3.7. Time Action of Insulin*, Three Multiple-Dose Daily Injections

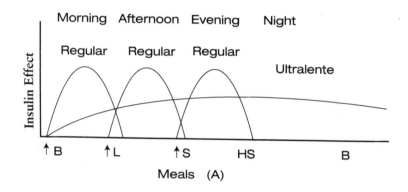

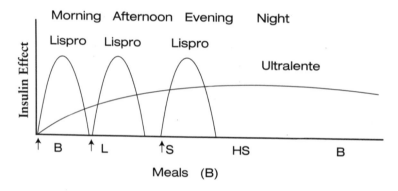

Idealized insulin effect provided by multiple-dose regimen providing basal long-acting (Ultralente) insulin and preprandial injections of short-acting insulin
A: Regular insulin
B: Rapid-acting insulin (lispro)

B = breakfast; L = lunch; S = supper; HS = bedtime snack; arrow = time of insulin injection, 30 minutes before meals
*Schematic representation only

*Source:* Reprinted with permission from Skyler.[2]

- Rapid-acting or short-acting insulin alone before breakfast, lunch, and dinner, and an intermediate-acting or long-acting insulin (NPH, Lente, Ultralente, or insulin glargine) at bedtime is another option. The pharmacokinetic properties of insulin glargine makes it an attractive basal insulin choice. Please note that this pharmacokinetic profile is not depicted.
- Rapid-acting or short-acting insulin with an intermediate-acting insulin in the morning before breakfast, rapid-acting or short-acting insulin alone before lunch and before the evening meal, and an intermediate-acting insulin at bedtime is illustrated in Figure 3.8A and B.

## Figure 3.8. Time Action of Insulin*, Four Multiple-Dose Daily Injections

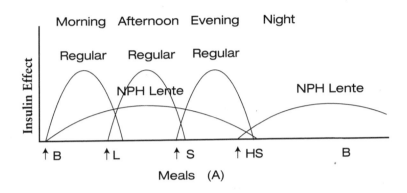

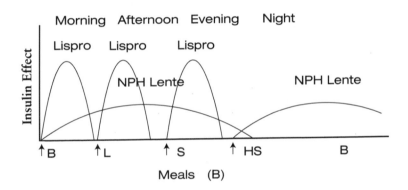

Idealized insulin effect provided by multiple-dose regimen providing basal intermediate-acting (NPH or Lente) at bedtime (HS) and before breakfast and preprandial injections of short-acting insulin.

A: Regular insulin

B: Rapid-acting insulin (lispro)

B = breakfast; L = lunch; S = supper; HS = bedtime snack; arrow = time of insulin injection, 30 minutes before meals

*Schematic representation only

- The rapid-acting or short-acting insulin provides postmeal glycemic control, while the intermediate-acting or long-acting insulin dose ensures a low, steady rate of insulin throughout the day.
- Four injections of short-acting insulin given about 6 hours apart may be indicated for some patients. This program may be effective during an illness or if ketoacidosis is imminent. Formulas for calculating dosages vary, but about one third of the total daily dose is given before breakfast, a slightly smaller amount at lunchtime, about 30% preceding the evening meal, and about 15% at midnight.

## Figure 3.9. Time Action of Insulin*, Pump Therapy

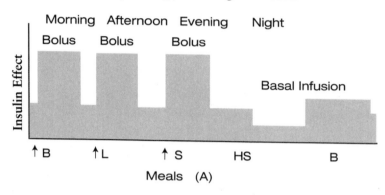

Pump Therapy with Regular Insulin

Pump Therapy with Lispro Insulin

Schematic representation of idealized insulin effect provided by pump therapy with either regular insulin (A) or lispro insulin (B). The insulin pump is programmed to deliver a determined rate of insulin throughout the day; prior to each meal, the patient activates the pump to deliver a bolus of insulin to control the glycemic response to food intake.

B = breakfast; L = lunch; S = supper; HS = bedtime snack; arrow = time of insulin injection, 30 minutes before meals
*Schematic representation only

*Source:* Reprinted with permission from Skyler.[22]

**E** Pump therapy is a continuous basal amount of insulin (0.5 to 1.0 U/hour) that is usually administered in addition to bolus doses given prior to meals (Figure 3.9).

## Pulmonary Insulin

**1** Recent technological advances have made it feasible to deliver insulin to the alveolar space where it is rapidly absorbed into the alveolar capillaries and disbursed throughout the systemic circulation.[29]

**A** Insulin administered via the pulmonary route in human studies has a soluble, rapid-acting formulation. However, in the future a pulmonary administration of longer acting insulin may also be possible.

**B** Two inhalation systems use different technology to deliver insulin via the pulmonary route.

- One system uses a fine-powdered formulation of insulin. The particle size is less than 5 μm in diameter. Particles of this size are able to reach the deep lung with slow, deep inhalation and they then pass a single cellular layer into the circulation. Insulin from this system will be available in "blister packs" and will remain stable at room temperature for up to 2 years. The device used to deliver the insulin is the size of a mechanical flashlight.

- The other system being evaluated in the US uses a handheld inhalation device that is regulated with microprocessors to produce a consistent dose using commercially available liquid insulins. Liquid insulin is inserted into the device and the aerosol delivers particles 2 to 3 μm in size directly to the alveoli.

**2** Several clinical trials have demonstrated the effectiveness, safety, and acceptability of inhaled insulin in persons with type 2 and type 1 diabetes.[30-32] At this time, inhaled insulin is not yet clinically available.

## Oral Antidiabetes Agents in the Management of Diabetes

**1** Currently, there are 6 chemical classes of oral agents available in the US for the management of diabetes.

**A** Sulfonylureas: first- and second-generation (insulin secretagogues)

**B** Benzoic acid derivative: repaglinide (insulin secretagogue)

**C** D-Phenylalanine derivative: nateglinide (insulin secretagogue)

**D** Biguanide: metformin (insulin sensitizer)

**E** Thiazolidinediones (glitazones): rosiglitazone and pioglitazone (insulin sensitizer)

**F** Alpha-glucosidase inhibitors: acarbose, miglitol (delay glucose absorption)

**2** These agents may be used as monotherapy for the treatment of type 2 diabetes, for treatment of secondary diabetes in individuals with substantial capacity for insulin production, or in combination with each other or with insulin.[33,34]

**3** Oral antidiabetes agents may be used in type 1 diabetes only as an adjunct to insulin therapy.

**4** These agents are not advised for use during preconception care or pregnancy (pregestational diabetes or gestational diabetes) or for children.

**5** Generally, monotherapy with any of these agents is associated with a reduction in HbA1c of approximately 0.5% to 1.5%.[35] This does not mean, however, that any agent will be equally efficacious for all patients; matching the pharmacologic action of a given agent with the patient's pathophysiologic basis(es) of hyperglycemia is a major determinant in therapeutic efficacy.

**6** When combination therapy is utilized (2 or more oral antidiabetes agents or an oral agent combined with insulin) an additive effect is observed, as demonstrated by a further decrease in HbA1c.[33,34]

    **A** Frequently used and/or well-studied combination therapies:
- Sulfonylurea with metformin
- Sulfonylurea with insulin
- Sulfonylurea with alpha-glucosidase inhibitor
- Glitazone with insulin
- Glitazone with sulfonylurea
- Glitazone with metformin
- Nateglinide with metformin

    **B** Less frequently used and/or less well-studied, or not-studied combination therapies:
- Triple combination therapy
- Metformin with alpha-glucosidase inhibitor
- Alpha-glucosidase inhibitor with insulin
- Repaglinide with metformin

## Sulfonylureas

**1** Available agents: Sulfonylureas can be classified as first- and second-generation oral hypoglycemic agents as shown in Table 3.5.[36] The first-generation agents are further divided into rapid-acting, intermediate-acting, and long-acting products.

**2** The pharmacologic actions of sulfonylureas include

    **A** Hypoglycemic agent: The major pharmacologic action has the potential to reduce blood glucose level below normal (ie, cause hypoglycemia).

    **B** Primary effect: Increases release of insulin from the pancreas, especially at the onset of therapy.

**3** They have the following pharmacokinetics:

    **A** Absorption is generally rapid, fairly complete, and unaffected by food except for short-acting glipizide, which is most effective when taken on an empty stomach.

    **B** Metabolism and excretion of these agents varies greatly. Most sulfonylureas are metabolized in the liver to active or inactive metabolites except for chlorpropamide, which is partially excreted unchanged in the urine. Biliary excretion is significant with glyburide and to a lesser extent with glipizide.[37]

**4** Significant contraindications or precautions to sulfonylurea therapy:

    **A** Not recommended for use during pregnancy, for breastfeeding women, or for children

    **B** Sulfonylurea hypersensitivity

    **C** Diabetic ketoacidosis

    **D** Severe infection

# Table 3.5. Oral Antidiabetes Agents

## Second-Generation Sulfonylureas

| Drug | Glyburide (DiaBeta®, Micronase®, Glynase Prestabs®) | Glipizide (Glucotrol®/Glucotrol XL®) | Glimepiride (Amaryl®) |
|---|---|---|---|
| Recommended dose | 1.25 to 10 mg single or divided dose; 0.75 to 12 mg (Glynase) | 2.5 to 20 mg single or divided dose; single dose for extended release (XL) | 1 to 4 mg single dose |
| Maximum dose | 20 mg; 12 mg (Glynase) | 40 mg; 20 mg (XL) | 8 mg |
| Half-life, h | Biphasic 3.2+10 | 3.5 to 6 | 2.5±1.2 |
| Onset, h | 1.5 | 1 | 2 to 3 |
| Duration, h | 24 | 12 to 16 | 24 |
| Metabolism/Excretion | 24% absorbed; completely metabolized in liver to nonactive derivatives; excreted in urine and bile 1:1 | Metabolized in liver to inactive metabolites; excreted primarily in urine | Completely metabolized via oxidative biotransformation to 2 major metabolites; metabolites excreted 60% renal and 40% hepatic elimination |
| Comments | 50 to 200 times more potent than first generation agents; no disulfiram-like reaction; caution in elderly | Glucotrol needs to be taken on an empty stomach; no disulfiram-like reaction; caution in elderly | Take with first main meal, once daily dosing; no disulfiram-like reaction |

## First-Generation Sulfonylureas

| Drug | Tolbutamide (Orinase®) | Tolazamide (Tolinase®) | Chlorpropamide (Diabinese®) |
|---|---|---|---|
| Recommended dose | 0.25 to 3.0 g divided doses | 0.1 to 1.0 g single or divided doses | 0.1 to 0.5 g single dose |
| Maximum dose | 2 to 3 g | 0.75 to 1.0 g | 0.5 g |
| Half-life, h | 5 to 7 | 7 | 24 to 48 |
| Onset, h | 1 | 4 to 6 | 1 |
| Duration, h | 6 to 12 | 10 to 14 | 72 |
| Metabolism/Excretion | Totally metabolized to inactive form; inactive metabolite excreted via kidney | Absorbed slowly; metabolite active but less potent than parent compound; excreted via kidney | Previously thought not to be metabolized, but recently found that metabolism may be quite extensive; significant percentage excreted unchanged via kidney |
| Comments | Most benign; least potent; short half-life, especially useful in kidney disease | Essentially no advantage over tolbutamide; said to be equally effective with less severe side effects | Longest duration; caution in elderly patients and those with kidney disease; disulfiram-like reactions may occur with alcohol; hyponatremia may be a problem |

Source: Adapted from Campbell and White.[16]

## Table 3.5. Oral Antidiabetes Agents (cont.)

### Nonsulfonylureas

| Drug | Repaglinide (Prandin®) | Nateglinide (Starlix®) | Metformin (Glucophage®) | Metformin Extended Release (Glucophage XR®) |
|---|---|---|---|---|
| Recommended dose | 0.5 to 4.0 before meals | 120 mg before meals | 500 to 850 mg tid or 1000 mg bid | 500 to 2000 mg once daily with evening meal |
| Maximum dose | 16 mg/day | 120 mg before meals | 2550 mg/day | 2000 mg/day |
| Half-life, h | 1 | 1.5 | 6 | 1.5 to 4.9 |
| Onset, h | 0.25 to 0.5 | Within 20 minutes | Not related to dose | Not related to dose |
| Duration, h | 2 to 3 | 2 to 3 hours | ~6 | up to 24 h |
| Metabolism/Excretion | Hepatic metabolism to inactive metabolites: <1% of parent drug excreted via kidney | Hepatic metabolism with approximately 16% of the parent compound excreted via the kidneys | Excreted unchanged in the urine | Excreted unchanged via the kidneys |
| Comments | Short duration; potential for accumulation is minimal; frequency of dosing dependent upon frequency of meals | Shortest duration; effect dependent on glucose levels; potential for accumulation is minimal; frequency of dosing, dependent on frequency of meals | Do not use in patients with renal or active liver disease | Same precautions as metformin |

| Drug | Pioglitazone (Actos®) | Rosiglitazone (Avandia®) | Acarbose (Precose®) | Miglitol (Glyset®) |
|---|---|---|---|---|
| Recommended dose | 15 to 45 mg daily | 2 to 8 mg daily | 25 to 100 mg tid | 25 to 100 mg tid |
| Maximum dose | 45 mg daily | 8 mg daily | 300 mg/day | 100 mg tid |
| Half-life, h | 16 to 24 | 103 to 158 | 2 | 2 to 3 |
| Onset, h | days | days | Immediate | Rapid |
| Duration, h | n/a | n/a | ~6 | Short |
| Metabolism/Excretion | Primarily hepatic metabolism | Extensive hepatic metabolism | <2% absorbed, metabolized in GI tract | Unchanged via kidney and feces |
| Comments | Monitor liver function tests every 2 months for first year, then periodically thereafter | 4 mg bid more effective than 8 mg daily; monitor liver function tests every 2 months for first year, then periodically thereafter | Take with first bite of meal for maximum effectiveness | |

*Source:* Adapted from Campbell and White.[36]

**E** Surgery, trauma, or other severe metabolic stressor

**F** Elderly, debilitated, or malnourished patients and patients with adrenal, pituitary, or hepatic insufficiency who are particularly susceptible to the hypoglycemic effects of glucose-lowering agents

**G** Refer to package labeling for specific agents for additional contraindications and precautions

**5** Adverse effects associated with sulfonylurea agents:

**A** Hypoglycemia is the most serious complication of sulfonylurea therapy. An age-related decline in renal function can contribute to susceptibility to hypoglycemia in the elderly.[38]

**B** Weight gain, probably secondary to increased insulin secretion

**C** Skin rashes in approximately 2% of users

**D** Gastrointestinal disturbances in approximately 5% of users

**E** Metabolic disorders such as a renal syndrome of inappropriate antidiuretic hormone (SIADH) can occur with the use of chlorpropamide. SIADH (ADH=vasopressin), manifested by hyponatremia and hypervolemia, occurs in about 4% of patients treated with chlorpropamide.

**F** Hepatic changes—abnormal hepatic function tests and icterus—are rare.

**G** Hematologic changes—thrombocytopenia, agranulocytosis, and hemolytic anemia—have been described with tolbutamide and chlorpropamide but appear to be very rare with second-generation sulfonylureas.

**6** *Treatment failure* occurs when an individual is insensitive to the effects of sulfonylureas.

**A** *Primary failure:* No response to the initial sulfonylurea therapy; occurs in 20% of patients.

**B** *Secondary failure:* No or diminished response to the sulfonylurea, after an initial therapeutic response; occurs in 5% to 10% of those individuals whose blood glucose initially responded to a given agent.

**7** Clinically important drug interactions with sulfonylurea agents are listed in Table 3.6.

**8** The role of sulfonylurea agents in the treatment of diabetes include

**A** Use as monotherapy only in type 2 diabetes or secondary diabetes with substantial capacity for insulin production.

• Typical candidate for initial sulfonylurea monotherapy: Has type 2 diabetes, without dyslipidemia, not overweight, and a fasting plasma glucose level >20 mg/dL above the target concentration.[39]

**B** Therapy initiated at a low, single daily dose, with gradual increases to reach glucose goals.

• Doses of the sulfonylurea preparations are listed Table 3.5. Although there is noticeable variance in the relative weight potency between first- and second-generation agents, the maximum hypoglycemic effect between these agents is similar.[40]

• Initial dosage may need to be adjusted for patients with hepatic or renal dysfunction.

• Use chlorpropamide with caution in patients who are elderly or have renal insufficiency because of the potential for accumulation.

## Table 3.6. Drug-Disease and Drug-Drug Interactions

| Interacting Drug | Drug-Disease (Intrinsic Effect) | Drug-Drug Interaction* | Net Effect on Blood Glucose | Notes |
|---|---|---|---|---|
| Allopurinol | No | Sulfonylureas and Meglitinide | ↑ | • Decreased renal tubular secretion of chlorpropamide |
| Androgens/anabolic steroids | Yes | — | ↑ | • Mechanism unknown |
| Anticoagulants, oral (Dicumarol) | No | Sulfonylureas and Meglitinide | ↑ | • Interfere with metabolism of tolbutamide, chlorpropamide |
| Asparaginase I | Yes | — | ↑[1] ↓[2] | 1. Hyperglycemia associated with inhibition of insulin synthesis<br>2. Hypoglycemia reported occasionally |
| Aspirin | Yes[3] | Sulfonylureas[4] and Meglitinide | ↑ | 3. Large daily doses (~4 gm/d): Increased basal and stimulated release of insulin<br>4. Displace sulfonylurea from protein binding; decrease urinary excretion of sulfonylurea |
| Beta-adrenergic antagonists | Yes | — | ↑ ↓ | • Both hypoglycemic and hyperglycemic response has been reported; may alter physiologic response to, and subjective symptoms of, hypoglycemia; may reduce hyperglycemia-induced insulin release or decrease tissue sensitivity to insulin |
| Calcium channel blockers | Yes | — | ↑ ↓ | • Hypoglycemia reported with verapamil<br>• Hyperglycemia reported with diltazem, nifedipine |
| Cholestyramine | No | TZD[5] and Acarbose[6] | ↓[5] ↑[6] | 5. Cholestyramine reduces absorption of coadministered drugs<br>6. Cholestyramine may enhance effects of acarbose; interactions may be avoided by administering cholestyramine 2 hr apart from other medications |
| Chloramphenicol | No | Sulfonylureas and Meglitinide | ↑ | • Decreased hepatic metabolism and/or protein-binding displacement of tolbutamide, chlorpropamide |
| Chloroquine | Yes | — | ↑ | • Mechanism unknown |

## Table 3.6. Drug-Disease and Drug-Drug Interactions (cont.)

| Interacting Drug | Drug-Disease (Intrinsic Effect) | Drug-Drug Interaction* | Net Effect on Blood Glucose | Notes |
|---|---|---|---|---|
| Cimetidine/possible other H₂ antagonists | No | Sulfonylureas,[7] Meglitinide and Metformin[8] | ↓ | 7. Increased absorption and/or decreased clearance of glipizide, glyburide, tolbutamide<br>8. Decreased renal tubular secretion of metformin; other drugs excreted via renal tubular transport *may* similarly interfere with metformin clearance. |
| Clofibrate | Yes[9] | Sulfonylureas[10] and Meglitinide | ↓ | 9. Intrinsic hypoglycemic effect: Mechanism unknown<br>10. Displace certain sulfonylureas from protein binding |
| Corticosteriods | Yes | | ↑ | • Increased gluconeogenesis; transient insulin resistance |
| Cyclosporine | Yes | | ↑ | • Inhibition of insulin secretion |
| Diazoxide | Yes | | ↑ | • Inhibition of insulin secretion |
| Dicumarol | No | Sulfonylureas and Meglitinide | ↓ | • Inhibits hepatic metabolism of tolbutamide, chlorpropamide |
| Disopyramide | Yes | — | ↓ | • Most susceptible: Elderly or patients with renal or liver impairment |
| Diuretics | Yes | — | ↑ | — |
| Estrogen products | Yes | — | ↑ | • Mechanism unknown |
| Ethanol | Yes | Sulfonylureas[11] and Meglitinide | ↑[12] ↓[13] | 11. Disulfiram-like reaction may also occur, especially with chlorpropamide; not noted with second-generation sulfonylureas<br>12. Chronic alcohol ingestion may increase metabolism of sulfonylurea; alcohol ingestion, especially with carbohydrate-based drink (beer, mixed drink) has caloric effect.<br>13. Intrinsic hypoglycemic effect; impairs gluconeogenesis and increases insulin secretion; effect is potentiated if alcohol consumed without food or in fasting state |

## Table 3.6. Drug-Disease and Drug-Drug Interactions (cont.)

| Interacting Drug | Drug-Disease (Intrinsic Effect) | Drug-Drug Interaction* | Net Effect on Blood Glucose | Notes |
|---|---|---|---|---|
| Fluoxetine | Yes | — | ↑↓ | • Hypoglycemia and hyperglycemia have been reported |
| Fluconazole | No | Sulfonylureas and Meglitinide | ↓ | • Reported interaction with glipizide |
| Gemfibrozil | Yes | — | — | — |
| Glyburide | Yes | Acarbose and Miglitol[14] | ↓ | 14. Miglitol reduces the area under the curve (AUC) and peak concentration of glyburide |
| Guanethidine | Yes | Sulfonylureas[15] and Meglitinide | ↓[16] | 15. Protein-binding displacement of certain sulfonylureas<br>16. Intrinsic glycemic effect |
| NSAIDS (non-steroidal anti-inflammatory drugs) | Yes[17] | Sulfonylureas[18] and Meglitinide | ↓ | 17. Possible intrinsic hypoglycemic effect<br>18. Protein-binding displacement (tolbutamide, tolazamide) |
| Isoniazid | Yes | — | ↑ | • Increases glycogenolysis |
| Ketoconozal | Yes | Pioglitazone | ↓ | • In vitro studies suggest that ketoconozal inhibits the metabolism of pioglitazone |
| Metformin | No | Alpha-glucosidase inhibitors | ↓ | • Acarbose reduces metformin bioavailability by ~35% when coadministered; separate doses to avoid |
| Monoamine Oxidase Inhibitors | Yes[19] | Sulfonylureas[20] and Meglitinide | ↓ | 19. May stimulate insulin secretion (beta-adrenergic stimulation) or may be secondary to hepatotoxicity<br>20. May interfere with metabolism of sulfonylurea |
| Nicotinic Acid (Niacin) | Yes | — | ↑ | • Dose dependent, when lipid-lowering doses are used<br>• Insignificant effect at vitamin supplement dose |
| Octreotide | Yes | — | ↑↓ | • Hypoglycemia and hyperglycemia have been reported |
| Oral contraceptives | Yes | Pioglitazone[21] and Rosiglitazone[22] | ↑ | 21. Pioglitazone has not be evaluated; however, caution should be used<br>22. No clinically significant effect on ethinyl estradiol or norethindrone |
| Pancrelipase/pancreatic enzymes | Yes | — | ↑ | • Do not administer these agents concurrently with acarbose |
| Pentamidine | Yes | — | ↑↓ | • Initially, hypoglycemia; hyperglycemia may occur days or even months after initiation of therapy |

## Table 3.6. Drug-Disease and Drug-Drug Interactions (cont.)

| Interacting Drug | Drug-Disease (Intrinsic Effect) | Drug-Drug Interaction* | Net Effect on Blood Glucose | Notes |
|---|---|---|---|---|
| *Phenothiazines* | Yes | — | | • Hypoglycemia observed with some phenothiazines, hyperglycemia with others |
| *Phenytoin* | Yes | — | | • Decreased insulin secretion |
| *Probenecid* | Yes[23] | Sulfonylureas[24] and Meglitinide | | 23. Intrinsic glycemic effect<br>24. Decrease urinary excretion of chlorpropamide |
| *Protease inhibitors* | Yes | — | | — |
| *Rifampin* | Yes[25] | Sulfonylureas[26] and Meglitinide | [26] [25] | 25. Possible intrinsic hypoglycemic effect<br>26. Increased metabolism of chlorpropamide, glyburide, tolbutamide |
| *Salicylates* | Yes[27] | Sulfonylureas[28] and Meglitinide | | 27. Large daily doses (~4 gm/d): Increase basal and stimulated release of insulin<br>~28. Displace sulfonylurea from protein binding; decrease urinary excretion of sulfonylurea. |
| *Sulfonamides, highly protein-bound* | No | Sulfonylureas and Meglitinide | | • Various effects upon chlorpropamide, tolbutamide kinetics: displacement from protein binding, decreased urinary excretion, and/or altered metabolism |
| *Tacrolimus* | Yes | — | | — |
| *Thyroid products* | Yes | — | | • Once euthyroid status is achieved, diabetes medications may need to be adjusted to compensate for glycemic effect of thyroid product |
| *Urinary Acidifiers* | No | Sulfonylureas and Meglitinide | | • Interfere with chlorpropamide excretion |

This listing is not intended to be inclusive. Before any new medication is initiated, consult the package labeling (insert) or other reference. In general, these interactions are based on moderate to severe clinical significance and/or possible or established documentation.

• Interactions with sulfonylureas, meglitinide, metformin, pioglitazone and rosiglitazone (both thiazolidinediones), alpha-glucosidase inhibitors, and insulin are listed.

**C** Combination therapy, or transition to insulin monotherapy, is considered when sulfonylurea therapy approaches the maximum dose. In most cases at one half the maximum dose, additional increases in dosage will not yield additional increases in therapeutic effect; this phenomenon is referred to as the "ceiling effect."
  - In many patients, half the recommended maximum dose of sulfonylureas may be as effective as maximum doses.[41]

**D** Compared with the first-generation agents, the second-generation sulfonylureas generally interact less frequently with other agents, elicit fewer significant adverse effects, and have alternate routes of excretion.

## Meglitinide Analogues

**1** Available agents are
  **A** Benzoic acid derivative: Repaglinide (Prandin®)
  **B** D-Phenylalanine derivative: Nateglinide (Starlix®)

**2** Meglitinides are hypoglycemic agents whose major pharmacologic action has the potential to reduce the blood glucose level to below normal.

## Repaglinide

**1** Repaglinide is a nonsulfonylurea agent, but shares many of the pharmacologic actions and adverse effects of sulfonylureas. It increases release of insulin from the pancreas; the effect is glucose-dependent and diminishes at low blood glucose concentrations.
  **A** Treatment with repaglinide is effective in well-controlled patients with type 2 diabetes[42] or in patients whose control is suboptimal.[43] Patients treated with repaglinide who missed or delayed a meal had less risk of hypoglycemia compared to treatment with longer acting sulfonylurea drugs.[42] Repaglinide also resulted in better glycemic control when combined with a glitazone than monotherapy with either agent alone.[44]
  **B** Repaglinide (Prandin) is available in 0.5-mg, 1-mg, and 2-mg dosage units.

**2** Pharmacokinetics include
  **A** Absorption from the GI tract is rapid and complete; food slightly decreases absorption.[45]
  **B** Protein binding and binding to serum albumin: >95%.
  **C** Rapid hepatic metabolism to inactive metabolites; half-life of the drug is approximately 1 hour. Less than 1% of the parent drug is excreted by the kidneys. Because of the short half-life, the potential for accumulation is minimal with normal dosing regimens.[45]

**3** Significant contraindications or precautions to repaglinide therapy:
  **A** Not recommended for use during pregnancy, for breastfeeding women, or for children
  **B** Diabetic ketoacidosis
  **C** Severe infection
  **D** Surgery, trauma, or other severe metabolic stressor
  **E** Impaired hepatic function. Use cautiously. Titrate doses upward very gradually, with careful monitoring, to detect accumulation of parent drug and/or metabolites.

**F** Elderly, debilitated, or malnourished patients and those with adrenal, pituitary, or hepatic insufficiency who are particularly susceptible to the hypoglycemic effects of glucose-lowering agents

**G** Refer to package labeling for additional contraindications and precautions

**4** Adverse effects associated with repaglinide therapy:

**A** Gastrointestinal disturbances in approximately 4% of users

**B** Upper respiratory infection or problems

**C** Arthralgia or back pain

**D** Headache

**E** Hypoglycemia (16% to 31%)

**5** Treatment failure occurs when an individual is insensitive to the effects of repaglinide.

**A** Primary failure: No response to the initial repaglinide therapy.

**B** Secondary failure: No or diminished response to repaglinide, after an initial therapeutic response.

**6** Clinically important drug interactions with repaglinide are listed in Table 3.6.

**7** Role of repaglinide in the treatment of diabetes mellitus:

**A** Use as monotherapy only in type 2 diabetes or secondary diabetes in individuals with substantial capacity for insulin production.

- Typical candidate for initial repaglinide monotherapy: Type 2 diabetes, without dyslipidemia, with or without renal failure, not overweight, and fasting plasma glucose level >20 mg/dL above the target concentration.

**B** Therapy initiated at a low, single daily dose, with gradual increases to reach glucose goals.

- Instruct patients to take 15 minutes (0 to 30 minutes) before each meal. The number of daily doses taken is determined by the number of meals eaten. The "meal-based" dosing frequency may offer advantages for patients who vary frequency of daily meals or for those who choose to eat only 2 meals a day and need to avoid persisting hypoglycemic activity between the meals.
- Initial dose for patients not treated previously with glucose-lowering drugs or with HbA1c <8%: 0.5 mg with each meal.[43]
- Initial dosage does not need to be adjusted for patients with renal dysfunction; however, upward titration should proceed cautiously.
- Initial dose for patients previously treated with glucose-lowering drugs and with HbA1c >8%: 1 or 2 mg with each meal.
- At 1-week intervals, each preprandial dose may be doubled, up to 4 mg, until desired effect is attained.
- Maximum dose: 16 mg daily.

**C** Combination therapy, or transition to insulin monotherapy, is considered when repaglinide therapy approaches the maximum dose.

---

## Nateglinide

**1** The major pharmacologic action of nateglinide is its potential to reduce the blood glucose level to below normal; however, its effects are linked to ambient glucose levels.[46,47] In combination with metformin, nateglinide decreased mealtime glucose excursions, whereas metformin affected fasting glucose concentrations.[48]

**A** Nateglinide is a D-phenylalanine (amino acid) derivative and is a very rapid-acting oral insulin secretagogue which stimulates insulin secretion when needed (postprandial) and then allows insulin concentrations to return to normal basal concentrations.[46,47]

**B** Nateglinide (Starlix®) is available in 60-mg and 120-mg tablets.

**2** Pharmacokinetics include

**A** The mean time to reach maximum concentrations of nateglinide after oral administration is 0.82 hours. High-fat meals reportedly result in a 12% increase in maximum concentration and a 52% reduction in the time to reach that concentration.[49]

**B** Metabolism is by extensive hepatic metabolism via cytochrome P450 enzymes, primarily by CYP3A4 and CYP2C9.[50]

**C** It is eliminated predominately by the kidneys (80% of the parent compound and metabolites). The average terminal half-life is an average of 1.5 hours.[50]

**3** Significant contraindications or precautions to D-phenylalanine derivatives are

**A** Not recommended for use during pregnancy, for breastfeeding women, or for children.

**B** Diabetic ketoacidosis

**4** Adverse effects associated with nateglinide include

**A** Mild hypoglycemia in approximately 2.4% of patients in clinical trials. There were no reports of hypoglycemia requiring third-party assistance or nocturnal hypoglycemia in the phase III trials (2400 patients).

**B** Dizziness in approximately 3.6% of users.

**C** Weight gain of <1 kg from baseline and is attenuated with the concomitant use of metformin.[48]

**5** No clinically important drug interactions with nateglinide have been identified to date.

**6** Role of nateglinide in the treatment of diabetes mellitus:

**A** To be used as monotherapy in patients with type 2 diabetes with a capacity for insulin production whose hyperglycemia cannot be adequately controlled by nutrition therapy and exercise and who have not been treated long-term with other antidiabetic agents. The usual initial and maintenance dose of nateglinide is 120 mg taken just before (1 to 30 minutes) meals. Titration of dose is not usually necessary. The 60-mg dose may be used in patients who are near their HbA1c goal.

**B** Combination oral therapy, or transition to insulin monotherapy, may be considered when nateglinide therapy is ineffective as monotherapy. The addition of nateglinide to a sulfonylurea results in no additional benefit and is therefore not recommended. Nateglinide is efficacious when used in combination with metformin. The usual initial and maintenance dose of nateglinide when used in combination with metformin is 120 mg taken just before (1 to 30 minutes) meals. Titration of dose is not usually necessary. The 60-mg dose may be used in patients who are near their HbA1c goal.

**C** Dose adjustment is not needed in the elderly, in patients with mild to severe renal insufficiency, or in patients with mild hepatic insufficiency.

## Biguanides

**1** Available agents include

**A** Metformin (Glucophage®) in 500-mg and 850-mg dosage units

**B** Metformin (Glucophage XR®) in 500-mg dosage unit

**C** Glyburide/metformin (Glucovance®) in 1.25/250-mg, 2.5/500-mg, and 5/500 mg dosage units.

**2** Biguanides have the following pharmacologic actions:

**A** They are not a hypoglycemic agent because their major pharmacologic action does not increase insulin secretion and thus does not increase the risk of hypoglycemia. These agents have proven to be an effective antihyperglycemic agent or an insulin sensitizer.[51-55]

• Frequently, there is a slight (2-kg to 5-kg) weight loss seen with metformin therapy; however, the actual cause of weight loss is not known.

**B** Primary effects include

• Reduces hepatic glucose production primarily by reduction in glycogenolysis.[56]

• Enhances insulin-stimulated glucose transport in adipose tissue and skeletal muscle, thus reversing or partially reversing insulin resistance.[51]

**C** Decreases intestinal absorption of glucose (minor effect).

**D** Causes a reduction in triglyceride concentrations of approximately 16%, in LDL cholesterol by approximately 8%, and in total cholesterol by approximately 5% and is associated with an increase in HDL cholesterol by approximately 2%.[51,53]

**3** Pharmacokinetics include

**A** The oral bioavailability is 50% to 60%. Food decreases the extent of bioavailability and slightly delays the absorption of metformin.

**B** Does not bind to liver or plasma proteins.

**C** Major excretion is by the kidneys, largely unchanged, through an active tubular process.

**4** Significant contraindications or precautions to metformin therapy:

**A** Generally not indicated during pregnancy, for breastfeeding women, or for children

**B** Renal dysfunction with serum creatinine levels ≥1.5 mg/dL in males or >1.4 mg/dL in females. Metformin is excreted renally and can accumulate in patients with renal dysfunction.

**C** Hepatic dysfunction (lactate metabolism is carried out in the liver)

**D** Acute or chronic lactic acidosis

**E** History of alcoholism or binge ingestion of alcohol

**F** Metformin should be temporarily withheld in any situation which would predispose the individual to acute renal dysfunction or tissue hypoperfusion, including

• Cardiovascular collapse

• Acute myocardial infarction

• Acute exacerbation of congestive heart failure

• Use of iodinated contrast media

• Major surgical procedure

**G** Refer to package labeling for additional contraindications and precautions[57,58]

**5** Adverse effects associated with metformin therapy:

**A** Metformin monotherapy is not associated with hypoglycemia.
- Patients using combination therapy (metformin with insulin or metformin with sulfonylureas [eg, Glucovance]) may experience hypoglycemia secondary to the hypoglycemic agent.

**B** Gastrointestinal effects in up to 30% of users: Abdominal bloating, nausea, cramping, feeling of fullness, diarrhea.[59]
- Usually self-limiting, transient (7 to 14 days), and can be minimized by taking the medication with food, starting with a low dose, and slow upward titration of dosage.

**C** Miscellaneous: Agitation, sweating, headache, and metallic taste.

**D** Associated with a reduction in vitamin $B_{12}$ levels, although no cases of anemia have been reported in the US.

**E** Lactic acidosis can occur with the administration of metformin but is rare (0.03 cases per 1000 patient years). Lactic acidosis is primarily associated with its use in patients who have contraindications to the drug or in cases of overdose.[60]

**6** Clinically important drug interactions with metformin are listed in Table 3.6.

**7** Role of metformin in the treatment of diabetes mellitus:

**A** Use as monotherapy only in type 2 diabetes or secondary diabetes with substantial capacity for insulin production.
- Typical candidate for initial metformin monotherapy: Type 2 diabetes, with dyslipidemia, with obesity or genetic factors favoring insulin resistance, and fasting plasma glucose level >20 mg/dL above the target concentration.[23]

**B** Therapy initiated at a low dose, with gradual increases to obtain desired control.
- Usual initial dose: Standard formulation—500 mg or 850 mg qd or 500 mg bid, with doses taken prior to a meal. Glucophage XR formulation—500 mg with the evening meal.[57]
- Titrate dose upward as tolerated (to GI effects) to reach glucose goals. Increases usually occur at 14-day intervals for the standard formulation and at 7-day intervals for the XR formulation.[57]
- Maximum daily dose: Standard formulation—2550 mg daily (850 mg tid) (note, however, that the greatest reduction in fasting plasma glucose is seen at 2000 mg/day (1000 mg bid) XR formulation—2000 mg daily in 1 or 2 doses.

**C** Combination therapy, or transition to insulin monotherapy, is considered when metformin therapy approaches the maximum dose.[61]

## Thiazolidinediones (TZDs)

**1** Available agents are
**A** Pioglitazone (Actos) available in 15-mg, 30-mg, and 45-mg tablets
**B** Rosiglitazone (Avandia) available in 2-mg, 4-mg, and 8-mg tablets

**2** TZDs have the following pharmacologic actions:
**A** They are not a hypoglycemic agent; the major pharmacologic action does not increase insulin secretion and thus does not increase the risk of hypoglycemia. These agents may best be described as an antihyperglycemic agent or insulin sensitizers. These drugs probably reduce insulin resistance and improve blood glucose levels via the stimulation of peroxisome-proliferator-activated receptor-gamma (PPAR-y).[62,63]

**B** They enhance insulin action at the receptor and postreceptor level in hepatic and peripheral tissues, thus reversing or partially reversing insulin resistance.

**3** Pharmacokinetics are
  **A** Both of these medications are well absorbed without regard to meals.
  **B** Both medications are extensively bound (>99%) to serum albumin.
  **C** Both drugs are extensively metabolized in the liver.
  **D** Metabolites and parent compounds are eliminated primarily in the feces with minor amounts in the urine.

**4** Significant contraindications or precautions to thiazolidinedione therapy include
  **A** Generally not indicated during pregnancy, for breastfeeding women, or for children.
  **B** Thiazolidinediones should be used with caution in patients with hepatic dysfunction. Rare cases of severe idiosyncratic hepatocellular injury have occurred with troglitazone. Serum transaminase levels should be monitored every 2 months during the first year of therapy and then periodically thereafter.
  **C** In premenopausal anovulatory women with insulin resistance, thiazolidinedione therapy may result in resumption of ovulation, with a subsequent risk of pregnancy.
  **D** TZDs are contraindicated in patients with NYHA class III and IV failure since their safety in this population has not been studied.
  **E** Refer to package labeling for additional contraindications and precautions.[64,65]

**5** Adverse effects associated with thiazolidinedione therapy are
  **A** Elevated hepatic enzymes. Rare cases of severe idiosyncratic hepatocellular injury occurred with troglitazone. It is not clear if this effect is a class effect or if it was specific to troglitazone. While the hepatic injury associated with troglitazone was generally reversible, rare cases of hepatic failure, including death, were reported, which prompted removal of this drug from the market.[63]
  **B** Plasma volume expansion, resulting in small reductions in hemoglobin, hematocrit, and neutrophil counts.
  **C** Weight gain is probably a class effect of the TZDs.
  **D** Both TZDs have been associated with mild to moderate edema.[63]
  **E** Other considerations include incidences similar to that of placebo: GI discomfort, headache, pharyngitis.
  **F** Small increases in HDL and LDL cholesterol may occur with rosiglitazone while reductions in triglycerides and elevations of HDL have been reported with pioglitazone. The clinical significance of the lipid effects of this class or drugs is unclear at this time.

**6** Clinically important drug interactions with thiazolidinediones are listed in Table 3.6
  **A** Rosiglitazone is metabolized by CYP2C9 and CYP2C8. In vitro studies have suggested that inhibition of these isoenzymes by rosiglitazone does not occur at concentrations usually encountered clinically. The isoenzyme CYP3A4, which is responsible for the metabolism of several drugs including erythromycin, calcium channel blockers, corticosteroids, and HMG-CoA reductase inhibitors, is also partially responsible for the metabolism of pioglitazone. However, specific studies evaluating these agents have not been carried out. Therefore, the possibility of altered safety or efficacy should be considered when using these agents with pioglitazone.

**7** Role of TZDs in the treatment of diabetes mellitus:

 **A** Use as monotherapy only in type 2 diabetes or secondary diabetes with substantial capacity for insulin production.[66,67]

 • Typical candidate for initial TZD monotherapy: Type 2 diabetes, with obesity or genetic factors favoring insulin resistance, and fasting plasma glucose level >20 mg/dL above the target concentration.

 **B** Therapy initiated at a low dose, with gradual increases to reach plasma glucose goals. Instruct patients to take with main meal of day for maximum absorption.

 • Usual initial dose: Rosiglitazone—2-mg bid or 4-mg qd; pioglitazone—15 to 30 mg qd.

 • Titrate dose upward until desired therapeutic effect is reached. Dose increases should not occur less often than 4 weeks.

 • Maximum recommended daily dose for rosiglitazone is 4 mg bid or 8 mg qd and for pioglitazone, 45 mg qd.

 **C** Combination therapy is considered when TZDs are ineffective at maximum dose.

## Alpha-Glucosidase Inhibitors

**1** Available agents are

 **A** Acarbose (Precose®) available in 25-mg, 50-mg, and 100-mg tablets

 **B** Miglitol (Glyset®) available in 25-mg, 50-mg, and 100-mg tablets

**2** Pharmacologic actions include

 **A** They are not hypoglycemic agents; the major pharmacologic action does not increase insulin secretion and thus does not increase the risk of hypoglycemia. This agent may best be described as an antihyperglycemic agent.

 **B** They inhibit alpha-glucosidase enzymes in the brush border of the small intestine[68] and pancreatic alpha-amylase,[69] leading to a reduction in carbohydrate-mediated postprandial blood glucose elevation.

 • Alpha-glucosidase enzymes (maltase, isomaltase, glucoamylase, and sucrase) hydrolyze oligosaccharides, trisaccharides, and disaccharides to glucose and other monosaccharides in the brush border of the small intestine.

 • Alpha-amylase hydrolyzes complex starches to oligosaccharides in the lumen of the small intestine.

 • Inhibition of these enzyme systems reduces the rate of digestion of starches and the subsequent absorption of glucose.

**3** Pharmacokinetics are

 **A** Oral bioavailability: Acarbose has a negligible absorption of unchanged drug, about 35% of the intestinal metabolites of acarbose are absorbed. Miglitol is almost completely absorbed.

 **B** Acarbose is metabolized within the GI tract by intestinal bacteria and by digestive enzymes. Excretion of absorbed acarbose and its metabolites is by the kidneys. Miglitol is excreted unchanged in the urine with any unabsorbed drug being eliminated in the feces.

 **C** Acarbose plasma levels are elevated in patients with creatinine clearance (CrCl) <25 mL/min, suggesting accumulation of acarbose. However, dosage adjustment in this setting is not feasible because acarbose acts locally.

**4** Significant contraindications or precautions to alpha-glucosidase inhibitor therapy:

   **A** Generally not indicated during pregnancy, for breastfeeding women, or for children.

   **B** Inflammatory bowel disease, colonic ulceration, or obstructive bowel disorders; chronic intestinal disorders of digestion or absorption; or any medical condition that might deteriorate with increased intestinal gas formation[69]

   **C** Acarbose is contraindicated in patients with cirrhosis of the liver

   **D** Acarbose is not recommended in patients with serum creatinine levels >2.0 mg/dL since studies have suggested increases in drug or metabolite plasma concentrations with renal dysfunction, and long-term studies have not been carried out in this population.[35] Neither agent is recommended in patients with creatinine clearances of <25 mL/min.[69]

**5** Adverse effects associated with alpha-glucosidase inhibitor therapy:

   **A** Alpha-glucosidase inhibitor monotherapy is not associated with hypoglycemia.[69]

   • Patients using combination therapy (alpha-glucosidase inhibitor with insulin or alpha-glucosidase inhibitor with sulfonylureas) may experience hypoglycemia secondary to the insulin or sulfonylurea.

   • Hypoglycemia in this situation can be managed with oral glucose (if the patient is conscious) or intravenous glucose or glucagon (if the patient is unconscious). Because these drugs blunt the digestion of complex sugars to glucose, oral sugar sources other than glucose or lactose (eg, glucose tablets, milk) are unsuitable for rapid correction of hypoglycemia.[69]

   **B** Gastrointestinal effects, occurring primarily at initiation of therapy or when dosage is increased, are diarrhea, abdominal pain, and flatulence (in one third to two thirds of patients).

   • Usually self-limiting, transient, and can be minimized by starting with a low dose and slow upward titration of dosage. Redistribution of the inhibited enzymes usually occurs after several weeks of therapy resulting in a mitigation of adverse effects.[69]

   **C** Elevation of serum transaminases (AST or ALT) has been observed in clinical trials in patients taking acarbose at a dose of 200 to 300 mg tid. Elevations in hepatic enzymes have only been observed in patients taking greater than 100 mg tid.[35]

**6** Clinically important drug interactions with alpha-glucosidase inhibitors are listed in Table 3.6.

**7** Role of alpha-glucosidase inhibitors in the treatment of diabetes mellitus:

   **A** Use as monotherapy only in type 2 diabetes or secondary diabetes with substantial capacity for insulin production.[70]

   • Typical candidate for initial alpha-glucosidase inhibitor monotherapy: Type 2 diabetes, with dyslipidemia or obesity, and symptoms suggesting—or blood glucose profile demonstrating—significant postprandial hyperglycemia.

   • Individuals demonstrating significant premeal hyperglycemia without a significant premeal-to-postmeal glucose rise would not be expected to respond optimally to alpha-glucosidase inhibitor monotherapy.

   **B** Therapy initiated at a low dose to minimize GI adverse effects, with gradual increases to reach glucose goals.

   • The usual initial dose is 25 mg qd. Instruct patients to take with the first bite of the meal for the drug to be effective.

- Titrate dose upward as patient tolerance (to GI effects) allows, until desired therapeutic effect is reached.[71] The following titrate doses can be used:
  Acarbose
  —25 mg qd for 2 weeks
  —25 mg bid for 1 to 2 weeks
  —25 mg tid for 4 to 8 weeks
  —Increase to 50 mg tid for 4 to 8 weeks
  —Maintenance dose: 50 or 100 mg tid (50 mg tid if patient <60 kg)
  —Maximum daily dose: 50 mg tid if patient <60 kg; 100 mg tid if patient >60 kg
  Miglitol
  —25 mg tid initially for 4 to 8 weeks
  —50 mg tid for 3 months
  —Increase to 100 mg tid, if tolerated and if needed
  **C** Combination therapy, or transition to insulin, should be considered when the maximum dose is reached.

## Amylin Agonists

**1** Amylin is a hormone secreted by the pancreatic beta cells in response to hyperglycemia; its secretion parallels that of insulin. The main mechanism of amylin is to inhibit gastric emptying and, to a lesser extent, suppression of glucagon secretion.[72]

**2** Pramlintide acetate (SYMLIN™) is a synthetic version of human amylin. Amylin Pharmaceuticals has submitted the drug to the FDA for approval to market SYMLIN as an adjunctive therapy to insulin. It must be injected and currently can not be combined with insulin.

**3** Clinical trials in patients with type 1 and type 2 diabetes indicate that pramlintide improves postprandial hyperglycemia and modestly improves HbA1c.[73,74]

## Use of Glucagon Injection for Severe Hypoglycemia

**1** The available agent is glucagon, which must be given by injection: 1 mg lyophilized powder in a single dose vial with 1 ml diluent contained in a disposable syringe/needle to allow rapid reconstitution of the powder and administration of the dissolved drug. This is the *Glucagon Emergency Kit*.
  **A** The dose is mixed by adding the diluent from the prefilled syringe in the emergency kit to the contents of the vial.
  **B** A 10-mg glucagon injection is commercially available, but is not intended for use as a glucose elevating agent; this product is used as a diagnostic aid in gastrointestinal examinations.

**2** Pharmacologic actions are
  **A** The primary effects are to raise blood glucose levels by accelerating hepatic glycogenolysis and stimulating hepatic gluconeogenesis.
  **B** Other effects are to stimulate catecholamine and insulin release.

**C** Glucagon is effective if adequate hepatic glycogen (stored glucose) is available, but may not be beneficial in patients with inadequate glycogen stores (eg, patients with alcoholic hepatic disease, starvation, adrenal insufficiency, or chronic hypoglycemia).

**3** Pharmacokinetics include
   **A** The bioavailability is 100% and it may be injected intramuscularly, intravenously, or subcutaneously.
   **B** It is degraded in the liver, kidney, and plasma. The plasma half-life is 3 to 6 minutes.

**4** Significant contraindications or precautions for glucagon:
   **A** Insulinoma: Marked hypoglycemia may occur following the initial increase in blood glucose
   **B** Pheochromocytoma: Marked hypertension may occur
   **C** Safety during pregnancy or for breastfeeding women is not known
   **D** Refer to package labeling for additional contraindications and precautions

**5** Adverse effects associated with glucagon use include
   **A** Nausea, vomiting (most common adverse effect)
   **B** Generalized allergic reactions including urticaria, respiratory distress, and hypotension

**6** Clinically important drug interactions with glucagon:
   **A** Oral anticoagulants: Hypoprothrombinemic effects may be increased, possibly with bleeding, which may occur after several days. Appears to be dose-related, and occurs minimally with a single 1-mg dose for hypoglycemia.

**7** Role of glucagon injection in diabetes mellitus:
   **A** Indicated for the treatment of severe hypoglycemia, in situations when the individual requires assistance from another person (see Chapter 7, Hypoglycemia, in Diabetes Management Therapies, for more information). Situations in which glucagon is indicated:
   • Patient is unconscious or uncooperative
   • Patient cannot take oral fluids
   • Emergency staff are not available to treat the hypoglycemia with an injection of 50% dextrose
   • If a hospitalized patient develops severe hypoglycemia, is unconscious, and an intravenous line is not running, glucagon may be administered until intravenous access can be obtained
   **B** Dosage is based upon patient's age and clinical condition:
   • Adults and children over 5 or 6 years of age (>20 kg): 1.0 mg SC or IM
   • Children under 5 years of age (<20 kg): 0.5 mg SC or IM
   • Infants: Should probably be given 0.25 mg SC or IM
   **C** Blood glucose response usually occurs in 5 to 20 minutes. If response is insufficient, an additional dose may be needed.
   • Liquids containing glucose are needed when the patient becomes conscious to restore hepatic glycogen stores and to prevent secondary hypoglycemia.

- Instruct patients to eat a snack containing carbohydrate when nausea subsides. The snack may need to be repeated because glycogen reserves can take 8 to 12 hours to be replenished. ✓

**D** Protect patients from injury or aspiration if convulsions occur. A common adverse effect of glucagon is nausea and possibly vomiting as the patient returns to consciousness.

---

## Use of Other Drugs in Diabetes Care

**1** A variety of drugs other than antihyperglycemic agents are commonly used in the care of people with diabetes.

**A** Medications are used for the treatment or prevention of the following complications of diabetes:
- Autonomic neuropathy
- Cardiovascular disease
- Problems of peripheral circulation
- Distal symmetric polyneuropathy
- Hyperlipidemia
- Nephropathy
- Periodontal disease
- Circulation abnormalities

**B** Medications are used for the treatment of the following conditions or diseases that occur frequently in people with diabetes:
- Hypertension
- Glaucoma
- Cataracts
- Hypothyroidism
- Infections (eg, vaginitis)
- Certain forms of joint disease

**C** Medications are used for the treatment of the following conditions or diseases that are unrelated to the diabetes:
- Colds
- Coughs
- Birth control/hormone replacement therapy
- Smoking cessation
- Arthritis
- Depression/anxiety
- Sunburn
- Acid indigestion
- Allergies
- Contact dermatitis
- Others

**2** Because of the number of drugs that may be used for various concurrent problems, it is important to examine the overall potential consequences when one or more drugs are added to or removed from the drug regimen for a person with diabetes (for more information, see chapters on complications in Diabetes and Complications).

## Potential Effects of Other Drugs

**1** Certain drugs have an effect on blood glucose levels. The following types of interactions can occur.

**A** A drug-disease or *pharmacodynamic interaction* is defined as a desirable or undesirable alteration of blood glucose level by a drug prescribed for a purpose other than its glycemic effect (Table 3.6). This interaction has an intrinsic physiologic effect.

**B** A *drug-drug interaction* is defined as a desirable or undesirable effect of a drug on the efficacy or toxicity on the antidiabetes drug(s) (Table 3.6).

**C** A *drug-food interaction* is defined as a desirable or undesirable effect of food on the efficacy or toxicity of the hypoglycemic or antidiabetes drugs(s) (Table 3.7).

**2** Certain drugs have an effect on the complications of diabetes.

**A** A complication or comorbid condition may be worsened when certain drugs are added to or removed from the overall diabetes treatment program.

**B** Potential effects can be best anticipated by carefully examining the pharmacologic action or adverse effects of a drug that are described in the package labeling (insert) or other therapeutic reference.

**C** The following are examples of drugs that have an effect on the complications of diabetes.

- An antacid with an adverse effect of constipation may aggravate constipation associated with diabetic autonomic neuropathy.
- An oral decongestant with vasoconstriction adverse effects may aggravate peripheral vascular problems such as intermittent claudication.
- An antihypertension medication with an adverse effect of impotence may worsen diabetes-related sexual dysfunction.

**3** Certain drug adverse effects have an impact on diabetes self-management (Table 3.8).

**A** Patients are taught to be attentive to particular signs and symptoms that may indicate impending hypoglycemia or hyperglycemia. In addition, certain procedures and aspects of diabetes care require the patient to be alert, coordinated, and capable of making self-management decisions. A drug that mimics a patient's usual warning signs of hypoglycemia or hyperglycemia, or one that impairs a patient's ability to perform necessary self-care tasks, may adversely affect glycemic control.

- Frequent urination or nocturia from initiation of diuretic therapy may be mistakenly interpreted as a symptom of hyperglycemia.
- Central nervous system adverse effects such as dizziness, headache, fatigue, weakness, loss of energy, or tingling of extremities may be mistaken for symptoms of hypoglycemia.
- Adverse effects of drowsiness, tiredness, lethargy, or depression could be mistaken for symptoms of hyperglycemia or may affect diabetes control by interfering with the patient's ability or desire to exercise or carry out other self-management activities.
- Blurred vision as an adverse effect of another agent may lead to a dosing error in insulin administration.
- Drug-induced night blindness may aggravate night blindness from previous retinal photocoagulation or autonomic neuropathy.

## Table 3.7. Drug-Food Interactions of Diabetes Medications

| | |
|---|---|
| *Sulfonylurea Agents* | • Administration of most sulfonylurea agents with food only slightly alters absorption characteristics.<br>• Patients are often advised to take these agents 1/2 to 1 hour prior to eating to allow the onset of action to occur more closely with the postprandial glucose rise.<br>• When sulfonylurea-induced gastric distress occurs, patients may be advised to take these agents with food to minimize stomach upset.<br>• Glipizide (short-acting) is the only sulfonylurea specifically recommended to be taken on an empty stomach. |
| *Repaglinide*<br>*Nateglinide* | • Food only slightly affects absorption; however, patients are advised to take repaglinide 15 minutes before eating so that the rapid action of the drug matches the timing of glucose rise following the meal. |
| *Metformin* | • Food decreases the extent of and slightly delays the absorption of metformin.<br>• Taking metformin with or after food is usually advised to reduce stomach upset. |
| *Thiazolidinediones* | • No significant interaction. |
| *Acarbose*<br>*Miglitol* | • No reported food interactions.<br>• Must be taken with the meal ("first bite of the meal") to attain optimal therapeutic effect. |
| *Insulin* | • Not applicable because insulin must be taken by injection.<br>• Timing of injection prior to eating may be an important factor in postprandial glycemic control.<br>• Lispro insulin is injected no more than 5 to 15 minutes prior to eating to avoid preprandial hypoglycemia. |

## Significance of Drug-Related Effects

1 Some problems have *major clinical significance*, which means an event is relatively well-documented (established documentation) and has the potential of being harmful to the patient.

2 Some problems have *moderate clinical significance*, which means more documentation is needed (possible documentation) and/or the potential harm to the patient is less.

3 Some problems have *minor clinical significance*, which means an event may occur but may be less significant because of poor documentation, minimal potential harm to the patient, or low incidence of the interaction.

## Table 3.8. Adverse Drug Effects Related to Diabetes

**Specific Drugs or Drug Classes** (see Table 3.6 for blood glucose effects)
Drugs within a drug class often share adverse effects, although to varying degrees. Certain drug classes warrant particular attention to effects that may have an impact upon complications or comorbidity conditions for specific patients.

| | |
|---|---|
| *Alpha-1 antagonists (prazosin, terazosin, doxazosin)* | Impotence; constipation (aggravates chronic constipation from autonomic neuropathy); diarrhea (aggravates diarrhea from autonomic neuropathy); dizziness, headache, weakness (may be confused for signs of hypoglycemia); blurred vision, drowsiness, xerostomia (may be confused for signs of hyperglycemia) |
| *Antihistamines, anticholinergic* | Contraindicated in neurogenic bladder (may occur in diabetic autonomic neuropathy); blurred vision; constipation, abdominal pain |
| *Antihypertensives in general* | Impaired sexual function; constipation (selected agents); orthostatic hypotension may occur in diabetic autonomic neuropathy |
| *Anti-inflammatory agents* | Nonsteroidal: Renal effects; hypertensive effects<br>Steroidal: Osteoporosis; hypertension; weight gain/increase in appetite may worsen diabetes control; diminished wound healing; thin fragile skin; glaucoma |
| *ß-blockers* | Mask signs/symptoms of hypoglycemia; impaired sexual function; reduced peripheral circulation and cold extremities |
| *Calcium channel blockers* | Constipation (selected agents aggravate chronic constipation from autonomic neuropathy); orthostatic hypotension (aggravate diabetes-related orthostatic hypotension); glycemic effects (selected agents) |
| *Chemotherapeutic agents* | Nausea, vomiting, stomatitis, anorexia, alterations in taste (makes diabetes nutrition therapy difficult or inconsistent); diarrhea |
| *Clonidine* | Urinary retention; constipation; diminished sexual function; orthostatic hypotension; nocturia, lethargy, xerostomia, drowsiness (may be confused for signs of hyperglycemia) |
| *Codeine (as cough suppressant) or opiate analgesics* | Constipation (aggravate chronic constipation from autonomic neuropathy) |
| *Diuretics* | Changes in lipid profile; total body potassium loss (unless potassium-sparing diuretic or formulation); diuresis mimics polyuria/nocturia which may interfere with use of these signs as a warning sign of hyperglycemia; diminished effectiveness in decreasing renal function; aggravate diabetes-related orthostatic hypotension |

## Table 3.8. Adverse Drug Effects Related to Diabetes (cont.)

| | |
|---|---|
| *Sorbitol, as compounding ingredient and/or sweetening agent* | Loose stools, diarrhea, flatulence (aggravate diarrhea from autonomic neuropathy) |
| *Sympathomimetics* | Hypertension; peripheral vasoconstriction |

**Specific Adverse Effects/Adverse Reactions**

The package labeling (insert) or product information usually provides a list of adverse effects by body system affected and in the order of frequency of occurrence. Certain adverse effects should arouse suspicions or raise questions about the potential for drug-related problems in patients with diabetes.

| | |
|---|---|
| *Gastrointestinal (GI)* | • Nausea, vomiting, constipation, diarrhea, bloating, gas: Additive problem with various forms of autonomic neuropathy<br>• Dry mouth: Could be mistakenly interpreted as a symptom of hyperglycemia |
| *Genitourinary (GU)* | • Impotence, failure to ejaculate, reduced libido: Additive problem with diabetes-related impotence |
| *Renal* | • Glycosuria listed as an adverse effect: Carefully read the package insert to ascertain if this adverse effect refers to a lowered threshold for glucose or an indication of hyperglycemia<br>• Frequent urination, nocturia, polyuria: Could be mistakenly interpreted as a symptom of hyperglycemia; could lead to hypovolemia and problems with orthostatic hypotension<br>• Elevations of creatinine or BUN: May pose problems in patient predisposed to renal dysfunction |
| *Central nervous system (CNS)* | • Dizziness: Additive problem with orthostatic hypotension, hypoglycemia<br>• Headache, fatigue, weakness, loss of energy, blurred vision, tingling of extremities: Could be mistakenly interpreted as symptom of hypoglycemia<br>• Drowsiness, tiredness, lethargy, depression: Could be mistaken for symptom of hyperglycemia; could affect diabetes control by interfering with ability and desire to exercise<br>• Numbness/tingling of extremities, paresthesias, neuropathy: Additive problem with diabetes-related neuropathy |
| *Dermatologic* | • Pruritus, rash, dry skin: Aggravate the dry skin and itching associated with peripheral neuropathy and venostasis |

## Table 3.8. Adverse Drug Effects Related to Diabetes (cont.)

| | |
|---|---|
| *Ophthalmic* | • Night blindness: May aggravate night blindness resulting from retinal photocoagulation |
| *General* | • Elevated cholesterol or triglyceride levels: May pose problems in patient predisposed to lipid disorders<br>• Hypoglycemia, hyperglycemia: May require adjustment of diabetes treatment plan<br>• Peripheral edema: Aggravate problems in patient with impaired peripheral circulation and venous return |

**4** It is important to note that the classification of "major" versus "minor" significance is not solely a matter of the degree of documentation. The individual patient characteristics must be considered in making this determination. For example, in the following situations the first would represent a problem of minor significance whereas the second could be major.

**A** A 37-year-old man with type 2 diabetes, who is relatively healthy otherwise, has been taking an oral hypoglycemic agent for the past 2 years. Today his provider has added a diuretic. If this individual experiences hypoglycemia during the first few days of diuretic therapy, it is unlikely that the potential diuresis, hypovolemia, or dizziness from the diuretic would exaggerate the dizziness/weakness of hypoglycemia to a dangerous state.

**B** An 87-year-old widow with type 2 diabetes, osteoporosis, sporadic nutrition and fluid ingestion, and occasional disequilibrium has been taking an oral hypoglycemic agent for the past 2 years. She lives alone. Today her provider has added a diuretic. If this patient experiences hypoglycemia at the same time she experiences dizziness from the diuretic, the drug-related problem may have major significance: a fall, broken hip, and no one in the house to render assistance.

## Caveats to Drug Interactions and Drug-Related Problems

**1** Drug interactions may be beneficial or detrimental. For example, using a drug with intrinsic hypoglycemic activity may be detrimental for a patient with hypoglycemia unawareness (drug-disease interaction and an effect on a diabetes complication).

**2** Drug interactions are not necessarily predictable because they do not always happen to all people.

**3** Drug interactions are usually dose dependent.

**4** A specific combination of interacting drugs can have a different interaction profile depending on the order in which the drugs are initiated.

    **A** Adding a diuretic to an established dose of sulfonylurea can reasonably be expected to raise the blood glucose level, thus lessening the apparent effectiveness of the sulfonylurea.

    **B** When a sulfonylurea is added to an established dose of a diuretic, the blood glucose would not be expected to rise further.

**5** The severity of an interaction is different for different people (variable responses) depending on the following individual variables:

    **A** Current metabolic control

    **B** Self-monitoring practices

    **C** Lability/stability of complications and concurrent conditions

    **D** Duration/dosage of proposed therapy

    **E** Potential for administration error

## Ways to Help Prevent, Minimize, or Prepare for Potential Drug-Related Problems

**1** Inform the patient if a drug-related problem is likely to occur and the usual signs and symptoms to watch for.

**2** If possible, inform the patient as to when the interaction/drug problem would be expected to occur. Some interactions may occur after the first dose while others may not occur until the problem drug has reached steady state or has accumulated in the body.

**3** Devise a strategy by which the patient can determine if the anticipated problem has occurred.

    **A** Recommend blood glucose monitoring at specific times of day or at more frequent intervals until the patient's response to the drug is established.

    **B** Stress the importance of additional monitoring or observation.

**4** Provide an action plan for the patient to use if the suspected drug-related problem has occurred. This action plan is based on the drug and the severity of the interaction/problem.

    **A** For problems of major clinical significance, instruct the patient to notify the provider as soon as possible. Specify whether the drug should be stopped or continued while attempting to reach the health professional.

    **B** For problems of moderate clinical significance, the problem may be resolved by making appropriate compensations. A member of the healthcare team may need to be contacted for assistance.

    **C** For problems of minor clinical significance, the problem is primarily an inconvenience or is self-limiting and does not generally require any specific action.

**5** Prepare a backup plan should problems arise. Determine alternatives the patient might use if the drug problem occurs.

## Self-Review Questions

**1** Describe the effects of insulin on fat, protein, and glucose utilization.

**2** List 4 categories of patients who are candidates for insulin therapy.

**3** What concentrations of insulin are available and which concentration is most commonly used in the United States?

**4** Describe the guidelines for insulin storage.

**5** Compare and contrast the sulfonylureas, meglitinides, biguanides, thiazolidinediones, alpha-glucosidase inhibitors, and D-phenylalanine derivatives as to adverse effects and contraindications.

**6** How should metformin therapy be initiated and titrated?

**7** How should acarbose therapy be initiated and titrated?

**8** Which antidiabetes oral medications must be taken with a meal ("first bite of the meal") to attain their therapeutic effect?

**9** Which antidiabetes oral medication is specifically recommended to be taken on an empty stomach?

**10** List the indications for use of glucagon.

**11** List 3 chronic complications of diabetes for which some type of pharmacologic therapy will be needed to prevent or treat that complication.

**12** Name the 2 complications or conditions associated with diabetes which may be aggravated by administration of certain oral decongestants (sympathomimetics).

**13** List 3 drugs with intrinsic hyperglycemic activity.

**14** List 3 drugs with intrinsic hypoglycemic activity.

**15** List 3 adverse effects of various drugs which may mimic symptoms of hypoglycemia and cause confusion in the perception of hypoglycemia.

**16** List 2 adverse effects of various drugs which may mimic symptoms of hyperglycemia and cause confusion in the perception of hyperglycemia.

**17** Define the following terms: (a) major clinically significant problem, (b) moderate clinically significant problem, (c) minor problem.

## Key Educational Considerations

**1** Oral antidiabetes agents are not a substitute for meal planning and exercise, but will work best when all aspects of therapy are combined.

**2** Many patients assume that sulfonylureas are "oral insulin" and become confused by what they hear about insulin.

**3** It is common for patients who take oral agents to believe that they have a "touch of sugar" or "mild diabetes." If this information is obtained as part of the educational assessment, it can prompt the educator to ask additional questions about the patient's perceptions and beliefs about diabetes and then to provide relevant content.

**4** The recognition and treatment of hypoglycemia is essential information for all patients taking insulin or insulin secretagogues.

**5** Teach patients to inform all healthcare providers about their diabetes and their medications so that the potential for drug interactions will be recognized.

**6** Address the potential problems of using alcohol with certain sulfonylureas with those patients for whom it is appropriate.

**7** The dosage of metformin or acarbose may be titrated over weeks in order to minimize adverse effects. Written dosage instruction handouts may help patients minimize adverse effects.

**8** Type 2 diabetes patients taking oral agents often assume that when they must start insulin, it is a signal that they are "getting worse" or that it is because they have not "followed the diet right." Explain that over time, the oral agents do not lower the blood glucose as well as they did originally.

**9** Type 2 diabetes patients who change from oral agents to insulin sometimes assume that they no longer have to be concerned about the amounts of food eaten because the insulin will regulate the blood glucose. It should be explained that the insulin is being started to meet the patient's physiologic insulin requirement, not to replace meal planning related to amounts, timing, and consistency of eating.

**10** Inform patients and families that with weight loss, nutrition changes, and/or increased physical activity some individuals may no longer require therapeutic agents (including insulin), although this is often temporary. However, that applies only to people with type 2 diabetes. The current treatment for type 1 diabetes requires lifelong insulin therapy.

**11** Most insulin-requiring individuals will need 2 or more daily insulin injections, often using 2 types of insulin in each injection to provide insulin in a more physiologic manner.

## Learning Assessment: Case Study 1

LR is a 22-year-old woman with type 1 diabetes that was diagnosed 5 years ago. She has cared for her diabetes with 2 insulin injections daily for the past 15 months as follows:
  AM: 20 units NPH insulin and 8 units regular insulin
  PM: 10 units NPH insulin and 4 units regular insulin

She has hypertension, for which she is taking 50 mg hydrochlorothiazide daily. She has also been taking an oral contraceptive for 3 months. Today she comes to the clinic expressing concern about her glucose levels. Her SMBG record averages for the past 3 weeks are as follows:

| SMBG Levels | 7 AM mg/dL (mmol/L) | 11 AM mg/dL (mmol/L) | 4 PM mg/dL (mmol/L) | 9 PM mg/dL (mmol/L) |
|---|---|---|---|---|
| *Previous month* | 107 (6.0) | 112 (6.2) | 129 (7.1) | 120 (6.6) |
| *Week 1* | 151 (8.3) | 168 (9.2) | 112 (6.3) | 176 (9.7) |
| *Week 2* | 158 (8.7) | 167 (9.2) | 142 (7.9) | 168 (9.2) |
| *Week 3* | 167 (9.2) | 172 (9.5) | 141 (7.8) | 171 (9.4) |

She reports that her activity, weight, and dietary intake are unchanged.

## Questions for Discussion

**1** What other information do you need?

**2** What possible explanations could be given for her blood glucose levels?

**3** What therapeutic options are available for LR?

## Discussion

**1** An initial review of these data suggests that further information is needed.

   **A** Your assessment reveals that LR's insulin administration routine is accurate, including storage of insulin, injection sites, timing, and technique.

   **B** She reports no significant change in her food intake or the introduction of new food products.

   **C** There has been no change in her activity level, daily habits, level of stress, or coping methods.

**2** Potential explanations are either the hydrochlorothiazide or the estrogen-containing contraceptive is causing a drug interaction that is inducing an increase in blood glucose level. LR has been taking hydrochlorothiazide for 3 years with no previous problem. The contraceptive has produced no problem thus far.

**3** A trial period of other medications for hypertension and/or contraception might be indicated.

   **A** Unless the HCTZ was specifically chosen for diuresis as well as antihypertensive effects (ie, the patient has problems with peripheral edema or other fluid accumulation) an angiotensin-converting-enzyme inhibitor (ACE inhibitor) is the drug of choice for hypertension in diabetes. Unlike HCTZ, an ACE inhibitor does not have a potential for causing hyperglycemia or lipid abnormalities.

   **B** A "low dose" contraceptive agent may be considered.

**4** Adjustments in insulin are also an option, such as

   **A** The evening dose of intermediate-acting insulin could be increased by 1 to 2 units, or LR could eat less carbohydrates for supper or exercise in the evening to reduce her 7 AM glucose concentration.

   **B** The AM regular insulin could be increased by 1 or 2 units, or LR could eat less carbohydrates for breakfast to reduce her 11 AM glucose concentration.

   **C** Evaluate the 9 PM level based on when LR eats her evening meal.

   **D** Her 4 PM level may be improved by reducing the morning glucose levels.

   **E** If LR is open to the idea of 3 daily injections, the evening dose could be changed to rapid-acting insulin or regular insulin at the evening meal and NPH at bedtime. Administering her NPH at bedtime would help to lower her fasting glucose.

**5** Any changes in insulin doses needs to be made slowly, and by altering 1 dose at a time.

## Learning Assessment: Case Study 2

AH is a 57-year-old male referred to the diabetes clinic for evaluation of his glycemic control. He was diagnosed with type 2 diabetes about 15 months ago. He remains overweight in spite of numerous attempts to lose weight. His fasting blood glucose concentrations have risen lately and range from 170 to 185 mg/dL (9.4 to 10.3 mmol/L) over the last few weeks. He complains of weakness, fatigue, increased urination, and increased thirst.

**Past Medical History**
Hypertension x 10 y
Type 2 diabetes mellitus

**Family History**
(+) Diabetes
(+) Hypertension

**Social History**
Smokes, ½ to 1 pack per day
Alcohol, none

**Current Medications**
Hydrochlorothiazide (HCTZ) 50 mg qd
KCl 40 mEq q AM
Propranolol 40 mg qid

**Physical Examination**
Weight 198 lb (90 kg), increase of 3 kg
Height 5'8"
BP 154/94 (previous BP ranged from 150/92 to 160/96)
Pulse 88 regular
RR 14

## Questions for Discussion

**1** How do the antihypertensive agents affect AH's blood glucose level?
**2** Which class of oral agent might be appropriate for AH?

## Discussion

**1** It would be appropriate to begin by substituting different drugs for those that worsen glucose tolerance (HCTZ and propranolol).
   **A** This patient's hypertension might be better treated with an ACE inhibitor or a calcium channel blocker.
   **B** If the HCTZ is discontinued or an ACE inhibitor is initiated the potassium supplement should probably be discontinued as well.

**2** The effects of HCTZ and propranolol on glucose tolerance may take a number of weeks to resolve. In the interim, his hyperglycemia should be treated with oral agents or low-dose insulin in order to relieve his symptoms. Metformin may be a good choice for

AH because he is overweight and probably insulin resistant. Metformin could lower his blood glucose levels, weight, and lipid levels (if elevated).

**3** Prior to initiation of any new therapy, evaluation for potential contraindications (particularly hepatic or renal dysfunction) or drug allergies is needed.

**4** Other considerations include cost, patient convenience, patient preference, and lifestyle concerns.

**A** Many of the sulfonylurea agents are available generically, which are generally less expensive than the brand or newer products.

**B** A once-a-day agent such as glyburide, glipizide long-acting, glimepiride, or pioglitazone may offer the advantage of being easier to take correctly and consistently.

**C** If hypoglycemia poses a particular risk for AH (eg, due to work or living situation), a nonhypoglycemic agent such as acarbose, metformin, or a thiazolidinedione may offer an advantage.

**D** The patient's willingness or ability to self-monitor blood glucose levels may influence the type of agent chosen or blood glucose goals.

**5** As the effects of the propranolol and HCTZ wane following their discontinuance, AH may no longer need an antidiabetes agent.

**6** Assess the patient's level of interest in meal planning for glucose control and referral to a dietitian.

## Learning Assessment: Case Study 3

MC is a 79-year-old female with type 2 diabetes who resides in a nursing home. You are the nursing home consultant. You notice that 10 days ago MC developed a urinary tract infection (UTI), which was initially treated with co-trimoxazole (Septra DS®). After the second dose of Septra DS, intense pruritus and a rash appeared on her arms and upper chest. The Septra was discontinued and ampicillin was prescribed. Diphenhydramine (Benadryl®) and a methylprednisolone dose pack (Medrol®) were given for the sulfonamide reaction.

Over the next several days, you notice that symptoms of increased urination, incontinence, and mental confusion are documented in the nursing notes. After reading the notes and talking with the staff, you learn that these observations were attributed to her advancing age and deteriorating mental status, so no action was taken.

You suspect that the changes observed are related to drug problems rather than changes in patient's mental status.

## Questions for Discussion

**1** What information would you need to help determine if this reaction is a drug-related problem?

**2** What possible explanations could be given for what has happened to MC?

**3** Assuming your suspicions are correct and MC has experienced a drug-related reaction, what recommendations could you make to resolve MC's problem?

**4** What could be done to prevent this from occurring in the future?

---

## Discussion

**1** The following information is needed to help determine the causes of MC's problem:

   **A** Current drug profile (Is she taking oral agents? Insulin? Have other drugs been recently initiated that would cause symptoms of polyuria or mental confusion?)

   **B** Recent blood glucose results (Have her blood glucose levels been increasing recently, and did the increase coincide with the onset of UTI symptoms? Did the blood glucose levels increase further when the steroid was initiated?)

   **C** Ongoing blood glucose patterns and HbA1c (Has chronic hyperglycemia predisposed this patient to infection?)

   **D** Description of MC's mental status during the period of the UTI and treatment

   **E** Lab results and vital signs to assess if the UTI is responding to therapy

   **F** Blood chemistries to assess for possible hyperglycemic hyperosmolar state (HHS)

**2** A urinary tract infection is an example of physical stress that can raise blood glucose concentrations (release of counterregulatory hormones). If MC's diabetes was previously poorly controlled or "brittle" (blood glucose fluctuating dramatically with changes in her meal plan, exercise, illness, stress), the hyperglycemic effect of illness would be more exaggerated.

**3** Subsequent hyperglycemic factors include the allergic reaction (causing endogenous release of corticosteroid) and the initiation of methylprednisolone (intrinsic hyperglycemic activity).

**4** The increased urination, incontinence, and mental confusion may be symptoms of the resulting hyperglycemia; depending upon severity of neurologic symptoms and blood chemistries, HHS may be developing.

**5** Diphenhydramine in an elderly person may substantially alter mental alertness or cause urinary retention resulting in overflow incontinence.

**6** The following measures can be taken to resolve MC's symptoms:

   **A** Assure adequate hydration.

   **B** Insulin may be needed temporarily in place of oral antidiabetes agents; if MC is already on insulin, doses need to be increased temporarily.

   **C** Monitor blood glucose more frequently until control is reestablished.

   **D** Continue to follow signs and symptoms of UTI to assure resolution of infection.

   **E** Discontinue diphenhydramine. Institute shorter-acting or nonsedating antihistamine if antipruritic agent still needed. Topical steroid creams may provide relief.

   **F** Discontinue methylprednisolone as soon as feasible. A slow taper is not necessary.

**7** The following preventive recommendations could be instituted:

   **A** The nursing home could establish standard policies regarding detection and management of acute loss of glycemic control in residents with diabetes.

- Blood glucose testing is essential even for residents with well-controlled diabetes. An increase in blood glucose levels often precedes the clinical manifestations of infection and may thus serve as a warning that illness may be developing.

**B** Blood glucose testing (at least qd or bid) is performed under the following conditions:

- When infection is suspected or confirmed, more frequent testing is needed until blood glucose results return to preinfection levels.
- Upon initiation of drugs with intrinsic hyperglycemic or hypoglycemic activity, more frequent testing is needed until the drug interaction is resolved.
- Upon initiation of drugs with potential adverse effects that mimic hyperglycemia or hypoglycemia, more frequent testing is needed until the patient's response to the drug is determined.

---

## References

**1** Fertig BJ, Simmons DA, Martin DB. Therapy for diabetes. In: National Diabetes Data Group. Diabetes in America. 2nd ed. Bethesda, Md: National Institute of Diabetes and Digestive and Kidney Diseases; 1995. NIH Publication 95-1468:519-540.

**2** Skyler JS. Insulin treatment. In: Lebovitz HE, ed. Therapy for Diabetes Mellitus and Related Disorders. 3rd ed. Alexandria, Va: American Diabetes Association; 1998:186-203.

**3** Howey DC, Bowsher RR, Brunelle RL, Woodworth JR. [Lys(B28), Pro(B29)]-human insulin, a rapidly absorbed analogue of human insulin. Diabetes. 1994;43:396-402.

**4** Ciofetta M, Lalli C, Del Sindaco P, et al. Contribution of postprandial versus interprandial blood glucose to HbA1c in type 1 diabetes on physiologic intensive therapy with lispro insulin at mealtime. Diabetes Care. 1999;22:795-800.

**5** Lalli C, Ciofetta M, Del Sindaco P, et al. Long-term intensive treatment of type 1 diabetes with the short-acting insulin analogue lispro in variable combination with NPH insulin at mealtime. Diabetes Care. 1999;22:468-477.

**6** Holleman F, Schmitt H, Rottiers R, Rees A, Symanowski S, Anderson JH Jr. Reduced frequency of severe hypoglycemia and coma in well-controlled IDDM patients treated with insulin lispro. The Benelux-UK Insulin Lispro Study Group. Diabetes Care. 1997;20:1827-1832.

**7** Brunelle BL, Llewelyn J, Anderson JH Jr, Gale EA, Koivisto VA. Meta-analysis of the effect of insulin lispro on severe hypoglycemia in patients with type 1 diabetes. Diabetes Care. 1998;21:1726-1731.

**8** Renner R, Pfutzner A, Trautmann M, Harzer O, Sauter K, Landgraf R, on behalf of the German Humalog–Pump Therapy Study Group. Use of insulin lispro in continuous subcutaneous insulin infusion treatment. Diabetes Care. 1999;22:784-788.

**9** Zinman B, Tildesley H, Chiasson JL, Tsui E, Strack T. Insulin lispro in pump therapy: results of a double blind crossover study. Diabetes. 1997:46:440-443.

**10** Home PD, Lindholm A, Hyllegerg B, Round P. Improved glycemic control with insulin aspart: a multicenter randomized double-blind crossover trial in type 1 diabetic patients. UK Insulin Aspart Study Group. Diabetes Care. 1998;21:1904-1909.

**11** Lindholm A, McEwen J, Riis AP. Improved postprandial glycemic control with insulin aspart. A randomized double-blind trial cross-over trial in type 1 diabetes. Diabetes Care. 1999;22:801-805.

**12** Mudaliar SR, Lindberg FA, Joyce M, et al. Insulin aspart (B28 asp-insulin): a fast-acting analogue of human insulin. Diabetes Care. 1999;22:1501-1506.

**13** Bode BW, Strange P. Efficacy, safety, and pump compatibililty of insulin aspart used in continuous subcutaneous insulin infusion therapy in patients with type 1 diabetes. Diabetes Care. 2001;24:69-72.

**14** Rosskamp RH, Park G. Long-acting insulin analogues. Diabetes Care. 1999;22(suppl 2):B109-B113.

**15** Lepore M, Kurzhals R, Pamjpanelli S, Fanelli CG, Bollli GB. Pharmacokinetics and dynamics of s.c. injection of the long-acting insulin glargine (HOE 901) in T1DM (abstract). Diabetes. 1999;48(suppl 1):A97.

**16** Raskin P, Klaff L, Bergenstal R, Halle J-P, Donley D, Mecca T. A 16-week comparison of the novel insulin analogue insulin glargine (HOE 901) and NPH human insulin used with insulin lispro in patients with type 1 diabetes. Diabetes Care. 2000;23:1666-1671.

**17** Rosenstock J, Schwartz SL, Clark CM, Park GD, Donley DW, Edwards MB. Basal insulin therapy in type 2 diabetes. 28-week comparison of insulin glargine (HOE 901) and NPH insulin. Diabetes Care. 2001;24:631-636.

**18** Hermansen K, Madsbad S, Perrid H, Kristensen A, Axelsen M: Comparison of the soluble basel insulin analog detemir with NPH insulin: a randomized open crossover trial in type 1 diabetic subjects on basal-bolus therapy. Diabetes Care. 2001;24:296-301.

**19** American Diabetes Association. Insulin administration (position statement). Diabetes Care. 2001(suppl 1):S94-S97.

**20** American Diabetes Association. Continuous subcutaneous insulin infusion (position statement). Diabetes Care. 2001(suppl 1):S98.

**21** Lantus Package Insert. Kansas City: Aventis; 2000.

**22** Bolognia JL, Braverman IM. Skin and subcutaneous tissues. In: Lebovitz HE., ed. Therapy for Diabetes Mellitus and Related Disorders. 3rd ed. Alexandria, Va: American Diabetes Association; 1998:290-303.

**23** White JR Jr, Hartman J, Campbell RK. Drug interactions in diabetic patients. Postgrad Med. 1993;93:131-139.

**24** Skyler JS, ed. Medical Management of Type 1 Diabetes. 3rd ed. Alexandria, Va: American Diabetes Association; 1998.

**25** Zimmerman BR, ed. Medical Management of Type 2 Diabetes. 4th ed. Alexandria, Va: American Diabetes Association; 1998.

**26** Jovanovic L, ed. Medical Management of Pregnancy Complicated by Diabetes. 3rd ed. Alexandria, Va: American Diabetes Association; 2000.

**27** Seigler DE, Olsson GM, Skyler JS. Morning versus bedtime isophane insulin in type 2 (non-insulin dependent) diabetes mellitus. Diabetic Med. 1992;9:826-833.

**28** Roach P, Yue L, Arora V. The Humalog Mix25 Study Group, Improved postprandial glycemic control during treatment with Humalog Mix25, a novel protamine-based insulin lispro formulation. Diabetes Care. 1999;22:1258-1261.

**29** White JR Jr, Campbell RK. Inhaled insulin: an overview. Clinical Diabetes. 2001;19:13-16.

**30** Cefalu WT, Gefland RA, Kourides LA. A three-month, multicenter clinical trial of therapy with inhaled insulin in type 2 diabetes mellitus (abstract). Diabetologia. 1998;41(suppl 1):A226.

**31** Weiss SR, Berger S, Cheng S, Kourides I, Landschultz W, Gefland R. Adjunctive therapy with inhaled insulin on type 2 diabetic patients failing oral agents: a multicenter phase II trial (abstract). Diabetes. 1998;48(suppl 1):A12.

**32** Skyler JS, Cefalu WT, Kourides IA, et al. Efficacy of inhaled insulin in type 1 diabetes mellitus: a randomized proof-of-concept study. Lancet. 2001;357:324-325.

**33** White JR Jr. Combination oral agent/insulin therapy in patients with type II diabetes mellitus. Clinical Diabetes. 1997;15:102-112.

**34** Mudaliar S, Henry RR. Combination therapy for type 2 diabetes. Endocr Pract. 1999;5:208-219.

**35** DeFronzo RA. Pharmacologic therapy for type 2 diabetes mellitus. Ann Intern Med. 1999;131:281-303.

**36** Campbell RK, White JR. Medications for the Treatment of Diabetes. Alexandria, Va: American Diabetes Association; 2000.

**37** Lebovitz HE. Insulin secretagogues: sulfonylureas and repaglinide. In: Lebovitz HE, ed. Therapy for Diabetes Mellitus and Related Disorders. 3rd ed. Alexandria, Va: American Diabetes Association; 1998;160-170.

**38** Halter JB. Geriatric patients. In: Lebovitz HE, ed. Therapy for Diabetes Mellitus and Related Disorders. 3rd ed. Alexandria, Va: American Diabetes Association; 1998:234-240.

**39** White JR Jr. The pharmacologic management of patients with type II diabetes mellitus in the era of new oral agents and insulin analogues. Diabetes Spectrum. 1996;9:227-234.

**40** Gerich JE. Oral hypoglycemic agents. N Engl J Med. 1989; 321:1231-1245.

**41** Stenman S, Melander A, Groop P, Groop LC. What is the benefit of increasing the sulfonylurea dose? Ann of Intern Med. 1993;118:169-172.

**42** Damsbo P, Clauson P, Marbury TC, Windfeld K. A double-blind randomized comparison of meal-related glycemic control by repaglinide and glyburide in well-controlled type 2 diabetic patients. Diabetes Care. 1999;22:789-794.

**43** Moses RG, Gomis R, Frandsen KB, Schlienger J-L, Dedov I. Flexible meal-related dosing with repaglinide facilitates glycemic control in therapy-naïve type 2 diabetes. Diabetes Care. 2001;24:11-15.

**44** Raskin P, Jovanovic L, Berger S, Schwartz S, Woo V, Ratner R. Repaglinide/troglitazone combination therapy. Improved glycemic control in type 2 diabetes. Diabetes Care. 2000;23:979-983.

**45** Prandin Package Insert. Princeton, NJ: Novo Nordisk; 1997.

**46** Kalbag JB, Walter YH, Nedelman JR, McLeod JF. Mealtime glucose regulation with nateglinide in healthy volunteers. Diabetes Care. 2001;24:73-77.

**47** Keilson L, Mather S, Walter YH, Subramanian S, McLeod JF. Synergistic effects of nateglinide and meal administration on insulin secretion in patients with type 2 diabetes mellitus. J Clin Endocrinol Metab. 2000;85:1081-1086.

**48** Horton ES, Clinkingbeard C, Gatlin M, Foley J, Mallows S, Shen S. Nateglinide alone and in combination with metformin improves glycemic control by reducing mealtime glucose levels in type 2 diabetes. Diabetes Care. 2000;23:1660-1665.

**49** Dunn CJ, Faulds D. Nateglinide. Drugs. 2000;60:607-615.

**50** Starlix Package Insert. East Hanover, NJ: Novartis Pharmaceuticals Corporation; 2000.

**51** Bailey CJ. Metformin: an update. Gen Pharmacol. 1993;24:1299-1309.

**52** DeFronzo RA, Goodman AM. Multicenter Metformin Study Group. Efficacy of metformin in patients with non-insulin-dependent diabetes mellitus. N Eng J Med. 1995;333:541-549.

**53** Wu MS, Johnston P, Sheu WHH, et al. Effects of metformin on carbohydrate and lipoprotein metabolism in NIDDM patients. Diabetes Care. 1990;13:1-8.

**54** Stumvoll M, Nurijhan N, Perriello G, et al. Metabolic effects of metformin on non-insulin-dependent diabetes mellitus. N Engl J Med. 1995;333:550-554.

**55** DeFronzo RA, Barzilai N, Simonson DC. Mechanism of metformin action in obese and lean non-insulin dependent diabetic subjects. J Clin Endocrinol Metab. 1991;73:1294-1301.

**56** Hundal RS, Krssak M, Dufour S, et al. Mechanism by which metformin reduces glucose production in type 2 diabetes. Diabetes. 2000;49:2063-2069.

**57** Glucophage, Glucophage XR Package Insert. Princeton, NJ: Bristol-Meyers Squibb Company; 2000.

**58** Glucovance Package Insert. Princeton, NJ: Bristol-Meyers Squibb Company; 2000.

**59** Dandona P, Fonseca V, Mier A, et al. Diarrhea and metformin in a diabetic clinic. Diabetes Care. 1983;6:472-474.

**60** Stang M, Wysowski DK, Butler Jones D. Incidence of lactic acidosis in metformin users. Diabetes Care. 1999;22:925-957.

**61** Aviles-Santa L, Sinding J, Raskin P. Effects of metformin in patients with poorly controlled, insulin-treated type 2 diabetes mellitus. Ann Intern Med. 1999;131:182-188.

**62** Saltiel AR, Olefsky JM. Thiazolidinediones in the treatment of insulin resistance and type II diabetes. Diabetes. 1996;45:1661-1664.

**63** Glitazones. In: White J, Campbell RK. Medications for the Treatment of Diabetes, Alexandria, Va: American Diabetes Association; 2000;71-86

**64** Actos Package Insert. Indianapolis: Eli Lilly; 1999.

**65** Avandia Package Insert. Philadelphia: SmithKline Beecham; 1999.

**66** Aronoff S, Rosenblatt S, Braithwaite S, Egan JW, Mathisen AL, Schneider RL, The Pioglitazone 001 Study Group. Pioglitazone hydrochloride monotherapy improves glycemic control in the treatment of patients with type 2 diabetes. Diabetes Care. 2000;23:1605-1611.

**67** Phillips LS, Grunberger G, Miller E, Patwadhan R, Rappaport EB, Salzman A, for the Rosiglitazone Clinical Trials Study Group. Once- and twice-daily dosing with rosiglitazone improves glycemic control in patients with type 2 diabetes. Diabetes Care. 2001;24:308-315.

**68** Santeusanio F, Compagnucci P. A risk-benefit appraisal of acarbose in the management of non-insulin-dependent diabetes mellitus. Drug Safety. 1994;11:432-444.

**69** Alpha-glucosidase inhibitors. In: White J, Campbell RK. Medications for the Treatment of Diabetes. Alexandria, Va: American Diabetes Association; 2000:57-70.

**70** Chiasson JL, Josse RG, Hunt JA, et al. The efficacy of acarbose in the treatment of patients with non-insulin-dependent diabetes mellitus. Ann Intern Med. 1994;121:928-935.

**71** Lebovitz H. Alpha-glucosidase inhibitors in treatment of hyperglycemia. In: Therapy for Diabetes Mellitus and Related Disorders. 3rd ed. Lebovitz HE, ed. Alexandria, Va: American Diabetes Association; 1998:176-180.

**72** Shmitz O, Nyholm B, Orskov L, et al. Effects of amylin and the amylin agonist pramlintide on glucose metabolism. Diabet Med. 1997;14(suppl 2):S19-S23.

**73** Thompson RG, Peterson J, Gottlieb A, et al. Effects of pramlintide, an analogue of human amylin, on the plasma glucose profiles in patients with IDDM: results of a multicenter trial. Diabetes. 1997;46:632-636.

**74** Thompson RG, Pearson L, Schoenfeld SL, et al. The pramlintide in type 2 diabetes group: pramlintide, a synthetic analogue of human amylin, improves the metabolic profile of patients with type 2 diabetes using insulin. Diabetes Care. 1998;21:987-993.

## Suggested Readings

American Diabetes Association Vital Statistics. Alexandria, Va: American Diabetes Association; 2000.

Bell DH, Mayo MS. Outcome of metformin-facilitated reinitiating of oral diabetic therapy in insulin-treated patients with non-insulin-dependent diabetes mellitus. Endocr Pract. 1997;3:73-76.

Bohannon NJ. Benefits of lispro insulin. Postgrad Med. 1997;101:73-80.

Fleming DR, Jacober SJ, Vandenberg MA, Fitzgerald JT, Grunberger G. The safety of injecting insulin through clothing. Diabetes Care. 1997;20:245-248.

Garber AJ, Duncan TG, Goodman AM, et al. Efficacy of metformin in type II diabetes: results of a double-blind, placebo-controlled, dose-response trial. Am J Med. 1997;103:491-497.

White J, Campbell RK. Medications for the Treatment of Diabetes, Alexandria, Va: American Diabetes Association; 2000.

White JR Jr, Campbell RK, Hirsch I. Insulin analogues. Postgrad Med. 1997;101:58-70.

Young DS. Effects of Drugs on Clinical Laboratory Tests. 4th ed. Washington, DC: American Association for Clinical Chemistry Press; 1995:274-281.

# Learning Assessment: Post-Test Questions

## Pharmacologic Therapies

**3**

**1** Insulin exerts all of the following effects on the body tissues except:
  **A** Stimulate entry of glucose into muscle cells for utilization as an energy source
  **B** Enhance fat storage
  **C** Promote breakdown of liver glycogen to maintain blood glucose levels
  **D** Stimulate entry of amino acids into cells enhancing protein biosynthesis

**2** When the pancreas is stimulated by an elevated blood glucose level, insulin enters the blood stream:
  **A** In equimolar quantities with proinsulin
  **B** In equimolar quantities with C-peptide
  **C** In equimolar quantities with glucagon
  **D** With a small amount of C-peptide

**3** Lispro and aspart insulin analogs are a:
  **A** Rapid-acting insulin which has an onset of action in 15 to 30 minutes, reaches a peak in 1 to 2 hours, and has a therapeutic duration of 3 to 4 hours
  **B** Long-acting insulin which has an onset of action in 4 to 6 hours, reaches a peak in 18 hours, and has a therapeutic duration of 24 to 36 hours
  **C** Intermediate-acting insulin which has an onset of 1 to 4 hours, reaches a peak in 8 hours, and has a therapeutic duration of 10 to 16 hours
  **D** Rapid-acting insulin which has an onset of 30 minutes to 1 hour, reaches a peak in 2 to 4 hours, and has a therapeutic duration of 6 to 8 hours

**4** MJ is planning a trip to Europe for 21 days. She asks how her insulin should be stored while traveling. Which of the following is the best advice for MJ?
  **A** "Carry ice packs to keep your insulin at 36°F to 46°F."
  **B** "Store your open insulin at room temperature for 7 days, after which time it must be discarded."
  **C** "Insulin may be stored at 59°F to 86 F for the entire trip provided it is used within 1 month."
  **D** "People with diabetes in all foreign countries use U-100 insulin, so there should be no difficulty obtaining insulin when traveling in Europe."

**5** A patient asks you if she can reuse her syringes and needles. Which of the following is the best answer?
  **A** "Needles and syringes should never be reused because of increased risk of infection."
  **B** "Needles and syringes may be used indefinitely since the new needles are thin and never become dull."
  **C** "Needles and syringes may be reused provided they are kept refrigerated."
  **D** "Syringes and needles can be reused. The needle should be safely recapped and the syringe should be stored at room temperature."

**6** A primary action of thiazolidinediones is to:
  **A** Decrease gluconeogenesis
  **B** Stimulate the beta cells of the islets of Langerhans to produce more insulin
  **C** Inhibit alpha-glucosidase
  **D** Enhance insulin-stimulated glucose transport into muscle cells

**7** The most acutely dangerous complication of sulfonylurea therapy is:
  **A** Weight gain
  **B** Skin rashes
  **C** Gastrointestinal disturbance
  **D** Hypoglycemia

**8** GW, a 70-year-old patient with type 2 diabetes, has a blood creatinine level of 3.0 mg/dL. Which of the following drugs is contraindicated for GW?
**A** Pioglitazone
**B** Glipizide
**C** Glyburide
**D** Metformin

**9** Thiazolidinediones should be used with caution in patients with:
**A** Hepatic dysfunction
**B** Renal dysfunction
**C** Hypoglycemia
**D** Dyslipidemia

**10** An oral agent for diabetes that may be especially useful in patients who have type 2 disease with elevated triglycerides and LDL cholesterol is:
**A** Glyburide
**B** Glimepiride
**C** Metformin
**D** Acarbose

**11** The role of exogenous glucagon is to:
**A** Stimulate hepatic glucose release
**B** Counteract hyperglycemia
**C** Delay gastric emptying
**D** Increase the postprandial glucose levels

**12** When should combination therapy for persons with type 2 diabetes be considered?
**A** Two years following diagnosis
**B** Only after a person develops 2 or more complications
**C** When sulfonylurea dose approaches half of the maximum dose
**D** When sulfonylurea dose is at the maximum dose

*See next page for answer key.*

# Post-Test Answer Key

## Pharmacologic Therapies

3

| | | | | |
|---|---|---|---|---|
| **1** | C ✓ | | **7** | D ✓ |
| **2** | B ✓ | | **8** | D |
| **3** | A ✓ | | **9** | A |
| **4** | C ✓ | | **10** | C |
| **5** | D ✓ | | **11** | A |
| **6** | D ✓ | | **12** | D |

# A Core Curriculum for Diabetes Education
Diabetes Management Therapies

## Monitoring

*Virginia Peragallo-Dittko, RN, MA, CDE*
*Diabetes Education Center*
*Winthrop-University Hospital*
*Mineola, New York*

## Introduction

**1** Regular monitoring is an essential component of any diabetes management program.

**2** *Monitoring* by the patient includes self-monitoring of blood glucose (SMBG), serum ketones, urine ketones, and urine glucose, if recommended.

**3** Monitoring of metabolic control by the healthcare team involves assessing glycosylated hemoglobin and fructosamine, reviewing blood glucose patterns, assessing growth and patterns of weight change, and monitoring the development and progression of long-term complications, including urinary protein measurements. This area of diabetes care clearly combines the diabetes educator's skills of management and education.

## Objectives

Upon completion of this chapter, the learner will be able to

**1** List factors that affect the accuracy of self-monitoring of blood glucose (SMBG) results.

**2** Describe the most common user error related to SMBG.

**3** Identify 3 critical uses of SMBG data by patients.

**4** Describe 2 ways that educators use SMBG results to teach an abstract principle of diabetes management.

**5** Identify 2 psychosocial adaptations related to SMBG.

**6** Identify the SMBG needs of special populations.

**7** Explain the measurement methods and target ranges for glycosylated hemoglobin, fructosamine, and urinary protein.

**8** List the indications for tests of ketonemia, ketonuria, and glycosuria.

**9** Identify how to use documentation of weight patterns as a monitoring tool.

## Self-Monitoring of Blood Glucose

**1** Self-monitoring of blood glucose is an important component of the treatment plan for patients with diabetes mellitus because it provides immediate feedback and data for the following:

**A** Achieving and maintaining specific glycemic goals.

**B** Preventing and detecting hypoglycemia and avoiding severe hypoglycemia.

**C** Adjusting care in response to changes in lifestyle of individuals who require pharmacologic therapy.

**D** Determining the need for insulin therapy in gestational diabetes mellitus.[1]

**E** Evaluating the glycemic response to physical activity and types and amounts of foods.

**2** Two types of blood glucose meters are used for SMBG: color reflectance meters and those that use sensor technology.

**A** With *reflectance meters*, the glucose in a drop of blood reacts with an enzyme on the test strip and changes the color of the strip. The meter accurately measures the color of the strip and gives a numeric readout. In general, the darker the test area, the higher the glucose content.

**B** *Sensor-type meters* measure the electronic charge generated by the reaction of the glucose and the enzyme.

**3** It is essential to ensure the accuracy of the blood glucose monitoring values because these values are used to make treatment decisions concerning medication dosage adjustment, food-intake or timing, and exercise timing.

**A** Blood glucose meters designed for home use are not completely accurate. The American Diabetes Association recommends that the performance goal for blood glucose meters should be a total error of less than 10% at blood glucose levels of 30 mg/dL to 400 mg/dL (1.7 mmol/L to 22.2 mmol/L), 100% of the time.[1] Many products do not meet this performance goal.

**B** *Accuracy* is defined as the "degree of conformity of a measure to a standard or true value." For blood glucose meters, the laboratory is the standard against which they are judged.

- The laboratory measures *venous blood glucose* and the meter measures *capillary blood glucose*. By the time blood reaches the veins, some of the glucose in the blood has been transferred to other tissues, so the blood flowing through the veins has less glucose than the blood flowing through the capillaries. After a fast of 8 or more hours, the difference between the level of glucose in capillary blood and in venous blood is very small. After a meal, the difference can be quite large, as blood glucose levels rise and the rate of glucose transfer into the tissue accelerates.

- Another consideration concerning the accuracy of blood glucose meters concerns the difference between whole blood glucose and plasma blood glucose. *Whole blood* is composed of plasma (serum) and 3 formed elements: red blood cells (erythrocytes), white blood cells (leukocytes), and platelets. The glucose content of red blood cells is about 20% less than the glucose content of plasma, due to the density of the red blood cells. Since whole blood consists of approximately equal portions of plasma and red blood cells, a mixture of the two would yield a glucose value about 11% to 15% lower than plasma alone as measured in the laboratory.

- While all meters use a drop of whole blood on the test strip, some read the plasma glucose level or have been programmed to calculate the plasma glucose level. A meter that provides plasma glucose levels will have results that are closer to the laboratory's results.

- Since a meter that reports whole blood values and a meter that reports plasma values will have different results for the same blood sample, the American Diabetes Association revised the suggested blood glucose treatment goals. When using a meter that reports whole blood glucose levels the target goal before a meal is between 80 mg/dL and 120 mg/dL (4.4 mmol/L and 6.7 mmol/L). When using a meter that reports plasma blood glucose, the target goal before a meal is between 90 mg/dL and 130 mg/dL (5.0 mmol/L and 7.2 mmol/L).[2]

**C** Potential sources of user error include inadequate blood sample, a soiled meter, an uncalibrated meter, or defective reagents.

- The reagents must be stored according to the manufacturer's guidelines to yield accurate results. These guidelines also refer to avoiding exposure to heat, cold, and humidity during shipping.

- Teach patients to check the expiration date of the reagents, especially when a mail-order shipment could include reagents that expire within a few months and need to be used immediately. Because reagents are costly, patients are commonly tempted to use expired reagents. This may lead to inaccurate readings.

- *Control solution* is a product that is provided by manufacturers to verify that the meter and reagent are working together properly. This underused method of verifying accuracy operates the same way that the patient monitors a drop of blood. Every manufacturer provides at least 1 control solution and some have low-, normal- and high-level control solutions to test the meter at extremes.
- Other factors that may influence the results of SMBG systems include variations in the hematocrit (newer systems are accurate with hematocrit ranges of 20% to 60%), altitude, environmental temperature and humidity, hypotension, hypoxia, and triglyceride concentrations.[1]
- Calibrating the meter is another way to ensure the most accurate results. Newer meter technology automatically calibrates the reagent with the meter, whereas older meter technology requires setting a code or inserting a chip or strip to calibrate the meter.
- With some reflectance meters, the blood sample intended for the strip may come in contact with the meter and soil the optic window. This will yield inaccurate results. The manufacturers provide instructions for cleaning the meter.
- User error is the most common reason for inaccurate results. Despite improvements in technology such as the inclusion of error codes, not putting enough blood on the reagent is frequently the cause of inaccurate results and errors in subsequent treatment decisions. Some meters have a feature that signals the user when the blood sample is not large enough to provide an accurate reading. Unfortunately, this feature creates a false sense of security because users assume that if they do not get the signal, they have given an adequate sample. The meter will only signal the user about a blood sample it cannot process, any other sample —even an inadequate one—will register a reading, but the reading will be inaccurate. Patients should be asked at every opportunity to demonstrate their technique for using their meters. This demonstration gives the educator an opportunity to verify technique, provide advice, or clean a soiled unit.
- Some patients have difficulty securing a drop of blood and may require guidance in choosing a lancing device or meter. Providing individualized guidance for each patient's needs minimizes waste of reagents and eases patient frustration with blood glucose monitoring.

**D** Patients should be taught specific directions for securing an adequate blood sample.[3] For example, when using the fingertips as a puncture site, the patient should be aware of the following procedures:
- Vigorously wash hands with warm water to increase circulation to fingertips.
- Try hanging the hand at your side for 30 seconds so the blood can pool in your hand.
- Shake the hand to be pricked as though you were shaking down a thermometer.
- Use a lancing device or endcap that will allow a deeper puncture.
- After your finger is punctured, gently milk the blood from the bottom to the tip of your finger until the blood drop is the correct size. Milking the finger works better than just squeezing the fingertips.

**E** Meters and strips have been designed to use the forearm, upper arm, or thigh as puncture sites. When using these sites for skin puncture, warm the site by gently massaging the skin for approximately 15 seconds or until warm.

## Table 4.1.  Patient Uses of SMBG Data

- Identifying and treating hypoglycemia
- Making decisions concerning food intake or medication adjustment
  when exercising
- Determining the effect of food choices or portions on blood glucose levels
- Pattern management
- Managing intercurrent illness
- Managing hypoglycemia unawareness

**4** Many patients are trained in the mechanics of using a meter but not how to use the data.  This inadequacy may be related to patient education.  Harris and associates[4] found that the frequency of monitoring was related to having attended a diabetes patient education class.  Diabetes patient education was associated with an almost threefold greater probability that subjects monitored their blood glucose at least once per day.

**A** The critical uses of SMBG data by patients are shown in Table 4.1.

**B** Self-monitoring of blood glucose provides reliable data for problem-solving and decision-making.
- While some decisions (eg, treating hypoglycemia or determining the need for a snack) require instantaneous feedback for decision-making, most decisions require reviewing numerous readings to identify a pattern (eg, adjusting medication dosages, changing the meal plan, or recognizing the impact of exercise).
- The memory feature of many meters is not intended to replace the logbook, but rather provide the option of recording readings at a later date.
- Although a written record and graph of blood glucose readings yields important information, jotting down comments or explanations can be more helpful for teaching the impact of certain decisions related to medication, exercise, or food.

**C** Educators and clinicians rely on SMBG to teach problem-solving skills, which are the essence of diabetes self-management, and complex management skills such as blood glucose pattern awareness and insulin dose adjustment (see Chapter 5, Pattern Management, in Diabetes Management Therapies, for examples).

**D** Diabetes educators use SMBG as the tool that links abstract principles of management with daily decision making.
- Educators can use blood glucose results to teach the concept of postexercise, late-onset hypoglycemia and the behaviors necessary to prevent this condition.
- Behavior change concerning food choices or portions is facilitated by relating the food or portion to the postprandial blood glucose result.[5,6]
- For patients with type 2 diabetes who are asymptomatic for hyperglycemia, the need for behavior change becomes personally relevant when they monitor and record blood glucose levels.

**E** Self-monitoring of blood glucose is used by educators to identify and influence psychosocial adaptations.
- Self-monitoring of blood glucose can influence self-efficacy.[7] For example, patients report increased confidence in their problem-solving abilities as a result of using SMBG.

- The act of monitoring can also hold emotional consequences when patients are confronted with an unacceptable number. This phenomenon, called *monitor talk*, can help identify psychosocial needs and direct future learning.[8] Educators can discourage value judgment and replace the notion of good and bad readings with the terms *in range* or *out of range*. Reference to blood glucose tests can be replaced with the terms *checks* or *measurements*.
- Identified barriers to monitoring include the discomfort of finger-sticks, elevated or labile readings, reminder of the diagnosis of diabetes, cost of reagents, and the inconvenience of record keeping. By identifying barriers, the educator can provide direction and support the patient's choice in using this valuable tool.
- Self-monitoring of blood glucose can be used to allay anxiety about hypoglycemia, especially parental anxiety, and is a critical tool for treating fear of hypoglycemia.[9]
- Although the influence of stress and stress management techniques on glycemic control is controversial, individuals may benefit from identifying a physical marker for their psychological distress.

**F** The frequency and timing of SMBG are determined by how the data will be used.
- More frequent monitoring is beneficial during insulin dose adjustment, whereas periodic postprandial checks may benefit someone with type 2 diabetes who is learning about the glycemic effect of food portions.
- Postprandial monitoring is an essential part of diabetes self-management. Research has demonstrated that any therapy targeted at lowering postprandial blood glucose will also lower HbA1c.[10] One of the most common barriers to postprandial monitoring is that patients frequently forget to check after a meal since there is no trigger to remind them.
- Monitoring schedules are based on the patient's needs, desires, and use of the data. Although some insurers and clinicians have not yet been convinced of the merit of SMBG for patients not treated with insulin, the value of SMBG cannot be overemphasized as a teaching tool, motivator, and reinforcer and as an aid in prescribing appropriate dosages of the various combinations of blood glucose lowering agents.

**G** Guidelines for teaching individuals how to use a blood glucose meter are listed in Table 4.2.

---

## Table 4.2. Guidelines for Teaching Individuals How to Use a Blood Glucose Meter

- Use universal precautions: change lancets, endcaps, and gloves for each patient.[11]
- Demonstrate how to check blood glucose using control solution first and then using the individual's blood.
- After demonstrating this technique, ask the individual to provide a return demonstration before teaching about control solution, calibration, cleaning, and using the logbook.
- Explain how to dispose of lancets in an appropriate sharps container.
- Evaluate the individual's technique at every opportunity.

**5** Educators are frequently asked to provide consultation regarding the choice of a meter for a hospital or other facility. Although the scientific literature contains numerous reports of the statistical accuracy of systems for SMBG, most determine accuracy in ways that may not be clinically useful for these settings. The Error Grid Analysis[12] provides a useful methodological contribution for evaluating accuracy of glucose meters and clinical relevancy of statistical data related to SMBG.

**6** Noninvasive blood glucose monitoring is now available. Noninvasive monitoring involves measuring the concentration of glucose in the blood without puncturing the finger to obtain a drop of blood.[13]

**7** Data management systems allow for downloading the memory stored in the meter to a remote computer (either directly or by modem) for plotting the results on a graph. These systems can be accessed via personal computer or the internet. Data summarization alone, however, does not identify the relationship that leads to the observed outcomes (eg, the 4 carbohydrate servings at breakfast that led to postprandial hyperglycemia).

**8** The Joint Commission for the Accreditation of Health Care Organizations (JCAHO) and the Health Care Financing Administration (HCFA) require hospitals and other facilities to have quality assurance programs for bedside blood glucose monitoring.[14] Proficiency testing, use of control solutions, staff training, and correlation studies comparing bedside results with hospital laboratory values are essential elements of the quality assurance process.
  **A** The Clinical Laboratory Improvement Act of 1988 (CLIA '88)[15] placed additional restrictions on blood glucose monitoring performed outside the hospital setting. Blood glucose meters must have verified accuracy, and the provider's office must complete additional paperwork and submit fees for a waivered test that provides exemption from the requirements.

**9** Certain populations of people with diabetes have unique needs relating to SMBG.
  **A** Elderly people with diabetes remain an underserved population despite the prevalence of diabetes in the elderly and the validity of SMBG as a management tool.
  • Age should not be the sole criterion for decisions concerning SMBG. The elderly are a heterogeneous population requiring personalized therapy and monitoring schedules.
  • Educators need to consider the unique needs of some elderly patients that may influence the choice of products, such as potential limitations in manual dexterity, slowed reaction time, or fluctuating vision[16] (for more information, see Chapter 4, Diabetes in Older Adults, in Diabetes in the Life Cycle and Research).
  **B** Children also have unique needs that influence product choice.
  • Children especially benefit from reagents that require a small sample size of blood and lancing devices that hide the lancet and minimize discomfort.
  • Parents benefit from meters that quickly yield results and store at least the last reading in the memory. This latter feature is particularly important because after a skin puncture, parents are focused on comforting their child and the meter may turn off before the parent can write down the result (for more information, see

Chapter 1, Diabetes During Childhood and Adolescence, in Diabetes in the Life Cycle and Research).

**C** Visually impaired persons with diabetes, including those with fluctuating vision to nonfunctional vision, need products that are fully accessible to the visually impaired person; current products fall short of this need. Equipment features that would be of benefit include tactile markings on the reagent; durable reagents not damaged by touching; clear speech output on a small, portable meter; and a method of consistent placement of the blood sample[17] (for more information, see Chapter 7, Eye Disease and Adaptive Education for Visually Impaired Persons, in Diabetes and Complications).

## Continuous Glucose Monitoring

**1** The *continuous glucose monitoring system* is designed to be worn by patients as a device similar to a cardiac Holter monitor. The system continuously and automatically monitors glucose values in subcutaneous tissue. The typical measurement period is up to 72 hours.

**A** The continuous glucose monitoring system is intended for diagnostic and prescriptive use and can be helpful to identify glycemic effects of food, exercise, and insulin; previously unrecognized hypoglycemia; proper insulin doses to match food absorption in gastroparesis; and effects of dialysis on glucose levels.

## Long-Term Monitoring of Metabolic Control

**1** Glycosylated hemoglobin (HbA1c), the most abundant minor hemoglobin component in the red blood cell, increases in proportion to the blood glucose level over the preceding 3 to 4 months in persons with diabetes. It is an accurate, objective measure of chronic glycemia in diabetes.

**A** *Glycosylation* occurs as glucose in the plasma attaches itself to the hemoglobin component of the red blood cell; this process is irreversible.

- The more glycosylation, the higher the values.
- Because the red blood cell has a life span of 120 days, this test reflects the blood glucose concentration over that period of time.
- The glycosylated hemoglobin does not reflect the simple mean but reflects the weighted mean over a long period of time.[18] The traditional idea that glycosylated hemoglobin reflects the simple mean and is referred to as the average of the blood glucose is inaccurate. For example, in a HbA1c measured on May 1, 50% of the HbA1c level is determined by the plasma glucose level during the preceding 1-month period (April), 25% of its level is determined by the plasma glucose level during the 1-month period before that (March) and the remaining 25% is determined by the plasma glucose level during the 2-month period before the past 2 months (February and January).

**B** Glycosylated hemoglobin can be measured by many different methods. Accurate interpretation requires knowledge of the method used to determine the glycosylated hemoglobin level, the component measured, and the normal range for the particular assay.[19]

- *Affinity chromatography* and *colorimetric assay methods* measure total glycosylated hemoglobin (GHb), including all fractions of the hemoglobin molecule:

HbA1a, HbA1b, and HbA1c.[19] Upper normal values of GHb may be in the range of 8% to 9%.

- Ion-exchange chromatography, high-performance liquid chromatography (HPLC), and immunoassay methods are used to measure HbA1c.[19] The normal value is usually in the range of 4% to 6%.
- Some laboratories measure total glycosylated hemoglobin, but they report the ADA treatment goal of <7% in the reference range column of the report instead of listing the actual reference range of up to 9%. This may have clinical relevance if healthcare providers compare values from different laboratories. A result of 7.8% would be considered out of range if the reference range is 4.0% to 6.0% and within range if the reference range was 5.0% to 8.0%.
- It has been suggested that all glycosylated hemoglobin assays be standardized and reported in values equivalent to the HbA1c as measured in the Diabetes Control and Complications Trial (DCCT).[20]
- Interfering factors (sickle-cell hemoglobin and other hemoglobinopathies) may affect measurement of HbA1c depending upon the method.[21]
- HbA1c measurement is not currently recommended for diagnosis of diabetes because of the lack of nationwide standardization of the HbA1c test.

**C** Regular measurements of HbA1c permit timely detection of departures from the target range. In the absence of well-controlled studies that suggest a definite testing protocol, the ADA Standards of Medical Care for Patients With Diabetes Mellitus[2] suggest glycosylated hemoglobin testing at least 1 or 2 times a year in patients with a history of stable glycemic control, and at least quarterly assessments in patients whose therapy has changed or who are in poor control.

**D** Glycemic targets should be individualized for each patient.

- The DCCT[20] conclusively demonstrated, however, that the risk of retinopathy, nephropathy, and neuropathy in patients with type 1 diabetes is reduced by intensive treatment regimens compared with conventional treatment regimens. These benefits were observed with an average HbA1c of 7.2% (normal range = 4.0% to 6.0%) in the intensively treated group of patients. The reduction in risk of these complications correlated continuously with the reduction in HbA1c produced by intensive therapy.[2]
- A glycosylated hemoglobin result within the nondiabetic reference range (Table 4.3) may reflect frequent hypoglycemia. The glycosylated hemoglobin is a strong indicator of blood glucose control when compared with SMBG results.

**E** Glycosylated hemoglobin is a teaching tool as well as a marker of metabolic control. If a patient monitors only fasting blood glucose levels and finds values in the normal range but has a HbA1c result of 9.8% (normal range = 4.0% to 6.0%), the educator can encourage the patient to monitor at other times of the day (especially postprandial readings) to uncover periods of elevated blood glucose and identify the factors that may be associated with the elevations.

**2** Glycosylated serum albumin (fructosamine), a glycated serum protein test, measures glycemic control over 2 to 3 weeks.[21] Normal ranges vary among the different methods of measurements. Fructosamine values are used in short-term follow-up of interventions that have been recently implemented to lower blood glucose[1] or when there is a discrepancy between HbA1c and the patient's reported blood glucose readings.

## Table 4.3. Glycemic Targets for Nonpregnant Individuals With Diabetes[2]

| Biochemical Index | Nondiabetic Reference Range | Goal | Suggested Action Range |
|---|---|---|---|
| HbA1c, % | 4.0 to 6.0 | <7.0 | >8.0 |

Action suggested depends on individual patient circumstances. Such actions may include enhancement of diabetes self-management education, co-management with a diabetes team, referral to an endocrinologist, change in pharmacological therapy, initiation of increased SMBG, or more frequent contact with the patient.

## Ketone Tests

**1** Monitoring for the presence of ketones remains an essential component of diabetes care. Patients with type 1 diabetes are ketosis-prone, whereas patients with type 2 diabetes are generally ketosis-resistant.

**A** Either blood or urinary ketones can be measured. Blood ketones can be measured using a special meter designed for home use and urinary ketones can be measured using a dipstick and matching the results to a color chart.

**B** Ketones should be tested routinely during illness by all patients with diabetes. Patients with type 2 diabetes can become ketotic during severe stress precipitated by infections or trauma.[23]

- Patients with type 1 diabetes should test ketones when their blood glucose is consistently elevated (>300 mg/dL [>16.7 mmol/L]). For patients using an insulin pump, ketonuria or ketonemia in the presence of hyperglycemia may indicate failure of the insulin delivery system.

- Pregnant women with diabetes (including gestational diabetes) are advised to monitor urinary ketones every morning. These measurements are useful for detecting inadequate food intake (starvation ketosis) and providing warning of impending metabolic decompensation (for more information, see Chapter 2, Pregnancy: Conception to Postpartum, in Diabetes in the Life Cycle and Research).[24]

- Urinary ketones also should be measured on a regular schedule in patients actively trying to lose weight by calorie restriction. Because ketones are a waste product of fat metabolism, ketonuria in the presence of euglycemia can indicate weight loss, not metabolic decompensation.

- Patents with type 1 diabetes who are restricting calories to lose weight require decreased dosages of insulin to prevent hypoglycemia. Too much of a reduction of insulin will result in hyperglycemia, ketonuria and, if not corrected, metabolic decompensation to ketoacidosis.

**C** Three ketone bodies are formed from the conversion of free fatty acids in the liver: acetoacetate, 3-ß-hydroxybutyrate and acetone.

- Urinary ketones are detected by the nitroprusside reaction in the treatment of acute diabetic ketoacidosis. The nitroprusside reagent predominantly reacts with acetoacetate and does not react with ß-hydroxybutyrate.

- Following the institution of insulin therapy, the concentration of acetoacetate increases and ß-hydroxybutyrate decreases. This shift accounts for the clinical observation that urine ketone test results may become more positive during the early phase of therapy and indicate clinical improvement rather than deterioration.

**D** Rapid enzymatic methods have been developed for the quantification of 3-ß-hydroxybutyrate levels in small-volume blood samples. These systems are designed for use at home and can measure 3-ß-hydroxybutyrate levels on finger-stick blood samples.[25]

## Table 4.4. Definitions of Abnormalities of Albumin Excretion

|  | 24-h collection, mg/24 h | Timed collection, µg/min | Spot collection, µg/mg creatinine |
|---|---|---|---|
| Normal | <30 | <20 | <30 |
| Microalbuminuria | 30 to 299 | 20 to 199 | 30 to 299 |
| Clinical albuminuria | ≥300 | ≥200 | ≥300 |

Because of variability in urinary albumin excretion, 2 of 3 specimens collected within a 3- to 6-month period should be abnormal before considering a patient to have crossed one of these diagnostic thresholds. Exercise within 24 hours, infection, fever, congestive heart failure, marked hyperglycemia, and marked hypertension may elevate urinary albumin excretion over baseline values.
*Source:* Reprinted with permission from American Diabetes Association.[2]

## Urine Tests

**1** The ability to detect low levels of albumin in the urine (*microalbuminuria*) represents an important advancement in the diagnosis and treatment of diabetic nephropathy. The presence of microalbuminuria represents an early phase of nephropathy and is important for prompt diagnosis and intervention.

**A** Annual urine protein screening in individuals with type 1 diabetes should begin at puberty and after 5 years' duration of diabetes. Because of the difficulty in precise dating of type 2 diabetes, urinary protein screening should begin at the time of diagnosis.[2]

**B** Screening for microalbuminuria can be performed by 3 methods: measurement of the albumin-to-creatinine ratio in a random spot collection; 24-hour collection with creatinine, allowing the simultaneous measurement of creatinine clearance; and timed (eg, 4-hour or overnight) collection (see Table 4.4).

**C** The albustix reagent does not screen for microalbuminuria because it does not become positive until the albumin excretion rate (AER) exceeds 300 mg/24 h (200 µg/min).

**D** In healthy individuals, small amounts of albumin can be found in the urine with a mean albumin excretion rate of 10 ± 3 mg/day (7 ± 2 µg/min).[26]

**E** Screening for microalbuminuria should be avoided if the patient has a urinary tract infection or hematuria, has recently performed strenuous exercise, is experiencing acute illness or fever, or is menstruating.[27]

**2** *Urine glucose testing* was the original method of monitoring glycemic control, but blood glucose monitoring is the preferred method. Urine glucose testing provides retrospective information and does not reflect current blood glucose. Urine glucose testing is used only if the patient is unable or unwilling to perform blood glucose monitoring or if the only goal is avoiding symptomatic hyperglycemia.[2]

**A** The results of urine glucose testing should be reported in percent values not plus (+) values for continuity of results from one method to another.

**B** The advantages of urine testing for glucose are that it is less expensive than blood glucose monitoring and is noninvasive.

**C** Urine testing for glucose offers several distinct disadvantages.

- Elevated renal thresholds (blood glucose >180 mg/dL [>10 mmol/L]) that occur with age and during pregnancy will give false negative results.
- Since urine testing gives a delayed picture of what is happening in the blood, it is not indicated in intensive diabetes management.[19]
- False results (negative or positive) may occur with ingestion of certain medications (cephalosporins, large amounts of ascorbic acid).
- Urine testing can be awkward to do especially when away from home.

## Assessment of Growth and Weight   *Do when going to use data*

**1** Monitoring also involves assessing of growth in children and weight in all patients with diabetes.

**2** Documentation of weight is considered another indicator for diabetes management.

**A** Weight gain may reflect improvement in glycemic control, increased caloric consumption, frequent episodes of hypoglycemia, fluid retention, and eating disorders, among other conditions.

**B** Similarly, weight loss may reflect elevated blood glucose levels, decreased caloric consumption, or eating disorders.

**C** Fluctuations in weight can occur depending upon the scale used and time of day.

## Summary

**1** Since self-monitoring of blood glucose is one of the essential tools of self-management, diabetes educators have the unique opportunity and responsibility to provide instruction concerning not only monitoring techniques but use of the data.

**2** Diabetes educators can also teach individuals to approach monitoring as feedback (ie, helpful information) rather than evaluation (ie, punishment).

**3** Teach individuals that the meaning of the results from the methods used to monitor metabolic control provides more than feedback; it reinforces their active role in self-management and their position as the center of the healthcare team.

## Key Educational Considerations

**1** A variety of meters are available for monitoring blood glucose, and each one is unique.

**A** It is important to carefully assess the patient's visual acuity and dexterity skills before recommending a specific meter. Let the patient practice using the meter. Demonstration meters and supplies are available from the manufacturer's representative.

**B** Diabetes educators are pivotal in guiding patients to select the meter that is most appropriate for them and one for which they easily can obtain supplies. Some insurers only reimburse for certain meters and reagents.

**2** Ask patients to bring their meters and all supplies to each visit. The meter can be cleaned, the reagents and control solution can be tested, codes can be verified, and an actual blood glucose measurement can be performed.

**3** Provide patients with the toll-free customer service number for the manufacturer of their meter. Experts are available at this number 24 hours per day to answer questions and provide assistance.

**4** Careful and safe disposal of used lancets is critical. Teach patients to dispose of used lancets in an appropriate sharps container (regulations vary from state to state). When monitoring blood glucose away from home, patients can place their used lancets in an empty pill container or 35-mm film canister.

**5** Consider the cost of supplies when patients decide the frequency of monitoring. Be familiar with local suppliers who charge reasonable prices. Refer patients to a social worker or community agency when appropriate.

**6** Some patients benefit from having a second meter that is compact, quick, and simple to use for easily checking their blood glucose level away from home or before driving. Blood glucose monitoring results will be most consistent if the same model of a meter is used all the time. If a patient chooses to use a different model to check the blood glucose before driving, for example, then those readings should either be omitted from the logbook or noted as resulting from a different meter.

**7** Postprandial monitoring is effective for teaching the impact of food portions on blood glucose levels. For example, a patient may choose a large portion of frozen yogurt and have an elevated blood glucose reading 2 hours later, whereas after a medium portion of frozen yogurt the postprandial reading may be in the goal range.

**8** Use patient records or logbooks that list glucose levels for a certain time of day in a linear and vertical fashion. This format allows simple visual interpretation of the results.

**9** Recording blood glucose levels on a graph, as well as having a numerical listing, provides a useful visual aid for teaching the concept of blood glucose patterns. Computer software marketed by meter manufacturers can be very helpful in providing graphs and other visual representations of the data.

**10** Actual blood glucose records of common patterns should be used when teaching self-management.

**11** Provide patients with the opportunity to practice testing for urinary or serum ketones during their teaching appointment.

**12** A supply sheet, signed by the healthcare provider, can be an effective organizational aid for the patient and the pharmacist and may serve as a prescription.

**13** Teaching the concept of glycosylated hemoglobin can be challenging. This test can be referred to as a "smart" blood test that represents blood glucose levels over the last 3 months. HbA1c can be thought of as a long-term monitoring method as opposed to the day-to-day self-monitoring measurements that are performed with a home meter.

**14** Avoid referring to HbA1c as an average of blood glucose levels. Besides being technically inaccurate, patients often confuse HbA1c with the average in their meter memory.

**15** The educator can use a picture of a pyramid or a thermometer to outline the various HbA1c levels and then demonstrate the goal range and the patient's most recent result. Ask patients what they think about the results and what they would like to do about it rather than offering judgments.

## Self-Review Questions

**1** List the factors that affect the accuracy of SMBG results.
**2** Describe the most common user error related to SMBG.
**3** List tips that can be followed to secure an adequate blood sample.
**4** Define the critical uses of SMBG data by patients.
**5** Describe ways educators can use SMBG to link the principles of diabetes management with daily decision-making.
**6** Describe common psychosocial adaptations related to SMBG.
**7** Describe how monitoring schedules are determined.
**8** Define a reliable method for evaluating the accuracy of blood glucose meters.
**9** List the elements of quality assurance regarding blood glucose meters.
**10** Describe the unique SMBG needs of the elderly, children, and visually impaired persons with diabetes.
**11** Define glycosylated hemoglobin and the target ranges.
**12** Define fructosamine and when this assessment is used.
**13** List the advantages and disadvantages of urine glucose testing.
**14** Describe what groups of patients should monitor for ketones.
**15** List 3 methods of screening for microalbuminuria and the target ranges.
**16** List when screening for microalbuminuria should be avoided.
**17** Describe the role of documenting weight changes in the management of diabetes.

## Learning Assessment: Case Study 1

AD sees the diabetes educator regularly following a visit with his physician. At each visit with the educator, he brings both of his meters (from 2 different manufacturers) and presents different scenarios concerning the discrepancies between the 2 meters or between the lab and each meter. He keeps no records and barely checks his blood glucose because "he is not confident of the results." The diabetes educator dutifully verifies the accuracy of the meters and spends the entire visit defending the meters. When reviewing the documentation of these visits, the diabetes educator realizes that there has been no diabetes education and looks to colleagues for advice.

## Questions for Discussion

**1** What are the dynamics of these visits?

**2** What are possible explanations for the patient's behavior?

**3** How can the educator alter the pattern of the visits?

**4** What content is generally included when teaching about blood glucose monitoring?

## Discussion

**1** AD may be using the meters as an effective smoke screen.

   **A** If AD organizes the visits around the meters, then nothing else is discussed. He may have lost confidence in the meters, but verifying accuracy and defending the meters is not helping him regain his confidence.

   **B** When interactions with patients become frustrating, reflecting on the experience and seeking the advice of colleagues often helps to bring a different perspective to the situation. As a result of her thoughts and discussions, the educator recognizes her role in perpetuating this pattern. While she knows she cannot change AD's behavior, she can change her own.

**2** To alter the pattern of visits, the educator decides to develop a specific plan of action. When making the plan, she realizes that she needs to be sure that it is designed to meet AD's needs and includes strategies that keep him in control of the visit, such as asking questions and seeking his options rather than just offering advice. The important thing is to create a different, more functional partnership with him.

   **A** Because this might represent avoidance behavior, the educator needs to assess what AD is trying to avoid in order to more effectively meet his needs. This task will no doubt be challenging, but one technique for inviting discussion is to say, "It seems like we spend all of our time on this topic and I am concerned that you are not getting what you need from me. Could we start with your other concerns?"

   **B** If he is unable to identify concerns, you could share the barriers to self-care that others have identified and ask if he has had similar experiences or if there are other things about his diabetes care that are hard for him.

   **C** Another option would be to ask AD if the physician made any treatment changes during the last visit, offer to review these changes with AD, and use them as a springboard for teaching new content. The issues surrounding monitoring still need to be discussed, but focusing on another area of AD's concerns may decrease frustration for him and the educator. Generally, once the patient's technique in using the meter has been assessed (including reagent storage, expiration date, etc.), teach how to record blood glucose readings, target ranges, and, most importantly, how to use the data.

## Learning Assessment: Case Study 2

JD is a 26-year-old male who was diagnosed with type 1 diabetes 6 months ago. He vacationed in another state and presented in the emergency department with a hypoglycemic seizure. His blood glucose log revealed readings that were either elevated or within range. This patient's goal was euglycemia and he would adjust his insulin dosages based on his premeal blood glucose readings. The evening before the seizure, he participated in a family meal that included large portions of food and alcohol. In anticipation of an elevated bedtime blood glucose, he injected extra units of rapid-acting insulin immediately before the meal and again before going to bed. His wife was so frightened by the seizure that she cannot sleep and encourages him to eat more at night to prevent hypoglycemia.

He returned for his follow-up visit with the diabetes educator a week after seeing his endocrinologist. In February, his HbA1c was 6.2% (reference range 4.0%-6.0%) and in May the HbA1c was 4.7% with the same reference range. The result was confirmed 1 week later. His endocrinologist congratulated him on the tight control. At the visit with the educator, his prelunch blood glucose was 102 mg/dL (5.7 mmol/L) using the educator's supplies and he demonstrated accurate technique.

## Questions for Discussion

1 What clues are provided by his story and the recent HbA1c result?

2 What does the educator still need to assess?

3 How can the educator help JD's wife?

## Discussion

1 A low HbA1c result is often achieved at the expense of frequent hypoglycemia. A low result should signal the educator to assess for the frequency and severity of hypoglycemia keeping in mind that many patients underreport the frequency of hypoglycemia if they successfully managed the episode. It would be helpful to assess JD's understanding of the impact of alcohol on the blood glucose, especially the hypoglycemic effects of alcohol. It would also be prudent to review JD's guidelines for deciding on a pre-meal dose of rapid-acting insulin.

2 Part of the assessment of the patient's technique involves checking the meter to see if it is soiled (when applicable) and inquiring about reagent storage. JD found the vial of strips that accompany his meter to be bulky so he decided to store them out of the vial. This practice yielded inaccurate results. Unfortunately, JD was adjusting his insulin based on inaccurate results.

3 JD's wife might be comforted when she learns that incorrect storage of the strips contributed to JD's hypoglycemic seizure. Since she did not attend the visit, the educator could arrange to meet with JD's wife or telephone her to listen to her concerns. If applicable, the educator could reinforce the safety guidelines for insulin adjustment and nighttime snacking as prevention of nocturnal hypoglycemia. The educator could also reinforce how excessive nighttime snacking would not serve JD's needs and may create conflict.

# References

**1** American Diabetes Association. Self-monitoring of blood glucose (consensus statement). Diabetes Care. 1994;18:81-86.

**2** American Diabetes Association. Standards of medical care for patients with diabetes mellitus (position statement). Diabetes Care. 2001;24(suppl 1):S33-S43.

**3** Peragallo-Dittko V. The lowdown on lancets and lancing devices. Diabetes Self-Manage. 1999;16(3):64-71.

**4** Harris MI, Crowe CC, Howie LJ. Self-monitoring of blood glucose by adults with diabetes in the United States population. Diabetes Care. 1993;16:1116-1123.

**5** Babione L. SMBG: the underused nutrition counseling tool in diabetes management. Diabetes Spectrum. 1994;7:196-197.

**6** Ahern JA, Gatcomb PM, Held NA, Petit WA, Jr, Tamborlane WV. Exaggerated hyperglycemia after a pizza meal in well-controlled diabetes. Diabetes Care. 993; 16:578-580.

**7** Rubin RR, Peyrot M, Saudek CD. The effect of a diabetes education program incorporating coping skills training on emotional well-being and diabetes self-efficacy. Diabetes Educ. 1993;19:210-214.

**8** Price MJ. Qualitative analysis of the patient-provider interactions: the patient's perspective. Diabetes Educ. 1989;15:144-148.

**9** Cox DJ, Irvine A, Gonder-Frederick L, Nowacek G, Butterfield J. Fear of hypoglycemia: quantification, validation and utilization. Diabetes Care. 1987;10:617-621.

**10** Bastyr III EJ, Stuart CA, Broddows RG, Schwartz S, Graf CJ, Zagar A, Robertson KE. Therapy focused on lowering postprandial glucose, not fasting glucose, may be superior for lowering HbA1c. Diabetes Care. 2000;23:1236-1241.

**11** American Association of Diabetes Educators. Position statement. Educating providers and persons with diabetes to prevent the transmission of bloodborne infections and avoid injuries from sharps. Diabetes Educ. 1997;23:401-403.

**12** Clarke WL, Cox D, Gonder-Frederick LA, Carter W, Pohl SL. Evaluating clinical accuracy of systems for self-monitoring of blood glucose. Diabetes Care. 1987;10:622-628.

**13** Klonoff DC. Noninvasive blood glucose monitoring. Diabetes Care. 1997;20:433-437.

**14** Walker EA. Quality assurance for blood glucose monitoring. Nurs Clin North Am. 1993;28:61-70.

**15** American Diabetes Association. CLIA guidelines implemented. Diabetes Rev. 1993; 1:130.

**16** Peragallo-Dittko V. Clinical and educational usefulness of SMBG with the elderly. Diabetes Spectrum. 1995;8:17-19.

**17** Bernbaum M, Albert SG, Brusca S, et al. Effectiveness of glucose monitoring systems modified for the visually impaired. Diabetes Care. 1993;16:1363-1366.

**18** Tahara Y, Shima K. Kinetics of HbA1c, glycated albumin, and fructosamine and analysis of their weight functions against preceding plasma glucose level. Diabetes Care. 1995;18;440-447.

**19** Farkas-Hirsch R, ed. Intensive Diabetes Management. 2nd ed. Alexandria, VA: American Diabetes Association; 1998: 128-131.

**20** The Diabetes Control and Complications Trial Research Group. The effect of intensive treatment of diabetes on the development and progression of long-term complications of insulin-dependent diabetes. N Engl J Med. 1993;329:77-86.

**21** Goldstein DE, Little RR. More than you ever wanted to know (but need to know) about glycohemoglobin testing. Diabetes Care. 1994;17:938-939.

**22** Negoro H, Morley JE, Rosenthal MJ. Utility of serum fructosamine as a measure of glycemia in young and old diabetic and non-diabetic subjects. Am J Med. 1988;85:360-364.

**23** Fajans SS. Classification and diagnosis of diabetes. In: Porte D, Jr, Sherwin RS, eds. Ellenberg and Rifkin's Diabetes Mellitus: Theory and Practice. 5th ed. Stamford, Ct: Appleton and Lange; 1997:357-372.

**24** Metzger BE, Phelps RL, Dooley SL. The mother in pregnancies complicated by diabetes mellitus. In: Porte D, Jr, Sherwin RS, eds. Ellenberg and Rifkin's Diabetes Mellitus: Theory and Practice. 5th ed. Stamford, Ct: Appleton and Lange; 1997: 887-915.

**25** Laffel L. Ketone bodies: a review of physiology, pathophysiology and application of monitoring to diabetes. Diabetes Metab Res Rev. 1999;15:412-426.

**26** DeFronzo RA. Diabetic nephropathy. In: Porte D, Jr, Sherwin RS, eds. Ellenberg and Rifkin's Diabetes Mellitus: Theory and Practice. 5th ed. Stamford, Ct: Appleton and Lange; 1997:971-1008.

**27** Morgensen CE, Vestbo E, Poulsen PL, et al. Microalbuminuria and potential confounders. Diabetes Care. 1995;18:572-581.

## Suggested Readings

**1** Peragallo-Dittko V. How accurate is your meter? Diabetes Self Manage. 2000;17(5): 78-85.

**2** Atkin SH, Dasmahapatra A, Jaker MA, Chorost MI, Reddy S. Finger-stick glucose determination in shock. Ann Intern Med. 1991;114:1020-1024.

**3** Wedman B, Michael SR. Tool chest: glycosylated hemoglobin models. Diabetes Educ. 1988;14:280-282.

For a listing of currently available meters, refer to Diabetes Forecast: Buyers Guide (Annual Issue) and Diabetes Self-Management.

# Learning Assessment: Post-Test Questions

## Monitoring 4

1 The most important benefit to patients of SMBG is:
   **A** It facilitates problem-solving and decision-making skills
   **B** It decreases the number of medical visits they make
   **C** It enables them to make medication adjustments based on a single reading
   **D** It may reveal psychosocial issues

2 What is a decision concerning diabetes control that can be made from a single blood glucose reading?
   **A** Adjustment of a patient's split insulin regimen
   **B** Treatment of a blood glucose reading less than 70 mg/dL
   **C** Understanding the impact of a daily walking program
   **D** Adjustment of meal plan

3 The most common SMBG user error is:
   **A** Failure to get an adequate blood sample
   **B** Improper storage of meter and equipment
   **C** Failure to calibrate the meter
   **D** Inadequate reporting of high and low BG values

4 Which of the following is not a factor that can affect the accuracy of SMBG systems?
   **A** Altitude
   **B** Temperature and humidity
   **C** Microalbuminuria
   **D** Hypoxia and hypotension

5 Glycosylated hemoglobin:
   **A** Represents an average blood glucose concentration within a defined period of time
   **B** Is a weighted mean over a relative period of time
   **C** Should be measured at the onset of symptoms and during each routine medical checkup
   **D** Is easily measured by a single method with a known range using a defined component

6 JG brings in her blood glucose monitor to a diabetes education session. She states that it has not worked properly since she purchased it through a mail-order discount device company. What would be the educator's first assessment step to determine the problem?
   **A** Demonstrate proper technique of the meter and give the patient a videotape of instructions
   **B** Use the glucose control solution to determine the meter's accuracy
   **C** Ask the patient to demonstrate SMBG using her meter
   **D** Get a venipuncture to determine the patient's random blood glucose level

7 The expiration date on JG's reagent strip container indicates that her strips are current. Could they still be a source of error in SMBG determinations?
   **A** No, reagent strips are extremely durable and rarely are a source of SMBG error
   **B** No, even expired reagent strips are commonly used by patients with diabetes
   **C** Yes, the manufacturer could print the date wrong
   **D** Yes, environmental changes in temperature and atmosphere could degrade strips

8 An effective approach for teaching patients how to use a blood glucose meter is:
   **A** Show how to calibrate the meter before demonstrating its use
   **B** Change your gloves every hour
   **C** Evaluate the patient's technique whenever hyperglycemia occurs
   **D** Teach the patient how to check the blood glucose before teaching meter cleaning and record keeping

**9**  Urine testing of ketones using the nitro-prusside reaction primarily measures which of the following ketone bodies?

**A** Acetone
**B** Acetoacetate
**C** ß-hydroxybutyrate
**D** Ketone

**10** The accuracy of blood glucose measured by a meter designed for home use can be influenced by all of the following except:

**A** Measurement of whole blood versus plasma
**B** Measurement of capillary versus venous blood after a meal
**C** Measurement using different finger-tips for puncture
**D** Measurement using strips stored outside of the package

*See next page for answer key.*

# Post-Test Answer Key

## Monitoring                                                                  4

1   A

2   B

3   A

4   C

5   B

6   C

7   D

8   D

9   B

10  C

# A Core Curriculum for Diabetes Education
Diabetes Management Therapies

## Pattern Management of Blood Glucose 5

*Deborah A. Hinnen, RN, MN, ARNP, BC-ADM, CDE*
*Via Christi Regional Medical Center*
*Wichita, Kansas*

*Diana W. Guthrie, RN, ARNP, FAAN, CDE*
*Professor Emeritus*
*University of Kansas School of Medicine*
*Wichita, Kansas*

*Belinda P. Childs, RN, MN, ARNP, CDE*
*Mid-America Diabetes Associates*
*Wichita, Kansas*

*Richard A. Guthrie, MD, CDE*
*Mid-America Diabetes Associates*
*Via Christi Regional Medical Center*
*University of Kansas School of Medicine*
*Wichita, Kansas*

## Introduction

**1** *Pattern management* is the application of a systematic analysis of data by both persons with diabetes and health professionals in the daily, weekly, and long-term management of blood glucose levels.

**2** It is often used with intensive management programs to achieve euglycemia with the ultimate goal of preventing the chronic complications of diabetes.[1-3]

**3** This chapter addresses pattern management as a way to analyze the data collected through self-monitoring of blood glucose (SMBG) in a logical and methodical manner, thus allowing carefully planned changes to the treatment program.

## Objectives

Upon completion of this chapter, the learner will be able to

**1** List concepts of pattern management.

**2** Identify strategies utilized in pattern management.

**3** Describe algorithms for making insulin adjustments.

**4** Describe changes in the timing of injections to accommodate specific situations (eg, travel, shift work).

**5** Identify that combination therapy may result from pattern analysis of and contribute to intensive diabetes management for patients with type 2 diabetes.

## Concepts of Pattern Management

**1** Pattern management is a comprehensive approach to blood glucose management that includes all aspects of current diabetes therapy.[4] While this approach is typically identified with intensive insulin therapy, pattern management can actually include utilization of many pharmacological combinations to improve glycemic control.

**2** Combinations of multiple oral agents can be used to address the specific pathophysiologic problems of insulin resistance, secretory defect, and excessive hepatic glucose production. This further enhances the opportunity to personalize and intensify diabetes management for persons with type 2 diabetes.

**3** Improvements in monitoring tools increase the potential for gathering the information necessary to appropriately apply medical nutritional therapy, exercise, and medications to attain blood glucose goals established by the individual with diabetes and the diabetes care team (see Chapter 4, Monitoring, in Diabetes Management Therapies, for recommended blood glucose goals for adults and Chapter 1, Diabetes During Childhood and Adolescence, in Diabetes in the Life Cycle and Research, for glucose goal ranges for children).

**4** Elements of pattern management include

**A** Self-identified desire to be an active participant in care

**B** Identification of personal blood glucose goals by the individual with diabetes and diabetes care team

**C** Self-adjustment of food intake, exercise, and medication to achieve goals

**D** Frequent SMBG to provide data for making adjustments

**E** Multiple injections of insulin, combinations of oral medications or oral medications and insulin, or insulin pump therapy

**F** Frequent interaction between individuals with diabetes and the diabetes care team

- Telephone, fax, and e-mail can be used to discuss glucose values between visits

**G** Self-management education, including

- Comprehensive and interactive coverage of the content areas identified by the National Standards for Diabetes Self-Management Education[5,6]
- The relationship of glucose levels, food, activity, and medications
- The impact of elements of control on personal glucose levels by prevention or prediction of needs
- Purpose, strategies, and value of pattern management for intensive therapy to achieve blood glucose goals
- Decision-making and problem-solving skills
- Personal diabetes and health-related supplies
- An understanding of personal belief systems related to the value of health and intensive diabetes management

**H** Support systems to provide emotional and management support

- Diabetes care team with on-call nursing support
- Family or care partners
- Support groups (ie, American Diabetes Association, clinic, hospital, education center)
- Other community diabetes educational activities and offerings such as counseling

## Strategies for Pattern Management

**1** Pattern management involves reviewing several days of glucose records and making adjustments in diabetes therapies based on trends, rather than reacting to a single, high or low blood glucose reading. Adding supplemental or sliding scale insulin at the time of the elevated glucose level solves the problem only for that particular point in time but does not prevent the problem from occurring again.

**2** If blood glucose readings are high (or low) for several days at a specific time, potential causes for the elevated (or low) levels are examined so the problem can be corrected. This method of managing diabetes has been used since the 1930s, originally with children and later among adults with type 1 and type 2 diabetes.[7-9]

**3** Pattern management includes a review of all parameters of intensive management (food, exercise, stress, and illness) not just insulin adjustment.[10] (Table 5.1)

**4** Timing of glucose monitoring is variable depending on the pharmacological therapy and glucose goals.

**A** SMBG is done at the peak effect of the medication so that the appropriate insulin or medication can be adjusted (see the Problem-Solving Practice section of this chapter for examples).

- Premeal glucose measurements are needed to monitor basal (or background) insulin dose(s) (eg, NPH, glargine, or Ultralente) and to determine the dose/timing of the premeal (bolus) insulin dose(s). (Tables 5.2, 5.3)

## Table 5.1. Questions to Ask When Evaluating Blood Glucose Readings

**1** Is there a pattern appearing upon examination of 3 to 5 days of blood glucose readings?

**2** Does something happen at the same time every day, such as an insulin reaction, high glucose after breakfast, etc.?

**3** Are there blood glucose readings representing all "times" of the day?

**4** Are there blood glucose readings representing the "peak" times of each medication (insulins and/or oral agents)?

**5** Are there readings to represent peak glucose readings after all meals?

**6** Are there "other notes" or "changes" such as meal times, carbohydrate or calorie variances, exercise changes, unusual hours of work or school, stress, illness, etc.?

**7** Is prevention of weight gain important for the patient? If so, consideration must be given to trying to reduce the use of hypoglycemic medications (ie, insulin or insulin secretagogues), especially if low blood glucose levels are occurring routinely.

- Two-hour postprandial (pp) glucose readings are needed to titrate rapid-acting (eg, lispro, aspart) insulin for multiple injections. (Tables 5.4, 5.5, 5.6)
- Two-hour postinjection SMBG readings are needed to titrate rapid-acting (lispro, aspart) insulin.
- The effectiveness of metformin, thiazolidinediones (TZDs), alpha glucosidase inhibitors, glipizide, repaglinide, nateglinide, and others is tested using 2-hour postprandial readings.

**B** Insulin pump therapy requires SMBG levels 4 to 6 times per day to determine the effectiveness of the basal dose and the amount of the bolus dose.

**C** Pregnancy requires frequent SMBG (eg, 5 to 6 times per day) in order to make the adjustments needed for tight blood glucose control (see Chapter 2, Pregnancy, in Diabetes in the Life Cycle and Research).

**D** During acute illness, premeal testing is needed to determine the need for and dose of any supplemental insulin.

**E** Elevated fasting glucose levels require 3 AM testing at least once a week to rule out the Somogyi (rebound) syndrome or the dawn phenomenon.

**F** Asymptomatic hypoglycemia requires regular testing on a daily basis, particularly at peak insulin times and before driving as a precaution for recognizing low blood glucose levels.

**G** Unusual schedules present special challenges where use of pattern management and evaluation can help to maintain blood glucose levels.

- Travel across time zones, working night or swing shifts, farming, business schedules, and college student schedules all can make blood glucose levels difficult to control. Food intake varies and may not always be able to be scheduled. Eating out makes it difficult to estimate carbohydrate content or calories. Exercise opportunities are also variable.
- Each situation requires flexibility and individual planning. Understanding medications and their actions, especially insulin action, is critical. Start with the

individual's plan and factor in special situations related to food intake, meal patterns, medication, and activity.

- SMBG is critical and may be required 6 to 8 times per day until insulin doses are adequately titrated and glucose goals are attained. SMBG should be done pre-meal, 2 hours postmeal, at bed time, and between 2 and 3 AM.
- If the individual is unable to eat (especially children) or is hypoglycemic, rapid-acting insulin may be given at the end of the meal.

**5** Objective summary assessment of glycemia is needed in addition to SMBG data.

   **A** Glycosylated hemoglobin (HbA1c) is measured quarterly until goals are reached and then at least 2 times per year.[5]

   **B** Glycosylated albumin (fructosamine) may be used for biweekly testing during pregnancy[11] and for others needing a more rapid assessment of overall glycemic control.

**6** Other insulin therapy options can include long-term algorithm approaches or sliding scales.

   **A** The *algorithm approach* to insulin therapy is used to provide variation in the usual insulin dose; supplemental insulins are often utilized. Algorithm approaches may be compensatory or anticipatory.

- *Compensatory insulin changes*—This supplement is additional insulin used to correct unusual hyperglycemia in response to an unanticipated event (eg, acute illness). Medical centers use different methods to determine the compensatory insulin dose.
- Some centers may develop an individualized table listing premeal blood glucose levels above (or below) target goal ranges, and the number of units of premeal rapid-acting or short-acting insulin that should be added (or subtracted) from the usual premeal insulin dose. For example, if the premeal glucose level is 50 mg/dL (2.7 mmol/L) higher than the target blood glucose goal, the individual is instructed to take an additional 1 unit of insulin. If there is a consistent pattern of increasing or decreasing insulin doses, a change is made in the insulin affecting that time period.
- Other centers may use other methods. An example of formulas used to compensate for a high blood glucose is the 1500 rule for short-acting insulin and the 1800 rule for rapid-acting insulin. Use of this formula provides a starting point for bringing down glucose elevations.
- 1500 rule: 1500 ÷ current total daily insulin dose = *sensitivity factor* (sensitivity factor defines how much a unit of insulin will lower blood glucose); supplemental dose = actual blood glucose minus goal blood glucose ÷ sensitivity factor. The 1800 rule (for rapid-acting insulins) is calculated in the same manner, substituting 1800 for 1500.
- *Anticipatory insulin changes*—This supplement is additional insulin administered before expected increases in carbohydrate intake. Various formulas are available for calculating carbohydrate-to-insulin ratios (see Chapter 1, Medical Nutrition Therapy for Diabetes, and Chapter 6, Insulin Pump Therapy and Carbohydrate Counting for Pump Therapy: Carbohydrate-to-Insulin Ratios, in Diabetes Management Therapies). One unit of rapid-acting or short-acting insulin per 10 to 15 g of carbohydrate is a common starting point.
- If the premeal glucose is low, the appropriate insulin dose (rapid-acting) may be decreased, given at the time the person eats, or given at the end of the meal.

**B** The sliding scale approach tries to solve the problem only for a particular point in time but does not prevent the problem from occurring again.
- Sliding scale doses are given in addition to the usual insulin dose. The supplements are given in relation to a range of preset blood glucose values.
- A typical sliding scale program suggests a preset amount of insulin based on glucose readings, regardless of age or weight. The result is often a roller coaster-like shift between hypoglycemia and hyperglycemia, a situation that does nothing to contribute to overall health or feelings of well-being for the patient.
- If a sliding scale is used, it should be based on past patterns of the individual patient.

## Combination Therapies

**1** In the 1980s, combination therapy was limited to insulin and sulfonylurea combinations. The recent availability of multiple oral agents for the treatment of type 2 diabetes has created many new therapeutic options.

**2** A common combination is initiating monotherapy with either a sulfonylurea or metformin and adding the other agent when the doses approach maximum therapeutic limits. This combination requires specific clinical considerations.
- **A** Careful patient selection regarding liver, renal, and respiratory function (thiazolidinediones and metformin)
- **B** Prevention of possible hypoglycemia with *insulin secretagogues* (sulfonylureas, repaglinide, nateglinide)
- **C** Need for postprandial SMBG for dose titration
- **D** Patient reporting excess flatulence or diarrhea
- **E** Guidelines as to when agents should be taken in relation to meals (eg, sulfonylureas are taken 30 minutes prior to the meal; metformin is taken with the meal to reduce gastrointestinal disturbances and enhance medication action).[12]

**3** Alpha glucosidase inhibitors may be added as a third agent or used as monotherapy; taking with meals enhances medication action and reduces gastrointestinal side effects.

**4** The first thiazolidinediones (TZD) was initially approved for use in combination with insulin.[13] Recent studies have demonstrated TZDs effectiveness for other indications.[14,15]
- **A** Because the time to therapeutic response can be 6 to 8 weeks, other agents may need to be available to control hyperglycemia.
- **B** After the glycemic benefit occurs, doses of insulin or other oral agents may be titrated downward.
- **C** TZDs appear to be more effective when used in combination with other agents (see Chapter 3, Pharmacologic Therapies, in Diabetes Management Therapies, for additional information).

**5** Repaglinide and nateglinide provide additional options for combination therapies with metformin and/or TZDs.

**6** Postprandial glucose monitoring will give the most information for dose titration for all oral agents except metformin.

## Table 5.2. Pattern Management—Premeal Monitoring

### Insulin (3 injections per day)

Lispro, aspart, or regular/NPH insulin (or 70/30 or 75/25), AM dose
Lispro, aspart, or regular insulin (or 70/30 or 75/25), PM dose
NPH insulin, bedtime dose

### Evaluate Blood Glucose (BG) Patterns

1. Adjust insulin based on 2- to 3-day BG patterns.
2. Determine which insulin is responsible for the pattern.
3. Adjust insulin 10% to 20%.
4. 2-hour pp blood glucose tests needed for lispro or aspart titration.
5. If using lispro or aspart, 1 injection of NPH insulin may not provide 24-hour basal coverage in insulinopenic patients.

*[handwritten margin note: inconsistent w/answer to case study Q19]*

*[handwritten margin note: duplicate]*

| AM | Below Target Blood Glucose | Above Target Blood Glucose |
|---|---|---|
| Dose affecting | *Bedtime NPH insulin* | *Bedtime NPH insulin* |
| | 1. Consider increasing carbohydrate content or calories of the evening snack | 1. Consider decreasing carbohydrate content or calories of the evening snack. |
| | 2. Determine if low blood glucose is occurring during or after exercise. | 2. Evaluate nocturnal hypoglycemia or hyperglycemia (check 3 AM BG). |
| | 3. Evaluate nocturnal hypoglycemia (check 3 AM BG). | 3. Evaluate nocturnal hypoglycemia (check 3 AM BG). |
| | 4. Consider decreasing bedtime NPH insulin. | 4. Consider increasing bedtime NPH insulin. |

| Midday Lunch | Below Target Blood Glucose | Above Target Blood Glucose |
|---|---|---|
| Dose affecting | AM *lispro, aspart, or regular insulin* | AM *lispro, aspart, or regular insulin* |
| | 1. Consider increasing carbohydrate content or calories of midmorning snack. | 1. Consider decreasing carbohydrate content or calories of the midmorning snack. |
| | 2. Determine if low blood glucose is occurring during or after exercise. | 2. Consider adjusting exercise times or adding exercise. |
| | 3. Consider decreasing AM lispro, aspart, or regular insulin. | 3. Consider increasing AM lispro, aspart, or regular insulin. |

| PM Supper | Below Target Blood Glucose | Above Target Blood Glucose |
|---|---|---|
| Dose affecting | AM *NPH insulin* | AM *NPH insulin* |
| | 1. Consider increasing carbohydrate content or calories of afternoon snack. | 1. Consider decreasing carbohydrate content or calories of the afternoon snack. |
| | 2. Determine if low blood glucose is occurring during or after exercise. | 2. Consider adjusting exercise times or adding exercise. |
| | 3. Consider decreasing AM NPH insulin. | 3. Consider increasing AM NPH insulin. |

| Bedtime | Below Target Blood Glucose | Above Target Blood Glucose |
|---|---|---|
| Dose affecting | PM *lispro, aspart, or regular insulin* | PM *lispro, aspart, or regular insulin* |
| | 1. Consider increasing carbohydrate content or calories of supper. | 1. Consider decreasing carbohydrate content or calories of supper. |
| | 2. Determine if low blood glucose is occurring during or after exercise. | 2. Consider adjusting exercise times or adding exercise. |
| | 3. Consider decreasing PM lispro, aspart, or regular insulin. | 3. Consider increasing PM lispro, aspart, or regular insulin. |

## Table 5.3. Pattern Management—Premeal Monitoring

### Insulin (4 injections per day)

Lispro, aspart, or regular insulin, AM dose
Lispro, aspart, or regular insulin, midday dose
Lispro, aspart, or regular insulin, PM dose
NPH or glargine insulin, bedtime dose or Ultralente, supper dose

### Evaluate Blood Glucose (BG) Patterns

1 Adjust insulin based on 2- to 3-day BG patterns.
2 Determine which insulin is responsible for the pattern.
3 Adjust insulin 10% to 20%.
4 2-hour pp blood glucose testing needed for lispro or aspart titration.
5 If using lispro or aspart, 1 injection of NPH insulin may not provide 24-hour basal coverage in insulinopenic patients.

| AM | Below Target Blood Glucose | Above Target Blood Glucose |
|---|---|---|
| Dose affecting | *Bedtime NPH or glargine insulin or supper Ultralente*<br>1 Consider increasing evening snack.<br>2 Evaluate nocturnal hypoglycemia (check 3 AM BG).<br>3 Consider decreasing bedtime NPH, glargine, or Ultralente insulin. | *Bedtime NPH or glargine insulin or supper Ultralente*<br>1 Consider decreasing evening snack.<br>2 Evaluate nocturnal hypoglycemia or hyperglycemia (check 3 AM BG).<br>3 Consider increasing bedtime NPH, glargine, or Ultralente insulin. |

| Midday Lunch | Below Target Blood Glucose | Above Target Blood Glucose |
|---|---|---|
| Dose affecting | AM *lispro, aspart, or regular insulin*<br>1 Consider increasing carbohydrate content or calories of midmorning snack.<br>2 Determine if low blood glucose is occurring during or after exercise.<br>3 Consider decreasing AM lispro, aspart, or regular insulin. | AM *lispro, aspart, or regular insulin*<br>1 Consider decreasing carbohydrate content or calories of the midmorning snack.<br>2 Consider adjusting exercise times or adding exercise.<br>3 Consider increasing AM lispro, aspart, or regular insulin. |

| PM Supper | Below Target Blood Glucose | Above Target Blood Glucose |
|---|---|---|
| Dose affecting | *Midday lispro, aspart, or regular insulin*<br>1 Consider increasing carbohydrate content or calories of the afternoon snack.<br>2 Determine if low blood glucose is occurring during or after exercise.<br>3 Consider decreasing insulin. | *Midday lispro, aspart, or regular insulin*<br>1 Consider decreasing carbohydrate content or calories of the afternoon snack.<br>2 Consider adjusting exercise times or adding exercise.<br>3 Consider increasing insulin. |

| Bedtime | Below Target Blood Glucose | Above Target Blood Glucose |
|---|---|---|
| Dose affecting | PM *lispro, aspart, or regular insulin*<br>1 Consider increasing carbohydrate content or calories of supper.<br>2 Determine if low blood glucose is occurring during or after exercise.<br>3 Consider decreasing PM lispro, aspart, or regular insulin. | PM *lispro, aspart, or regular insulin*<br>1 Consider decreasing carbohydrate content or calories of supper.<br>2 Consider adjusting exercise times or adding exercise.<br>3 Consider increasing PM lispro, aspart, or regular insulin. |

## Table 5.4. Pattern Management—2 Hours Postmeal Monitoring

### Insulin (2 injections per day)

Lispro, aspart, or regular insulin/NPH AM dose
Lispro, aspart, or regular insulin/NPH PM dose

### Evaluate Blood Glucose (BG) Patterns

1 Adjust insulin based on 2- to 3-day BG patterns.
2 Determine which insulin is responsible for the pattern.
3 Adjust insulin by 10% to 20% of total daily dose.
4 2-hour pp blood glucose testing needed for lispro or aspart titration.
5 If using lispro or aspart, 1 injection of NPH insulin may not provide 24-hour basal coverage for insulinopenic patients.

| 2-h pp Breakfast | Below Target Blood Glucose | Above Target Blood Glucose |
|---|---|---|
| *Dose affecting* | AM *lispro, aspart, or regular insulin* | AM *lispro, aspart, or regular insulin* |
| | 1 Consider increasing carbohydrate content or calories of breakfast. | 1 Consider decreasing carbohydrate content at breakfast. |
| | 2 Determine if low blood glucose is occurring during or after exercise. | 2 Consider adjusting exercise times or adding exercise. |
| | 3 Consider decreasing AM lispro, aspart, or regular insulin. | 3 Consider giving regular injection 45 minutes before meal. |
| | | 4 Consider increasing AM lispro, aspart, or regular insulin. |

| 2-h pp Lunch | Below Target Blood Glucose | Above Target Blood Glucose |
|---|---|---|
| *Dose affecting* | AM *NPH insulin* | AM *NPH insulin* |
| | 1 Consider increasing carbohydrate content or calories of lunch. | 1 Consider decreasing carbohydrate content or calories of lunch. |
| | 2 Determine if low blood glucose is occurring during or after exercise. | 2 Consider adjusting exercise times or adding exercise. |
| | 3 Consider decreasing AM NPH insulin. | 3 Consider increasing AM NPH insulin. |

| 2-h pp Supper | Below Target Blood Glucose | Above Target Blood Glucose |
|---|---|---|
| *Dose affecting* | PM *lispro, aspart, or regular insulin* | PM *lispro, aspart, or regular insulin* |
| | 1 Consider increasing carbohydrate content or calories of supper. | 1 Consider decreasing carbohydrate content or calories of supper. |
| | 2 Determine if low blood glucose is occurring during or after exercise. | 2 Consider adjusting exercise times or adding exercise. |
| | 3 Consider decreasing PM lispro, aspart, or regular insulin. | 3 Consider giving regular injection 45 minutes before meal. |
| | | 4 Consider increasing PM lispro, aspart, or regular insulin. |

## Table 5.5. Pattern Management—2 Hours Postmeal Monitoring

### Insulin (3 injections per day)

Lispro, aspart, or regular/NPH insulin, AM dose
Lispro, aspart, or regular insulin, PM dose
NPH insulin, bedtime dose

### Evaluate Blood Glucose (BG) Patterns

1 Adjust insulin based on 2- to 3-day BG patterns.
2 Determine which insulin is responsible for the pattern.
3 Adjust insulin 10% to 20%.
4 2-hour pp blood glucose testing needed for lispro or aspart titration.
5 If using lispro or aspart, 1 injection of NPH insulin may not provide 24-hour basal coverage for insulinopenic patients.

| 2-h pp Breakfast | Below Target Blood Glucose | Above Target Blood Glucose |
|---|---|---|
| Dose affecting | AM *lispro, aspart, or regular insulin* <br> 1 Consider increasing carbohydrate content or calories of breakfast. <br> 2 Determine if low blood glucose is occurring during or after exercise. <br> 3 Consider decreasing AM lispro, aspart, or regular insulin. | AM *lispro, apart, or regular insulin* <br> 1 Consider decreasing carbohydrate content or calories at breakfast. <br> 2 Consider adjusting exercise times or adding exercise. <br> 3 Consider giving regular injection 45 minutes before meal. <br> 4 Consider increasing AM lispro, aspart, or regular insulin. |

| 2-h pp Lunch | Below Target Blood Glucose | Above Target Blood Glucose |
|---|---|---|
| Dose affecting | AM *NPH insulin* <br> 1 Consider increasing carbohydrate content or calories of lunch. <br> 2 Determine if low blood glucose is occurring during or after exercise. <br> 3 Consider decreasing NPH insulin. | AM *NPH insulin* <br> 1 Consider decreasing carbohydrate content or calories of lunch. <br> 2 Consider adjusting exercise times or adding exercise. <br> 3 Consider increasing NPH insulin. |

| 2-h pp Supper | Below Target Blood Glucose | Above Target Blood Glucose |
|---|---|---|
| Dose affecting | PM *lispro, aspart, or regular insulin* <br> 1 Consider increasing carbohydrate content or calories of supper. <br> 2 Determine if low blood glucose is occurring during or after exercise. <br> 3 Consider decreasing lispro, aspart, or regular insulin. | PM *lispro, aspart, or regular insulin* <br> 1 Consider decreasing carbohydrate content or calories of supper. <br> 2 Consider adjusting exercise times or adding exercise. <br> 3 Consider giving regular injection 45 minutes before meal. <br> 4 Consider increasing PM lispro, aspart, or regular insulin. |

## Table 5.6.  Pattern Management—2 Hours Postmeal Monitoring

### Insulin (4 injections per day)

Lispro, aspart, or regular insulin, AM dose
Lispro, aspart, or regular insulin, midday dose
Lispro, aspart, or regular insulin, PM dose
NPH or glargine insulin, bedtime dose or Ultralente, supper dose

### Evaluate Blood Glucose (BG) Patterns

**1** Adjust insulin based on 2- to 3-day BG patterns.
**2** Determine which insulin is responsible for the pattern.
**3** Adjust insulin 10% to 20%.
**4** 2-hour pp blood glucose testing needed for lispro or aspart titration.
**5** If using lispro or aspart, 1 injection of NPH insulin may not provide 24-hour basal coverage for insulinopenic patients.

| 2-h pp Breakfast | Below Target Blood Glucose | Above Target Blood Glucose |
|---|---|---|
| *Dose affecting* | AM *lispro, aspart, or regular insulin* | AM *lispor, aspart, or regular insulin* |
| | **1** Consider increasing carbohydrate content or calories of breakfast. | **1** Consider decreasing carbohydrate content or calories at breakfast. |
| | **2** Determine if low blood glucose is occurring during or after exercise. | **2** Consider adjusting exercise times or adding exercise. |
| | **3** Consider decreasing AM lispro, aspart, or regular insulin. | **3** Consider giving regular injection minutes before meal. |
| | | **4** Consider increasing AM lispro, aspart, or regular insulin. |

| 2-h pp Lunch | Below Target Blood Glucose | Above Target Blood Glucose |
|---|---|---|
| *Dose affecting* | *Midday lispro, apart, or regular insulin* | *Midday lispro, aspart, or regular insulin* |
| | **1** Consider increasing carbohydrate content or calories of lunch. | **1** Consider decreasing carbohydrate content or calories of lunch. |
| | **2** Determine if low blood glucose is occurring during or after exercise. | **2** Consider adjusting exercise times or adding exercise. |
| | **3** Consider decreasing midday lispro, aspart, or regular insulin. | **3** Consider giving regular injection 45 minutes before meal. |
| | | **4** Consider increasing midday lispro, aspart, or regular insulin. |

| 2-h pp Supper | Below Target Blood Glucose | Above Target Blood Glucose |
|---|---|---|
| *Dose affecting* | PM *lispro, aspart, or regular insulin* | PM *lispro, aspart, or regular insulin* |
| | **1** Consider increasing carbohydrate content or calories of supper. | **1** Consider decreasing carbohydrate content or calories of supper. |
| | **2** Determine if low blood glucose is occurring during or after exercise. | **2** Consider adjusting exercise times or adding exercise. |
| | **3** Consider decreasing PM lispro, aspart, or regular insulin. | **3** Consider giving regular injection 45 minutes before meal. |
| | | **4** Consider increasing PM lispro, aspart, or regular insulin. |

## Problem-Solving Practice

This section is designed to provide practice in pattern management through the evaluation of blood glucose logs and determination of problems, possible causes, and options for adjustments. Use the following as a guide for all of these situations.

Goals when well: Blood glucose levels in target range without significant hypoglycemic episodes; no ketones.

1   Monitor fasting and 2-hour postprandial blood glucose levels.
2   Analyze records once or twice per week.
3   For type 1 diabetes, aim for 75% to 85% in the target range; for type 2 diabetes, aim for 95% to 100% in the target range. *Seems high*
4   Increase or decrease food as the first change. *wrong*
5   Evaluate exercise amount and timing.
6   Change insulin dose in amounts of 1 + 2 units or 10%.
7   Evaluate sites and timing of injections.
8   Evaluate the need for stress management.
9   If blood glucose levels are erratic due to Somogyi (rebound) syndrome, consider decreasing insulin dose by ~10%.

## Sean

Type 1 diabetes
- Breakfast—12 units lispro/8 units NPH
- Lunch—3 units lispro
- Supper—14 units lispro
- Bedtime—11 units NPH
- 2600 calories—3 meals, 1 snack

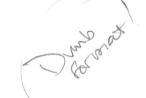

| Time | Mon | Thurs | Sun |
|---|---|---|---|
| Fasting | 100 mg/dL | 110 mg/dL | 103 mg/dL |
| After breakfast | 322 | 284 | 250 |
| Before lunch | | | |
| After lunch | 280 | 246 | 150 |
| Before supper | | | |
| After supper | 148 | 131 | 133 |
| Changes | | | |
| Food | +2 milk | pancakes, OJ | +1 toast |
| Insulin/Medication | | | |
| Reactions | | | |
| Activity | ↑ | | |
| Remarks | 7 PM football | | |

Key:  Food changes/time          Activity                    Reaction/Illness
        +1 = 1 extra CHO (15 g)     ↑ increased activity     M = mild     S = severe
        −1 = 1 less CHO (15 g)      ↓ decreased activity     Mo = moderate

## Problem

- Pattern of high blood glucose levels after breakfast and lunch

## Possible Causes

- Too much carbohydrate at breakfast/lunch
- Not enough insulin before breakfast/lunch

## Options

- Consider changing something in routine before the high tests:
    —Decrease total carbohydrate at breakfast/lunch
    —Include exercise
    —Increase lispro insulin before breakfast/lunch

## Ethel

Type 2 diabetes
- Glipizide 10 mg bid
- Metformin 1000 mg bid
- 1400 calories

| Time | Mon | Wed | Sat |
|---|---|---|---|
| Fasting | 72 mg/dL | 60 mg/dL | 71 mg/dL |
| After breakfast | 100 | 53 | 67 |
| Before lunch | | | |
| After lunch | 64 | 55 | 90 |
| Before supper | | | |
| After supper | 80 | 66 | 91 |
| Changes | | | |
| Food | +1/2 OJ | +1/2 milk | +1/2 honey |
| Insulin/Medication | | | |
| Reactions | 2:30 PM M | 9:15 AM M | 11:30 AM M |
| Activity | | Usual | Usual |
| Remarks | Yardwork | Picking beans | |

Key:  Food changes/time      Activity                  Reaction/Illness
        +1 = 1 extra CHO (15 g)   ↑ increased activity    M = mild    S = severe
        −1 = 1 less CHO (15 g)    ↓ decreased activity    Mo = moderate

## Problem

- Reactions too often throughout the day

## Possible Causes

- Too much medication
- Inadequate carbohydrate or total food intake

*inadequate Rx of hypoglyc.*

## Options

- Consider decreasing sulfonylurea until blood glucose is >100 mg/dL postprandially (individuals who do not want to gain weight) or
- Increase food 100 to 200 calories (individuals who want to gain weight). Example: 100 calories = 1½ CHO or 1½ meat. Distribute throughout the day.  *Bad answers*
- If individual was taking insulin, decrease doses by 10% overall.

*↳ only backgrd since PP ok*

## Mark (college student)

Type 1 diabetes
- Breakfast—34 units 70/30
- Supper—6 units R
- Bedtime—11 units NPH
- 2900 calories—3 meals, 3 snacks

| Schedule | Tues | Thurs | Sat |
|---|---|---|---|
| Fasting | 106 mg/dL | 110 mg/dL | 117 mg/dL |
| After breakfast | 175 | 341 | 148 |
| Before lunch | | | |
| After lunch | 151 | 150 | 229 |
| Before supper | | | |
| After supper | 135 | 153 | 210 |
| Changes | | | |
| Food | No change | No change | No change |
| Insulin/Medication | | | |
| Reactions | | | |
| Activity | Usual | Usual | Usual |
| Remarks | | | |

Key:  Food changes/time        Activity                    Reaction/Illness
      +1 = 1 extra CHO (15 g)   ↑ increased activity        M = mild     S = severe
      −1 = 1 less CHO (15 g)    ↓ decreased activity        Mo = moderate

## Problem

- Erratic blood glucose levels

## Possible Causes

- Injection sites
- Stress
- Somogyi (rebound, over insulinization)

## Options

- No change in dose, as 75% are less than 180 mg/dL postprandially
- Consider changing insulin regimen to rapid-acting insulin premeal for greater food flexibility

## Melissa

Type 1 diabetes
• Breakfast—3 units lispro/2 units Ultralente
• Lunch—2 units lispro
• Supper—4 units lispro/2 units Ultralente
• 1800 calories

| Schedule | Thurs | Sat | Sun |
|---|---|---|---|
| Fasting | 110 mg/dL | 150 mg/dL | 163 mg/dL |
| After breakfast | 132 | 191 | 198 |
| Before lunch | | | |
| After lunch | 163 | 161 | 185 |
| Before supper | | | |
| After supper | 128 | 230 | 236 |
| Changes | | | |
| Food | | | |
| Insulin/Medication | | | |
| Reactions | | | |
| Activity | Usual | Usual | Usual |
| Remarks | | | |

Key:    Food changes/time          Activity                        Reaction/Illness
        +1 = 1 extra CHO (15 g)     ⬆ increased activity      M = mild     S = severe
        –1 = 1 less CHO (15 g)      ⬇ decreased activity      Mo = moderate

## Problem

• Gradual increase in overall blood glucose levels

## Possible Causes

• Out of "honeymoon" stage
• Illness
• Pregnancy
• Puberty
• Insulin losing potency
• Increased stressors at work, school, or home

*(handwritten notes: weekend different schedule/ eats/activity than week. but is "usual" for her. Don't do by call!)*

## Options

• For adults: Consider decreasing food intake 100 to 200 calories and/or increase exercise. However, most women with type 1 diabetes eat at least 1800 calories.
• For children or adults: Consider increasing insulin 1 to 2 steps or 10% overall. Try this dose for 2 to 3 days. Increase again if blood glucose is still high. If 3 dose adjustments do not decrease blood glucose levels, instruct patient to call the diabetes care team.

## Mary

Type 2 diabetes
- Actos 45 mg (for 1 week)
- 1600 calories

| Schedule | Tues | Thurs | Sat |
|---|---|---|---|
| Fasting | 314 mg/dL | 288 mg/dL | 301 mg/dL |
| After breakfast | 282 | 214 | 285 |
| Before lunch | | | |
| After lunch | 296 | 322 | 274 |
| Before supper | | | |
| After supper | 252 | 297 | 244 |
| Changes | | | |
| Food | Birthday party 8 PM | Church lunch | Very careful |
| Insulin/Medication | X | X | After breakfast |
| Reactions | | | |
| Activity | Shopping | | |
| Remarks | | Tired | |

Key:  Food changes/time     Activity     Reaction/Illness
    +1 = 1 extra CHO (15 g)    ↑ increased activity    M = mild    S = severe
    −1 = 1 less CHO (15 g)    ↓ decreased activity    Mo = moderate

## Problem

- Blood glucose levels are too high

## Possible Cause

- TZD not taken long enough ✓

## Options

- Consider adding another oral glucose-lowering medication
- Consider adding sulfonylurea or insulin for 4 to 6 weeks, then reevaluate

## John

Type 2 diabetes
- AM—20 mg glucotrol, 1000 mg metformin
- PM—20 mg glucotrol, 1000 mg metformin
- 1800 calories

| Schedule | Mon | Wed | Sat |
|---|---|---|---|
| Fasting | 180 mg/dL | 192 mg/dL | 219 mg/dL |
| After breakfast | 145 | 154 | 138 |
| Before lunch | | | |
| After lunch | 162 | 143 | 121 |
| Before supper | | | |
| After supper | 129 | 116 | 95 |
| Changes | | | |
| Diet | 2000 | | |
| Insulin/Medication | X | X | X |
| Reactions | | | |
| Activity | Work at airplane factory | Work | "honey do" list and football |
| Remarks | | | |

*Not taking medications* (handwritten annotation)

Key:  Food changes/time  Activity  Reaction/Illness
+1 = 1 extra CHO (15 g)  ↑ increased activity  M = mild    S = severe
−1 = 1 less CHO (15 g)  ↓ decreased activity  Mo = moderate

## Problem

- High fasting blood glucose levels

## Possible Cause

- Inadequate medication in evening or at bedtime to prevent dawn phenomenon

## Options

- Assure individual the high fasting glucose levels are not because he/she ate too much at dinner or during the evening. Explain that food eaten is used or stored in 4 to 5 hours. Explain how the liver releases excessive glucose in the early morning hours if adequate insulin is not available.
- Consider adding bedtime NPH insulin dose
- Consider splitting supper meds

## Summary

**1** Diabetes therapy in the next century will become more specific to the physiologic or genetic problems leading to hyperglycemia.

**2** New agents are emerging that allow treatment of the specific cause of the hyperglycemia from insulin resistance to hepatic glucose output or beta cell secretory defects.

**A** Insulin analogs allow very precise treatment based on lifestyles and variables in eating and exercise routines.

**B** Insulin pump therapy is changing due to use of these insulin analogs.

**3** The success of this complex therapy depends on the skill and expertise of the educator in presenting and verifying understanding of self-management skills for the individual with diabetes.

**4** Practitioners will require continuing education, protocols, and support from diabetes experts if these new therapies are to be effective for improving patient outcomes and quality of life.

## Key Educational Considerations

**1** Pattern management can be used by both type 1 and type 2 patients. Careful assessment of the patient's readiness to participate actively in such a program is critical to the success of pattern management.

**2** Comprehensive self-management education is essential to achieve success in pattern management techniques. Particular emphasis for education includes

**A** Monitoring and recording blood glucose results

**B** Medications and appropriate blood glucose testing times to validate efficacy

**C** Medical nutrition therapy

**D** Exercise

**E** Hypoglycemia

**F** Sick-day care

**G** Team care

**H** Psychosocial implications

**I** Role of individual with diabetes in self-management

**3** Engage individuals with diabetes in problem-solving situations during instruction to teach pattern recognition and application of appropriate options.

**4** Assure individuals with diabetes that they will be able to access their healthcare team when necessary to establish confidence that self-initiated changes can be made safely.

## Self-Review Questions

**1** If a patient's fasting blood glucose levels are elevated, what would you do to determine the cause?

**2** If you determined that a patient's elevated fasting glucose level is due to low blood glucose levels during the night, what therapy changes could be made?

**3** If a patient is taking the maximum dose of an oral sulfonylurea and insulin therapy is recommended, what other options might you suggest?

**4** If a patient has persistently elevated glucose readings at midmorning or prelunch, what adjustment could be made?

**5** If a patient's presupper glucose level is elevated, what options are available to improve that blood glucose?

## Learning Assessment: Case Study 1

KS, a 14-year-old adolescent with type 1 diabetes, is going to try out for volleyball. Her games are at 5:30 PM. KS takes her insulin (70/30) at 4:30 PM, eats dinner, and then plays volleyball. However, KS is having low blood glucose levels during every game. Her fasting glucose levels (at 7 AM) are always above 170 mg/dL. She usually takes her morning injection of 70/30 insulin at 7:30 AM.

## Questions for Discussion

**1** What are reasons for KS's elevated fasting glucose levels?

**2** What could you suggest that would provide increased flexibility and help KS meet her glycemic goals?

## Discussion

**1** KS has a hectic schedule and would likely benefit from splitting the evening 70/30 injection into rapid-acting or short-acting insulin at suppertime and NPH at 10 PM. Her suppertime insulin and supper meal could be after the volleyball game.

**2** Giving the NPH at 10 PM would shift its peak to early morning. That single change may correct her elevated fasting level. If not, the bedtime NPH dose could be increased by 1 to 2 units every 2 to 3 days until the fasting blood glucose levels are within range.

**3** The rationale behind KS's current use of 70/30 insulin must be explored as there may be personal, emotional, or developmental issues in conflict with KS's pursuit of other options that are available for improved glycemic control. A switch to the new 75/25 mix (lispro instead of the regular insulin in 70/30) would allow her to take her morning injection and eat immediately.

## Learning Assessment: Case Study 2

SA is taking 40 mg of glipizide. Her doctor tells her she could stop taking this medication if she could lose 75 lb. At her annual physical last week, the doctor said her laboratory values were good, except for her fasting blood glucose of 248 mg/dL, and her HbA1c was 11.3%. He recommends insulin injections, but SA does not want to give herself injections.

## Questions for Discussion

**1** What do you say to SA about the advice to lose 75 lb?

**2** Are there other oral agents that might be effective?

**3** What lab work is needed prior to initiating TZD or metformin?

## Discussion

**1** Explain to SA that improving blood glucose is more important than losing weight. Even if individuals lose 75 lb most individuals cannot maintain that level of weight loss long-term. However, even a weight loss of 10 lb can be helpful. Explain to SA the progressive nature of type 2 diabetes and the need to change medical therapies.

**2** SA might be a candidate for metformin. If her creatinine is <1.4 mg/dL, she might start with 500 mg at breakfast, with weekly increases of 500 mg at supper, then twice daily until she reaches the clinically therapeutic dose of 2000 mg/day or until she reaches her blood glucose goals.

**3** SA may also be a candidate for adding a TZD if her liver function studies are within normal limits. However, it may take 6 to 8 weeks at starting doses to obtain full glycemic response.

**4** Repaglinide before meals may also be a consideration in lieu of glyburide. While similar to a sulfonylurea, it differs by increasing first-phase insulin release for patients who still have endogenous insulin producing ability.

# References

**1** The Diabetes Control and Complications Trial Research Group. The effect of intensive treatment of diabetes on the development and progression of long-term complications in insulin-dependent diabetes mellitus. N Engl J Med. 1993;329:977-986.

**2** UK Prospective Diabetes Study (UKPDS) Group. Intensive blood-glucose control with sulphonylureas or insulin compared with conventional treatment and risk of complications in patients with type 2 diabetes (UKPDS 33). Lancet. 1998;352:837-853.

**3** Ohkubo Y, Kishikawa H, Araki E, et al. Intensive insulin therapy prevents the progression of diabetic microvascular complications in Japanese patients with non-insulin-dependent diabetes mellitus: a randomized prospective 6-year study. Diabetes Res Clin Pract. 1995;28:103-117.

**4** Hirsch I. Implementation of intensive diabetes therapy for IDDM. Diabetes Rev. 1995;3:288-307.

**5** American Diabetes Association. National standards for diabetes self-management education programs. Diabetes Care. 2001;24(suppl 1):S126-S133.

**6** Guthrie DW, Guthrie RA, eds. Nursing Management of Diabetes Mellitus. 4th ed. New York: Springer; 1997.

**7** Jackson RL, Kelly HG. Growth of children with diabetes mellitus in relationship to level of control of the disease. J Pediatr. 1946;29:316.

**8** Jackson RL, Guthrie RA. Physiologic Management of Diabetes in Children. New York: Medical Examination Publishers; 1986:80-157.

**9** Shagan BP. Does anyone here know how to make insulin work backwards? Why sliding-scale insulin coverage doesn't work. Practical Diabetol. 1990;9(3):1-4.

**10** Guthrie DW, Guthrie RA. Approach to management. Diabetes Educ. 1990;16:401-406.

**11** American Diabetes Association. Tests of glycemia in diabetes (position statement). Diabetes Care. 2001;24(suppl 1):S80-S82.

**12** Childs BP, Guthrie RA, Carr M, McDaniel J, Rhiley D. Incorporating new diabetes oral agents into clinical practice. Diabetes Spectrum. 1996;9:266-268.

**13** Saltiel AR, Olefsky JM. Thiazolidinediones in the treatment of insulin resistance and type II diabetes. Diabetes. 1996;45:1661-1664.

**14** Aronoff S, Rosenblatt S, Braithwaite S, Egan JW, Mathisen AL, Schneider RL, The Pioglitazone 001 Study Group. Pioglitazone hydrochloride monotherapy improves glycemic control in the treatment of patients with type 2 diabetes. Diabetes Care. 2000;23:1605-1611.

**15** Phillips LS, Grunberger G, Miller E, Patwadhan R, Rappaport EB, Salzman A, for the Rosiglitazone Clinical Trials Study Group. Once- and twice-daily dosing with rosiglitazone improves glycemic control in patients with type 2 diabetes. Diabetes Care. 2001;24:308-315.

## Suggested Readings

Avignon A, Radauceanu A, Monnier L. Nonfasting plasma glucose is a better marker of diabetic control than fasting plasma glucose. Diabetes Care. 1997;20:1822-1826.

Bell D, Ovalle F, Shadmany S. Postprandial rather than preprandial glucose levels should be used for adjustment of rapid-acting insulins. Endocrine Practice. 2000;6:477-478.

Bergenstal R, Pearson J, Pearson T. Pattern Control: A Guide for Adjusting Your Insulin Dose. Minneapolis: IDC Publishing; 1997.

Brackenridge BP. Carbohydrate gram counting: a key to accurate meal-time boluses in intensive diabetes therapy. Practical Diabetol. 1992;11(2):22-28.

Brewer, KW, Chase HP, Owen, S, Garg, SK. Slicing the pie. Correlating HbA1c values with average blood glucose values in a pie chart form. Diabetes Care. 1998;21:209-212.

Brunelle BL, Llewelyn J, Anderson JH, Gale EA. Meta-analysis of the effect of insulin lispro on severe hypoglycemia in patients with type 1 diabetes. Diabetes Care. 1998;21:1726-1831.

Farkas-Hirsch R, ed. Intensive Diabetes Management. 2nd ed. Alexandria, Va: American Diabetes Association; 1998.

Hermansen K, Madsbad S, Perrild H, Kristensen A, Axelsen M. Comparison of the soluble basal insulin analog detemir with NPH insulin: a randomized open crossover trial in type 1 diabetic subjects on basal-bolus therapy. Diabetes Care. 2001;24:296-301.

Hirsch IB. Technological advances in diabetes care. Where are we going? Diabetes Spectrum. 1996;9:225-250.

Home PD, Lindholm A, Hylleberg B, Round P. Improved glycemic control with insulin aspart: a multicenter randomized double-blind crossover trial in type 1 diabetic patients. UK Insulin Aspart Study Group. Diabetes Care. 1998;21:1904-1909.

Howey DC, Bowsher RR, Brunelle RL, Woodworth JR. [Lys(B28), Pro(B29)]-human insulin. A rapidly absorbed analogue of human insulin. Diabetes. 1994;43:396-402.

Kalbag JB, Walter YH, Nedelman JR, McLeod JF. Mealtime glucose regulation with nateglinide in healthy volunteers: comparison with repaglinide and placebo. Diabetes Care. 2001;24:73-77.

Koivisto VA, Tuominen JA, Ebeling P. LisPro Mix25 insulin as premeal therapy in type 2 diabetic patients. Diabetes Care. 1999;22:459-462.

Lalli C, Ciofetta M, Del Sindaco P, et al. Long term intensive treatment of type 1 diabetes with the short-acting insulin analog lispro in variable combination with NPH insulin at mealtime. Diabetes Care. 1999;22;468-477.

Lindholm A, McEwen J, Riis AP. Improved postprandial glycemic control with insulin aspart. A randomized double-blind cross-over trial in type 1 diabetes. Diabetes Care. 1999;22:801-805.

Lebovitz HE, ed. Therapy for Diabetes Mellitus and Related Disorders. 3rd ed. 1998. Alexandria, Va: American Diabetes Association; 1998.

Pampanelli S, Torlone E, Talli C, et al. Improved postprandial metabolic control after subcutaneous injection of a short-acting insulin analog in IDDM of short duration with residual pancreatic b-cell function. Diabetes Care. 1995;18:1452-1459.

Peragallo-Dittko V. Tight control: a guide to getting started. Diabetes Self-Manage. 1996;13(5):20-24.

Pieber TR, Brunner GA, Schnedl WJ, Schattenberg S, Kaufmann P, Krejs GJ. Evaluation of a structured outpatient group education program for intensive insulin therapy. Diabetes Care. 1995;18:625-630.

Roach P, Yue L, Arora V. Improved postprandial glycemic control during treatment with Humalog Mix25, a novel protamine-based insulin lispro formulation. Diabetes Care. 1999;22:1258-1261.

Sawin CT. Action without benefit: The sliding scale of insulin use. Arch Intern Med. 1997;157:489.

Tuttleman M, Lipsett L, Harris MI. Attitudes and behaviors of primary care physicians regarding tight control of blood glucose in IDDM patients. Diabetes Care. 1993;16:765-772.

Ziegher O, Kolopp M, Louis J, Musse JP, Paris A, Debry G, Crouin P. Self-monitoring of blood glucose and insulin dose alteration in type I diabetes mellitus. Diabetes Res Clin Pract. 1993;21:51-59.

# Learning Assessment: Post-Test Questions

## Pattern Management of Blood Glucose 5

1 Components of an intensive diabetes management program can include:
   A Generalized glycemic goals that follow a preestablished pattern
   B Interaction with the healthcare team 2 to 3 times a year
   C Self-monitoring of blood glucose levels when symptoms occur
   D Self-management education and reliable support systems

2 The main reason to use an algorithmic approach to insulin therapy is to:
   A Increase insulin dosages by 10% to 20% to avoid hyperglycemia
   B Provide flexibility in usual insulin dosages to maintain euglycemia
   C Decrease insulin dosages by 10% to 20% to avoid hypoglycemia
   D Avoid using a meal plan and offset eating as desired

3 An adult with previously controlled diabetes has been experiencing hyperglycemia with blood glucose values over 225 mg/dL 2 hours after every meal for the past 2 weeks. Which would be the best initial action for the diabetes educator to take?
   A Evaluate food consumption of the person, especially protein intakes
   B Encourage more vigorous aerobic exercise be done by the individual
   C Assess all areas of diabetes self-management
   D Check the appearance and expiration date of the individual's insulin

4 Effectiveness of lispro insulin is best determined by measuring:
   A Premeal glucoses
   B Fasting glucoses
   C 2-hour postprandial glucoses
   D 3 AM glucoses

5 Pattern management of blood glucose levels involves reviewing:
   A Several days of glucose records and making changes in the diabetes management program when a problem persists
   B Sporadic glucose records and making corrections in the diabetes management program after problems have occurred
   C Glycosolated hemoglobin values and making adjustments in diabetes management before the onset of long-term complications
   D Fasting serum glucose values and making modifications in diabetes management before a problem surfaces

6 One reason sliding scale insulin administration is less desirable as a pattern management approach is:
   A It is based on patient's current weight
   B It varies according to patient's food intake
   C It may contribute to rapid shifts in glucose levels
   D It may confuse patients trying to remember amount of insulin to administer

7 Pattern management for an adult with type 2 diabetes is likely to be:
   A Testing only fasting and premeal blood glucose levels
   B Analyzing records once or twice a week
   C Testing urine for ketones
   D Sliding scale plan to cover blood glucose shifts

**8** Which of the following statements about combination therapy is most accurate?

**A** Addition of TZD to existing therapy produces a therapeutic response within a week

**B** Combination therapy improves glycemic control in persons with type 1 diabetes

**C** When oral agents are combined, the medications should be taken 1 hour before meals

**D** Individuals starting combination therapy will need to monitor postprandial blood glucose levels

**9** Examples of SMBG data that can be useful for managing blood glucose levels and making changes to the treatment plan include all of the following except:

**A** Using premeal testing to determine regular insulin dose for multiple injections

**B** Testing at 3 AM at least once a week when fasting glucose levels are elevated

**C** Testing daily for people who have asymptomatic hypoglycemia

**D** Using premeal testing before administering a supplemental insulin bolus during acute illness

*See next page for answer key.*

# Post-Test Answer Key

## Pattern Management of Blood Glucose

**5**

| | | | | |
|---|---|---|---|---|
| **1** | D | | **6** | C |
| **2** | B | | **7** | B |
| **3** | D | | **8** | D |
| **4** | C | | **9** | C |
| **5** | A | | | |

# A Core Curriculum for Diabetes Education
Diabetes Management Therapies

---

## Insulin Pump Therapy and Carbohydrate Counting for Pump Therapy: Carbohydrate-to-Insulin Ratios

*Insulin Pump Therapy*
*Ann Marie Brooks, RN, CDE*
*St. Marks Hospital Diabetes Center*
*Salt Lake City, Utah*

*Carbohydrate Counting for Pump Therapy: Carbohydrate-to-Insulin Ratios*
*Karmeen Kulkarni, MS, RD, BC-ADM, CDE*
*St. Marks Hospital Diabetes Center*
*Salt Lake City, Utah*

# Introduction

**1** Insulin pump therapy, also known as continuous subcutaneous insulin infusion (CSII), is a valuable asset in attaining normoglycemia.

**2** Studies such as the Diabetes Control and Complications Trial (DCCT)[1] and the United Kingdom Prospective Diabetes Study (UKPDS)[2] have shown conclusively that glycemic control is essential for preventing diabetes complications.

**3** Both the American Diabetes Association[3] and the American Association of Diabetes Educators[4] have position statements supporting the use of insulin pump therapy.

**4** The benefits and limitations of insulin pump therapy must be considered in determining the appropriateness of this type of therapy for a patient.

**5** Proper patient selection is critical to the success of insulin pump therapy. Specific criteria and ethical considerations are part of the selection process.

**6** Currently 5 insulin pumps are approved for use in the US. Each pump offers unique features that can serve as a guide in determining the best model to meet a patient's needs.

**7** A number of steps are involved in initiating successful pump therapy. The diabetes educator plays an important role in this process.

**8** Follow-up and fine-tuning are essential elements of successful pump therapy and achieving patient goals.

**9** Insulin therapy should be integrated into the usual eating and exercise habits of the person with diabetes.[5] Insulin pump therapy provides an excellent means of achieving this goal.

**10** Carbohydrate counting involving carbohydrate-to-insulin ratios is used to implement medical nutrition therapy for insulin pump therapy.

# Objectives

Upon completion of this chapter, the learner will be able to

**1** State the indications for patient use of insulin pump therapy.
**2** Explain the limitations of insulin pump therapy.
**3** Identify selection criteria for pump candidates.
**4** Identify insulin pumps that currently are available in the US.
**5** Describe how to fine-tune pump therapy.
**6** State the skills necessary for using carbohydrate counting for insulin pump therapy and how to evaluate a patient's understanding of and ability to use carbohydrate counting.
**7** Explain how carbohydrate counting is useful for pattern management.

## Insulin Pump Therapy

**1** The number of insulin pump users, or "pumpers," is increasing rapidly each year. According to the manufacturers of insulin pumps, there currently are an estimated 127 000 insulin pump users in the US. This number is relatively low considering that there are over 1 000 000 patients with type 1 diabetes. The number of type 2 patients with pumps is proportionally smaller.

**2** Insulin pump therapy can help patients achieve near-normal blood glucose levels. The Diabetes Control and Complications Trial Research Group (DCCT) conclusively demonstrated the beneficial effects and impact of optimal glycemic control, which changed the way that diabetes is treated.[6]

**3** The earliest model of the insulin pump weighed several pounds and looked like a backpack. Current models weigh as little as 3 ounces and can be worn on a belt like a pager or hidden under clothing.

  **A** The insulin pump is a miniature computer that mimics the functioning of the human pancreas as it delivers short-acting or rapid-acting insulin in 2 ways:
- Basal or metabolic/background insulin is preprogrammed to match pancreatic insulin release patterns.
- Bolus insulin doses are given to cover food intake or to correct a high blood glucose level. The bolus can be given all at once to cover a high-carbohydrate meal or over time to mimic the insulin release needed for a more slowly digested meal.

  **B** The insulin is delivered via an infusion set that is placed just under the skin into the subcutaneous tissue, usually into the abdomen. The infusion site is changed about every 72 hours, relieving the patient of frequent injections with a syringe.

## Benefits of Pump Therapy

**1** Insulin pump therapy provides one means of helping patients improve their glycemic control, which has been shown to reduce the long-term complications of diabetes.

**2** Immediate improvement in blood glucose levels is possible with insulin pump therapy.[7]

  **A** Insulin dosing with an insulin pump can be precise to within one tenth of a unit.

  **B** Differences in absorption from various sites is reduced.

  **C** Incidence of absorption loss from the site depot is reduced.

  **D** Continuous delivery improves insulin absorption.

  **E** Dawn phenomenon effects are easier to manage with insulin pump therapy because the basal rate can be increased to accommodate the rise in insulin requirements that occurs during the early morning hours.

**3** Insulin pump therapy provides an improved safety profile.

  **A** The fear of nocturnal hypoglycemia can be minimized when basal rates are reduced during the period of low physiological requirements.[8]

  **B** Patients experience greater safety while operating machinery or an automobile due to an increased ability to modify insulin delivery patterns.

**C** Patients are better able to make adjustments for sick days by using a temporary basal rate that matches their changed needs.

**4** Insulin pump therapy can increase lifestyle flexibility and patient satisfaction.
  **A** Food/meals can be customized to fit patient schedules and preferences.
  • The need for forced snacking is reduced.
  • Motivated patients who desire weight loss may find it easier with insulin pump therapy. Initially, however, improved glycemia may promote some weight gain.
  • Patients have a flexible schedule of variable food choices.
  • There are fewer problems with picky eaters, such as children, because the bolus can be given after the food consumption has been determined.
  **B** Patients can exercise more safely because basal rates can be reduced during the activity, or the basal delivery can even be suspended.
  **C** The increased flexibility makes it easier for pump wearers to travel. Once the destination is reached, the clock on the pump can be changed and all of the former settings are retained.
  **D** Schedule changes can be accommodated. Many pump wearers find the insulin pump useful for shift work or other kinds of unpredictable life situations.

## Limitations of Pump Therapy

**1** There are also drawbacks to or limitations of insulin pump therapy for patients.
  **A** There is a high learning curve associated with pump therapy; some patients are unable to master the learning curve.
  **B** Successful adaptation to pump therapy may take months; some individuals give up before realizing success.
  **C** Being connected to a pump is a visual reminder of having a chronic disease.
  **D** Technical failures do not occur with insulin and syringes but are possible with a pump.
  **E** There may be an increased risk of ketosis when only rapid-acting or short-acting insulin is available.
  **F** Some patients experience problems with skin irritation and infections. The special adhesive patches and occlusive dressings may irritate some types of skin.
  **G** Site changes require 3 to 10 minutes and may interrupt a busy schedule.
  **H** Some patient populations, such as children, may require assistance from a caregiver.

**2** Many physicians and other healthcare providers are unfamiliar with pump therapy and may be unable to provide needed patient support.

**3** The cost of an insulin pump is usually over $5000 and supplies are about $1000 to $1500 per year. Insurance companies typically cover only about 80% of pump expenses. Because coverage varies from state to state and from plan to plan, this needs to be checked on an individual basis. Reimbursement for diabetes education to support the patient is also variable. (See Chapter 8, Payment for Diabetes Education, in Diabetes Education and Program Management.)

**4** Many of these problems can be overcome, and motivated patients are usually successful.

## Medical Indications for Pump Therapy

**1** The need to improve overall glycemic control is a common indication for insulin pump therapy.

**A** Tighter blood glucose control has been shown to reduce the incidence of diabetic complications. The DCCT[1] and the UKPDS[2], as well as the Kumamoto[9] studies, have demonstrated that well-controlled blood glucose levels reduced complications for patients with type 1 as well as for patients with type 2 diabetes.

**B** Insulin pump therapy can improve outcomes and prevent deterioration of existing diabetes complications.

- Bolus options may help the patient with gastroparesis avoid postprandial high and low blood glucose readings.
- Patients who achieve normoglycemia may experience an improvement in neuropathy.
- Patients with diabetic foot ulcers may have an improved chance of healing.
- Patients may have an improved sense of energy and well-being.

**2** Insulin pump therapy has been shown to reduce the incidence of hypoglycemia, even for patients with tighter control.[8]

**A** Exercise-induced hypoglycemia is easier to prevent because the basal rate can be reduced, eliminated, or suspended. There is less risk that long-acting insulin will cause an unexpected dip in glucose levels.

**B** Nocturnal hypoglycemia can be controlled and the naturally occurring reduction in the need for insulin (typically between midnight and 3 AM) can be anticipated.[8]

**3** To control the dawn phenomenon, the basal rate can be increased to adjust for the hormone-mediated predawn increase in blood glucose.

**4** Insulin sensitivity, which is typically seen in smaller adults and children, can be managed more easily with insulin pump therapy. Basal rates as low as 0.1 unit per hour are possible; with dilution, even more minute basal rates are possible.

**5** Insulin pump therapy would benefit appropriate women with type 1 diabetes during pregnancy.[10] Problems with hypoglycemia may occur during the first 20 weeks of pregnancy, such as nausea and vomiting of food after an insulin injection is given. With the pump, the patient could use a bolus dose on a bite-by-bite basis. In addition, tight control has been found to improve maternal and fetal outcomes.[11]

**6** A variable lifestyle and changing work and activity schedules are handled more smoothly with insulin pump therapy.

**A** People who must travel frequently find they have better control with insulin pump therapy. They may change the clock on the pump once they arrive at the new destination. They may also make small corrections or adjustments more easily as they encounter changes in meal times and sleep times.

**B** People who perform shift work find insulin pump therapy beneficial in adjusting to variable patterns of eating and sleeping.

**C** Pump patients find they can have a more flexible lifestyle, including sleeping late, snacking, missing or delaying meals, or losing weight.

**7** Insulin-requiring patients with type 2 diabetes may benefit from pump therapy, enjoying greater flexibility in their lifestyle and the benefits of tight control.[12]

## Successful Pump Candidates

**1** Motivation is the most important ingredient for success. In addition, the successful pump candidate must be able to handle a variety of tasks and responsibilities.

**A** Patients must overcome the learning curve associated with new therapy, equipment, and problem-solving situations. They must be able to troubleshoot problems, keep records, and adjust insulin.

**B** Emotional maturity is essential for effective problem solving and acceptance of the disease. It is generally thought that the average child would be able to manage the basic operations of an insulin pump by the age of 10. However, decisions regarding the use of an insulin pump by children should be made on a case-by-case basis. Emotional maturity may not be related to age.[13]

**C** Testing and record keeping are vital to success with insulin pump therapy.

**D** Patients must master carbohydrate counting, which involves the use of carbohydrate-to-insulin ratios and is used to implement nutrition therapy for optimal pump therapy. They must know how to determine the correct amount of insulin for a bolus dose based on the foods they have chosen. Patients must be able to weigh or estimate portions accurately, and make adjustments for high-fat or high-fiber foods. Without carbohydrate counting, the benefits and flexibility of insulin pump therapy are greatly reduced and pump therapy is of little value over the traditional approach of using fixed meals and insulin doses.

**E** Insulin therapy should be integrated into the usual eating and exercise habits of the person with diabetes.

**F** Patients need sufficient dexterity to be able to operate the pump.

**G** Visually impaired patients can successfully use insulin pump therapy but will require increased education and motivation.

**H** If the pump wearer lacks the competence to handle this type of therapy (eg, a child or mentally challenged person), a motivated and continually accessible caregiver is necessary.

**I** Financial resources are necessary for using pump therapy. Most candidates rely on insurance, which generally covers about 80% of the cost. Highly motivated patients tend to be more successful in securing financial support.

## Contraindications to Pump Therapy

**1** Unrealistic expectations, such as thinking that insulin pump therapy will cure diabetes, will lead to failure using pump therapy.

**2** Severe depression or other serious psychological disorders are incompatible with successful insulin pump therapy. Patients have been known to use the device to harm themselves.

**3** Inability or unwillingness to calculate bolus doses is a contraindication for insulin pump therapy, with the noted exception of when a caregiver performs all or most of the functions.

**4** A history of poor compliance and healthcare practices, such as failure to perform self-monitoring of blood glucose, keep appointments, and weigh and estimate portions, will signal failure.

**5** Intense needle phobia will make it difficult, if not impossible, to use and benefit from insulin pump therapy.

**6** Denial of the disease and fear of diabetes exposure are contraindications because the pump is a visible reminder of the reality of having diabetes.[14]

**7** Educators need to be cautious in referring patients for pump therapy because negative outcomes hurt other candidates. Insurance companies look at failure rates and may deny pumps to appropriate candidates. Many companies have tightened eligibility requirements for insulin pump therapy to include 4 to 6 months of meticulous blood glucose records. Insurance companies may also increase copayments, thus making it more difficult for responsible candidates.

## Selecting an Insulin Pump

**1** Once the candidate for insulin pump therapy and his/her support team have decided to proceed, the process of selecting a pump begins in earnest.

**2** The physician or educator may have suggestions as to the best model to meet the patient's unique needs.

**3** There currently are 5 insulin pumps approved for distribution in the US. Others are in clinical trials and pending FDA approval.
  **A** The Animas pump has 2 models, the R-1000 and R-1000A. Features include menu-driven programming, 3-minute basal delivery, backlighting, multiple languages, waterproofing, and fashion covers.
  **B** The Dahedi pump is waterproof for surface activities, has a keypad for people with visual impairment, and is the smallest available pump at 2.8 ounces.
  **C** The Disetronic D-Tron pump features waterproofing for surface activities, 5 bolus alternatives, variable profiles, menu-driven programming, 3-minute basal delivery, backlighting, and occlusion detection.
  **D** The Disetronic H-Tron Plus pump is water resistant for surface activities; it has tactile buttons and 3-minute basal pulses; and it includes 2 pumps for the price of 1.
  **E** The Mini-Med 508 pump features 3 sets of basal rates, multiple bolus options, remote programming capability, multiple profiles, child blocking, a watertight design, and backlighting; it is menu driven.

## Obtaining the Chosen Model

**1** An insulin pump requires a doctor's prescription.

**2** Insurance companies require a letter of medical necessity from the physician.

**3** Once the insurance company is notified of the patient's desire for insulin pump therapy, it assesses the letter of medical necessity as well as the patient's history. Blood glucose records and other records may be required.

**4** After authorization has been granted, the patient, educator, or insurance company contacts a vendor who handles the chosen insulin pump.

**5** The patient and the medical team—physician, educators, and other healthcare professionals—schedule pump training and follow-up visits. The patient may wear the pump and initially use normal saline to become familiar with the mechanics and elements of daily living with the pump.

**6** Most pumps come with a training video that helps users become familiar with the mechanics of using the pump and demonstrates insertion techniques.

**7** At one time, patients stayed in the hospital for a day or more when pump therapy was initiated. Currently, most pump starts are performed on an outpatient basis. Because the training sessions may last only a few hours, greater effort and preparation on the part of the patient is required.

## Getting Started with Pump Therapy

**1** Patient education is crucial to success with insulin pump therapy.

**2** The patient needs to master the mechanics of the selected model.

**3** A carbohydrate-to-insulin ratio is calculated based on the patient's weight and current insulin dose. The effectiveness of this ratio is reflected in a comparison of preprandial and postprandial blood glucose levels. Some practitioners prefer a flat result, or no increase in blood glucose after a meal, while others prefer a 30 to 40 mg/dL (1.7 to 2.2 mmol/L) increase after a meal to prevent the need for snacking before the next meal. Patients may not have the same carbohydrate ratio for all meals because needs and insulin requirements may vary during the day.

**4** The education team, including the pump candidate, determines a reasonable target blood glucose level. Insulin bolus adjustments are based on this target, which might be 100 mg/dL (5.6 mmol/L) for patients in tight control. Patients who have not experienced tight glucose control might need to start with a higher target. A pregnant woman might have a target of 80 mg/dL (4.4 mmol/L).

**5** A correction factor, or sensitivity factor, is also an important consideration. The patient adds or subtracts insulin from the meal bolus based on how much 1 unit of insulin might be expected to decrease the blood glucose level. A formula can be used such as the one in the Insulin Pump Therapy Handbook,[15] or even more importantly, from patient input. The following example shows how a correction factor is used. The patient's target is 100 mg/dL, correction factor is 40.
- If the premeal blood glucose level is 140 mg/dL, add 1 unit to the meal bolus.
- If the premeal blood glucose level is 60 mg/dL, subtract at least 1 unit and give the bolus with the meal.

**6** The basal profile or rate is vital for insulin pump therapy. About 50% of the insulin requirement is reflected in the basal or background rate. Most patients require more than 1 rate. Insulin pumps currently offer 12 to 48 basal rates or profiles. These profiles begin at midnight and can be programmed to adjust for nocturnal hypoglycemia, dawn phenomena, or any routine physiological change.

   **A** Patient weight and current insulin use guide the clinician in establishing basal rates; clinicians often start by reducing current use by 25%.

   **B** Fasting blood glucose levels and readings between meals reflect the efficacy of the basal rates.

   **C** Some pump models offer up to 4 basal routines, such as for weekends, sick days, or exercise days.

   **D** Most pumps offer temporary basal rates for unusual circumstances, such as for surgery, exercise, or illness.

   **E** Basal profiles can reflect unique patient needs. Some patients may require more insulin in the early morning hours and some at the dinner hour. Other patients require little or no insulin at night or a reduction during the late afternoon.

   **F** Lispro insulin is frequently used with insulin pump therapy.[3,16] Insulin aspart may prove valuable in insulin pump therapy as well.[17]

**7** The healthcare team helps the pump candidate select an appropriate infusion site and an appropriate infusion set.

   **A** Most patients select a site on the abdomen. Absorption is usually best in this area and the sites are less obtrusive; sites in the arms, thighs, buttocks, and breasts are also used successfully. Scars, or scar tissue, such as seen with lipodystrophy, prevent even insulin absorption and should be avoided, as well as the area immediately around the umbilicus.

   **B** The tip of the infusion cannula must be in subcutaneous or fatty tissue. In some very thin patients the subcutaneous is just a compartment or layer between the dermis and the muscle. These individuals must roll and pinch up the skin to locate the correct site area.

   **C** The site is prepared by cleansing the skin thoroughly in a circular motion from the inside to the outside. Patients may develop an allergy to cleansers that are too harsh. Many patients cover the site with an occlusive dressing or tape and then insert the infusion set.

   **D** Infusion sets are available in a wide variety of styles, features, and prices. Most are interchangeable between the various brands of pumps. Some sets can be disconnected at or near the site to facilitate bathing, swimming, or intimate moments. Others must remain in place at all times. The sets should be changed every 2 to 3 days. A plugged, infected, or misplaced site must be changed at once.

   **E** MiniMed Technologies makes an insertion device that can be used to insert one of its infusion sets. This works well for patients with vision or dexterity problems.

**8** The insulin pump therapy candidate must be able to troubleshoot pump problems. Without long-acting insulin, diabetic ketoacidosis can develop more rapidly. Patients must be able to

   **A** Adjust for and prevent hypoglycemia or hyperglycemia.

   **B** Deal with alarms, batteries, and mechanical or site problems.

   **C** Understand sick-day management.

**D** Understand exercise adjustments and precautions.

**E** Know when to test and how to interpret the results. When insulin pump therapy is initiated, patients may need to test at 2 to 3 AM for a while to be able to understand the correct nocturnal insulin requirements.

**F** Locate a dependable source for insulin pump supplies. They must still carry insulin and syringes for emergencies.

**G** Have reasonable expectations because success requires time and patience in mastering the learning curve.

## Follow-Up: The Key to Success

**1** Insulin pump therapy is most successful when the patient has support from a multidisciplinary team. The patient, physician, and educators (nurse and dietitian) can assess patient records and responses. This ongoing follow-up and reassessment help the patient achieve individualized goals. Life itself—needs, habits, and activities—changes and evolves constantly. This is reflected in changing insulin requirements and a need for continuous fine-tuning.

## Looking Ahead

**1** Glucose sensors reflect a breakthrough in technology. The sensor is placed under the skin just like an infusion set and it checks blood glucose every 5 minutes for 3 days. The patient returns the device to the physician at the end of the 3 days and the blood glucose data are downloaded to a computer so the data are analyzed.

**A** This device helps identify physiological glucose patterns that were previously unknown to the patient and healthcare team. The information can be used to better determine basal rates, insulin ratios, etc. Even patients in tight control may experience glucose excursions of which they are unaware.

**B** Glucose sensors, which currently are available on a limited basis, may one day provide a closed-loop system in which glucose is sensed and insulin is released in response, mimicking the functioning of the human pancreas. This technology offers patients the hope of tight control over their lifetime.

**2** A Diaport system offers further hope of normoglycemia. In this system, which currently is undergoing safety trials in the US and Europe, a port that is placed in the peritoneal cavity automatically senses glucose levels.

## Key Educational Considerations for Pump Therapy

**1** Insulin pump therapy has been shown to be an effective tool for helping patients with diabetes achieve better glycemic control.

**2** Insulin pump therapy has many advantages, including lifestyle flexibility, reduction of hypoglycemia, and prevention of dawn phenomenon (hyperglycemia).

**3** Disadvantages include cost, risk of diabetic ketoacidosis, and a comprehensive learning curve.

**4** Patients must be selected carefully to ensure success with insulin pump therapy.

**5** A number of different insulin pumps are currently available, and they offer a variety of features.

**6** The pump candidate selects a pump and an infusion set to match personal needs.

**7** Insurance companies usually cover 80% of the costs of insulin pump therapy, although some cover 100%.

**8** Carbohydrate-to-insulin ratios, basal rates, and target/correction factors help patients achieve tight control safely.

**9** Patient success is facilitated by a team approach. Frequent follow-up is vital to maximize insulin pump use.

---

## Self-Review Questions on Pump Therapy

**1** State the indications for and limitations of insulin pump therapy.
**2** What are the characteristics of successful insulin pump therapy patients?
**3** Identify contraindications to insulin pump therapy.
**4** What insulin pumps are currently available in the US?
**5** What steps are necessary to obtain an insulin pump?
**6** State the key educational requirements for pump therapy patients.
**7** What are the most vital elements for continuing success with insulin pump therapy?

---

## Learning Assessment: Pump Therapy Case Study 1

Jared, age 22, has asked his physician for an insulin pump to "fix" his diabetes. He has heard about the pump and is adamant about having one. Jared has had type 1 diabetes since he was 11 years old. He tests his blood glucose level occasionally and takes his insulin when he remembers. Jared's current HbA1c is 14.2%. He has microalbuminuria and complains of increasing numbness in his feet. His family is pressuring the diabetes team to "stop the complications." Jared's insurance company requires 4 months of glucose testing records before reimbursing for an insulin pump, but he has thus far not produced the records. Twice he failed to show up for his carbohydrate counting session. Either Jared or his mother calls the diabetes team almost daily, and they believe the team is letting Jared down.

---

## Questions for Discussion

**1** Is Jared an appropriate candidate for insulin pump therapy? Why or why not?
**2** What are the obligations of the diabetes team in helping this patient obtain an insulin pump?
**3** What could Jared do to change this situation?

## Discussion

**1** At the present time Jared is not an appropriate insulin pump therapy candidate. His glycemic control would not likely improve with an insulin pump, and he might be even more likely to experience an episode of diabetic ketoacidosis because he would no longer be using any long-acting insulin.

**2** Jared has not learned carbohydrate counting so he would not be able to match his insulin dose with his carbohydrate intake.

**3** Jared has been unwilling to submit the blood glucose records that the insurance company requires before approving reimbursement for an insulin pump. The insurance company's rules protect patients, the company, and the healthcare team.

**4** The team has tried to help Jared achieve better control. He must make the effort to change his situation. He may need psychiatric help or counseling to accomplish this goal.

**5** If Jared fails to use his insulin pump properly and requires additional hospitalization, his failure may influence the availability of the program and benefits for other candidates.

**6** Jared can change this situation. He can start doing regular blood glucose testing, keep records, and attend a carbohydrate counting session. He also can begin taking multiple daily insulin injections. Performing these tasks in a responsible manner may then qualify Jared for insulin pump therapy and the chance to benefit from this type of therapy.

## Learning Assessment: Pump Therapy Case Study 2

Denise, age 27, and her husband are planning a pregnancy. Denise has had type 1 diabetes since the age of 15. She has had laser surgery for background retinopathy but has not experienced any other known complications. She manages her diabetes with insulin injections 3 times daily: 20 units NPH and 6 units regular insulin in the morning, 6 units regular insulin at dinner, and 12 units NPH at bedtime. Denise tests her blood glucose 3 times a day. She weighs 130 lb and is 5 ft 5 in tall. Her current HbA1c is 7.6%. Her physician would like her to have tighter control before becoming pregnant, and he has recommended an insulin pump.

## Questions for Discussion

**1** What kind of preparation will Denise need before she begins insulin pump therapy?
**2** What HbA1c level would be optimal for pregnancy?
**3** How might Denise's insulin need change during pregnancy?

## Discussion

**1** Denise will need to master carbohydrate counting as part of her preparation for insulin pump therapy. She can see a diabetes educator and begin this process at once.

**2** She will want to change her insulin regimen to multiple daily injections (MDI), possibly using Ultralente and lispro, to match her insulin and carbohydrate intake.

**3** Denise will need an eye exam if she has not had one is the last 6 to 9 months to ensure the stability of her retinopathy. Some physicians may also require a 24-hour urine clearance test.

**4** She will need to check her blood glucose level at least 4 times daily to facilitate the MDI and provide better glucose management data for her diabetes team.

**5** The physician or educator may help Denise choose her insulin pump. She will require alternative infusion sites once she is pregnant as her abdomen enlarges.

**6** The HbA1c goal for Denise will be below 7.0%, preferably closer to 6.0%, during her pregnancy.

**7** She will need close contact with her diabetes management team throughout her pregnancy because throughout her pregnancy because her basal insulin needs will change (increase) as her pregnancy progresses.[18]

## Pump Therapy References

**1** Diabetes Control and Complications Trial Research Group. The effect of intensive treatment of diabetes mellitus on the development and progression of long-term complications in insulin-dependent diabetes. N Eng J Med. 1993;329:977-986.

**2** UK Prospective Diabetes Study (UKPDS) Group. Intensive blood-glucose control with sulphonylureas or insulin compared with conventional treatment and risk of complications in patients with type 2 diabetes (UKPDS 33). Lancet. 1998;352:837-853.

**3** American Diabetes Association. Continuous subcutaneous insulin infusion (position statement). Diabetes Care. 2001;24(suppl 1):S98.

**4** American Association of Diabetes Educators Position Statement. Continuous subcutaneous insulin infusion pump users. Diabetes Educ. 2000;23:397-398.

**5** American Diabetes Association. Nutrition recommendations and principles for people with diabetes mellitus (position statement). Diabetes Care. 2001;24(suppl 1):S44-S47.

**6** Skylar J. Introduction. In: Fredrickson L, ed. Insulin Pump Therapy Book. Sylmar, Calif: MiniMed Technologies;1995:3-8.

**7** Mecklenburg RS, Benson EA, Benson JW Jr, et al. Long-term metabolic control with insulin pump therapy. N Engl J Med. 1985;313:465-468.

**8** Bode BW, Steed RD, Davidson PC. Reduction in severe hypoglycemia with long-term continuous subcutaneous infusion in type 1 diabetes. Diabetes Care. 1996;19:324-327.

**9** Ohkubo Y, Kishikawa H, Araki E, et al. Intensive insulin therapy prevents the progression of diabetic microvascular complications in Japanese patients with non-insulin dependent diabetes mellitus: a randomized prospective 6-year study. Diabetes Resources Clin Pract. 1995;8:113-117.

**10** Jovanovich-Peterson L, Peterson C, Coustan D, et al. A randomized clinical trial of the insulin pump vs. intensive conventional therapy in diabetic pregnancies. JAMA. 1986;255:631-636.

**11** Jornsay D. Pregnancy and continuous insulin infusion therapy. Diabetes Spectrum. 1998;11:26-32.

**12** Jennings A, Lewis K, Murdoch S, Talbot J, Bradley C, Ward J. Randomized trial comparing continuous subcutaneous insulin infusion and conventional therapy in type 2 diabetic patients poorly controlled with sulfonylureas. Diabetes Care. 1991;14:738-744.

**13** Slipper F, deBeaufort C, Bruining G, et al. Psychological impact of continuous subcutaneous insulin infusion therapy in non-selected newly diagnosed insulin dependent (type I) diabetic children: evaluation after 2 years of therapy. Diabetic Med. 1990;16:273-277.

**14** Tannenberg R. Candidate selection. In: Fredrickson L, ed. Insulin Pump Therapy Book. Sylmar, Calif: MiniMed Technologies;1995:21-30.

**15** Fredrickson L, ed. Insulin Pump Therapy Book. Sylmar, Calif: MiniMed Technologies; 1995.

**16** Zinman B, Tildesley H, Chiasson J-L, Tsui E, Strack T. Insulin lispro in CSII: results of a double-blind cross over study. Diabetes. 1997;46:440-443.

**17** Bode B, Strange P. Efficacy, safety, and pump compatibility of insulin aspart used in continuous subcutaneous insulin infusion therapy in patients with type 1 diabetes. Diabetes Care. 2001;24:69-72.

**18** Drexler A. Pump therapy in preconception and pregnancy. In: Fredrickson L, ed. Insulin Pump Therapy Book. Sylmar, Calif: MiniMed Technologies;1995:145-150.

## Suggested Readings on Pump Therapy

American Diabetes Association. Preconception care of women with diabetes (position statement). Diabetes Care. 2001;24:S66-S68.

Davidson P. Bolus and supplemental insulin. In: Fredrickson L, ed. Insulin Pump Therapy Book. Sylmar, Calif: MiniMed Technologies;1995:59-70.

Glucose Sensor. Sylmar, Calif: MiniMed Corporation;1999. Publication D9195869.

Grossman J. Successful management of type 2 diabetes: are the benefits worth the costs? Practical Diabetol. 1999;June:12-22.

Insulin Pump Therapy Series. Reprint 5. Minneapolis, Minn: Disetronic Medical Systems; 1998. (Readers will find the entire series of 15 pamphlets helpful.)

MiniMed Corporation. Selected abstracts from the 17th International Diabetes Federation Congress (Glucose Sensors), Mexico City, Mexico, 2000.

Special resource guide. Diabetes Forecast. 2001;Jan:58-67.

### Notes

Insulin pumps and supplies vary in price, as do amounts of insurance reimbursement. Readers may check with local vendors, the manufacturers, and local insurance carriers.

Thank you to the insulin pump manufacturers for providing synopses of pump features.

## Carbohydrate Counting for Pump Therapy: Carbohydrate-to-Insulin Ratios

**1** Early research on continuous subcutaneous insulin infusion (insulin pump therapy) demonstrated that premeal insulin boluses were related solely to carbohydrate intake while basal insulin could be adjusted according to fasting blood glucose levels.[1] Additional research documented the relationship of carbohydrate to bolus insulin doses.[2,3] Mixed meals (carbohydrate plus protein and fat) were shown to have very little effect on carbohydrate-based bolus insulin doses.

**A** Recent research confirmed that the amount of the carbohydrate in the meal determines the premeal (bolus) doses of insulin and that insulin should be adjusted accordingly.[4,5] Algorithms based on grams of carbohydrate are effective.[4]

**B** The glycemic index, fiber, fat, and caloric content of the meal do not effect the premeal (bolus) insulin doses.[4,5]

**C** This finding is further supported by the DCCT, which showed that individuals on intensive insulin therapy who adjusted their premeal insulin doses based on the carbohydrate content or food exchange had a lower HbA1c of 0.5% (P <0.03).[6,7]

**D** This research provided the documentation for using of carbohydrate-to-insulin ratios.

**2** There are 3 steps involved in using carbohydrate-to-insulin ratios:

**A** Identifying the anticipated carbohydrate intake at meals and snacks.

**B** Accurately determining the carbohydrate intake based on grams of carbohydrate or carbohydrate choices (15-g equivalents or carbohydrate exchanges), or a combination of grams and choices.

**C** Administering a rapid-acting or short-acting premeal insulin dose based on a predetermined carbohydrate-to-insulin ratio.[8]

**3** Certain prerequisites for patients are necessary before they move to this level of carbohydrate counting and implementing carbohydrate-to-insulin ratios:

**A** Mastery of the basic understanding of carbohydrate counting and the relationship between food, physical activity, and blood glucose levels. This knowledge is necessary for individuals to effectively manage their diabetes and is sometimes referred to as Level 1 and Level 2 Carbohydrate Counting.[9] For more information, see the section on carbohydrate counting in Chapter 1, Medical Nutrition Therapy for Diabetes, in Diabetes Management Therapies.

**B** Demonstrated proficiency in self-adjustment and supplementation of insulin. *Intensive insulin therapy* is defined as multiple daily injections (MDI) or use of insulin pump therapy.

**C** Being able to adjust insulin doses to meet blood glucose goals while consistently using food, blood glucose levels, and insulin records for at least 1 to 2 weeks to determine carbohydrate-to-insulin ratios.

- A *carbohydrate-to-insulin (C:I) ratio* is based on matching the carbohydrate content of food to be eaten with rapid-acting or short-acting insulin. A C:I ratio can be different for different people. For example, weight and physical activity influence the calculation of the C:I ratio. In addition, C:I ratios may vary from meal to meal based on insulin requirements. Therefore, the C:I ratio is always individualized.

**4** An outline of a possible protocol for determining carbohydrate-to-insulin ratios using carbohydrate grams is shown in Figure 6.1.

## Figure 6.1. Procedure for Determining Carbohydrate-to-Insulin Ratios Using Carbohydrate Grams

**Case Example:** Prior to RO starting on an insulin pump, RO goes through the procedure listed below for determining the carbohydrate-to-insulin (C:I) ratio based on premeal doses of lispro. RO has kept food, activity, and blood glucose records for 2 weeks. Based on a consistent intake of carbohydrate (CHO) and appropriate insulin adjustments to meet target blood glucose levels, you observe the following:

> Breakfast: 8 units lispro insulin for 65 g CHO
> Lunch: 6 units lispro insulin for 65 g CHO (50 g for lunch, 15 g for midafternoon
>     snack)
> Dinner: 7 units lispro insulin for 75 g CHO

Use this information and follow the steps below to calculate RO's carbohydrate-to-insulin ratio.

**1** Record the grams (g) of carbohydrate that are consistently eaten at each meal based on blood glucose and food records.

Breakfast ___65___ g        Lunch __50+15__ g        Dinner ___75___ g

**2** Record meal doses of lispro insulin that consistently meet target blood glucose levels.

Breakfast ___8___ units        Lunch ___6___ units        Dinner ___7___ units

**3** For each meal, determine the carbohydrate grams per unit of insulin by dividing total carbohydrate grams for each meal by the number of units of lispro insulin.

Breakfast = B      Lunch = L        Dinner = D

CHO g = _____        B____ = ____        L____ = ____        D____ = ____

units lispro insulin g/unit        g/unit        g/unit        g/unit

**4** If the answers to step 3 vary from each other by no more than 1 g of carbohydrate, add together the 3 answers and divide by 3 to get the average grams of carbohydrate per unit of insulin.

B_____ + L_____ + D_____ = _____ total g/unit ÷ 3 = _____

average g/unit

The appropriate carbohydrate-to-insulin ratio is _____ g/unit.

**5** If the answers to step 3 vary from each other by more than 1 g of carbohydrate, and you and the rest of the diabetes healthcare team agree that your basal insulin doses are well adjusted, use the answers to step 3 as carbohydrate-to-insulin ratios for each meal.

The appropriate carbohydrate-to-insulin ratios are

B _____ g/unit        L _____ g/unit        D_____ g/unit

**6** To make insulin adjustments for consuming more or less carbohydrate, add the total carbohydrate and divide by the appropriate carbohydrate-to-insulin ratio.

Total carbohydrate g _____ ÷ g/unit (ratio) _____ = _____units lispro

**Practice:** RO is going to eat a larger-than-usual dinner of a total of 90 g of carbohydrate. Using step 6, calculate how much insulin will be needed for this meal.

*Source:* Adapted with permission from the American Diabetes Association. Carbohydrate Counting: Using Carbohydrate/ Insulin Ratios. Alexandria: American Diabetes Association, 1995.

## Figure 6.2. Procedure for Determining Carbohydrate-to-Insulin Ratios Using Carbohydrate Choices (or Exchanges)

**Case Example:** RO has kept food, activity, and blood glucose records for 2 weeks. Based on a consistent intake of carbohydrate (CHO) and appropriate insulin adjustments to meet target blood glucose levels, you observe the following:

    Breakfast: 8 units lispro insulin for 4 CHO choices
    Lunch: 6 units lispro insulin for 4 CHO choices
    Dinner: 7 units lispro insulin for 5 CHO choices

Use this information and follow the steps below to calculate RO's carbohydrate-to-insulin ratio.

**1**  Record the meal doses of lispro insulin that consistently meet target blood glucose levels based on blood glucose and food records.
    Breakfast _____units      Lunch _____units      Dinner _____units

**2**  Record the number of carbohydrate choices that are consistently eaten at each meal.
    Breakfast_____      Lunch_____      Dinner_____
    CHO choices           CHO choices           CHO choices

**3**  For each meal, determine the units of lispro insulin per carbohydrate choice by dividing the number of units by the number of carbohydrate choices.
    units lispro insulin ÷ CHO Choices =
    CHO choices = _____ units/CHO choice

    Breakfast _____units/CHO choice
    Lunch     _____units/CHO choice
    Dinner     _____units/CHO choice

**4**  If the answers to step 3 are different for one or more meals, use more than 1 ratio. The appropriate carbohydrate-to-insulin ratios are as follows:
    B _____ L _____ D _____units/CHO choice

**5**  To make insulin adjustments for consuming more or less carbohydrate choices, add the total carbohydrate choices and multiply by the ratio units/CHO choice.
    Total CHO choices _____ x _____units/CHO choice = _____units lispro insulin

**Practice:** RO is going to eat a larger-than-usual dinner of a total of 6 carbohydrate choices. Using step 5, calculate how much insulin will be needed for this meal.

*Source:* Adapted with permission from the American Diabetes Association. Carbohydrate Counting: Using Carbohydrate/ Insulin Ratios. Alexandria: American Diabetes Association, 1995.

**A** The grams-per-unit ratio is obtained by dividing the grams of carbohydrate consistently consumed at a given meal by the number of units of rapid-acting or short-acting insulin needed to meet blood glucose goals.

**B** To adjust insulin for more or less than the usual carbohydrate intake, the total grams of carbohydrate to be consumed are divided by the carbohydrate-to-insulin ratio. For example, a patient who consistently has 60 g of carbohydrate at a meal and requires 6 units of rapid-acting or short-acting insulin to achieve target blood glucose levels would have a ratio of 10 g of carbohydrate per 1 unit of insulin. To adjust insulin dose for an intake of 80 g of carbohydrate, divide the 80 g by 10 to obtain the appropriate insulin requirement, which would be 8 units.

**5** An outline of a procedure for determining carbohydrate-to-insulin ratios using carbohydrate choices, or exchanges, is shown in Figure 6.2.[3]

**A** The units-per-carbohydrate-choice ratio is obtained by dividing the number of units of rapid-acting or short-acting insulin needed to meet blood glucose goals by the number of carbohydrate choices consistently consumed at a given meal.

**B** To adjust the insulin dose for consuming more or less than the usual carbohydrate choices, multiply the number of carbohydrate choices by the units-per-carbohydrate-choice ratio. For example, a patient who consistently consumes 6 carbohydrate choices at a meal and requires 9 units of regular insulin to achieve target blood glucose levels would have a ratio of 1.5 units per carbohydrate choice. To adjust the insulin dose for an intake of 8 carbohydrate choices, multiply the 8 carbohydrate choices by 1.5 to obtain the appropriate insulin requirement, which would be 12 units.

**6** Additional information to be considered when using carbohydrate-to-insulin ratios, which applies to both rapid-acting and short-acting insulins, includes the following:

**A** Patients may have more than 1 carbohydrate-to-insulin ratio.[10-12] For example, a patient may have a ratio of 10 g of carbohydrate to 1 unit of insulin at breakfast and a ratio of 15 g to 1 unit at lunch and dinner.

**B** Carbohydrate-to-insulin ratios may change with changes in body weight or level of physical activity.

**C** Portion control is important to assure precise matching of insulin doses with anticipated carbohydrate intake.[13]

**D** The increased flexibility of carbohydrate intake for meals and snacks while working to improve glycemic control can place patients at risk for weight gain. Reducing fat and total calorie intake and/or increasing physical activity can help maintain desired weight.

**E** With the shorter duration of action of rapid-acting insulin, the dose taken with the preceding meal may not provide adequate coverage of between-meal snacks. Snacks may need to be omitted, a lower carbohydrate snack may be needed, or an insulin bolus may be necessary at the time of a larger snack.

**F** Because fat slows down gastric emptying time,[14] a delay in the timing of the pre-meal rapid-acting or short-acting insulin may be necessary to match the peak of the insulin with the peak postprandial blood glucose response. However, the addition of fat does not change the area under the glucose curve.[3]

• If the pump has a square, dual, or extended wave bolus feature, the pump can be programmed to deliver the bolus dose over a specific amount of time. This feature is used for high-fat meals, and the adjustments are based on clinical observations.

**G** Dietary fiber generally is not digested and absorbed like other carbohydrates.[15] Therefore, paying attention to the fiber content in high-fiber foods (those containing 5 or more grams of dietary fiber) can help patients more accurately match the insulin dose with the available carbohydrate. (Subtracting the dietary fiber grams from the total carbohydrate grams equals the available carbohydrate grams.)

**H** Patients may identify specific carbohydrate foods or meals that produce blood glucose responses greater or less than anticipated. Such responses require changes in the carbohydrate-to-insulin ratios or timing of premeal insulin delivery, based on clinical observation in some insulin pump therapy patients.[16,17] For example, eating pizza may require additional insulin.[16]

- Meals that are high in slowly absorbed carbohydrate (eg, cooked dried beans) may require delivery of premeal short-acting insulin closer to the consumption time or delivery of rapid-acting insulin after consumption to match the peak insulin activity with the postprandial blood glucose peak.

## Key Educational Considerations for Carbohydrate Counting for Pump Therapy

**1** The individual needs to understand insulin adjustment and supplementation before introducing a new element that requires making a specific insulin dose adjustment such as carbohydrate-to-insulin ratios.

**2** After determining individual carbohydrate-to-insulin ratios, provide ample opportunities for the patient to complete paper-and-pencil exercises that simulate situations in which insulin adjustments would be needed for meals or snacks that are larger or smaller than usual. Examples can include a weekend brunch, pizza party, or a light lunch.

**3** Assess the patient's ongoing ability to accurately estimate carbohydrate amounts. If portion control or estimating skills are questionable, the patient may need to review the basics of carbohydrate counting and continue practicing skills from those levels.

**4** Periodically review the patient's food, blood glucose, and physical activity records to ascertain appropriate use of carbohydrate-to-insulin ratios.

**5** Monitor the patient's weight. If weight gain is a problem, emphasize portion control, limiting calories, protein, and fat intake and using weight-management behaviors.

## Self-Review Questions on Carbohydrate Counting

**1** List 3 prerequisites for determining carbohydrate-to-insulin ratios.

**2** What are 2 primary principles of using carbohydrate-to-insulin ratios?

**3** Explain how to calculate carbohydrate-to-insulin ratios using the carbohydrate gram method.

**4** Explain how to calculate carbohydrate-to-insulin ratios using the carbohydrate choice method.

**5** How much insulin would be needed to cover 90 g of carbohydrate for someone using a carbohydrate-to-insulin ratio of 15 g of carbohydrate per 1 unit of insulin?

**6** How much insulin would be needed to cover 7 carbohydrate choices for a person using 1 unit of insulin per carbohydrate choice?

**7** Why do patients using carbohydrate-to-insulin ratios also need to be concerned about intake of dietary fat?

## Learning Assessment:
## Carbohydrate Counting Case Study

RO is a 31-year-old female who has had type 1 diabetes for 5 years with no complications except for trace microalbuminuria. She and her husband are interested in starting a family within the next year. Her HbA1c was 8.6% to 9% on the last 2 tests (normal = 4.4% to 6.1%). Her preconception blood glucose goals are preprandial 70 to 100 mg/dL and postprandial at 1 h <140 mg/dL and at 2 h < 120 mg/dL. RO's blood glucose levels have ranged between 50 and 250 mg/dL for the past month. Her insulin regimen is 8 units NPH and 9 units lispro at breakfast, 8 units lispro at lunch, 10 units lispro at dinner, and 9 units NPH at bedtime. She has been advised to test her blood glucose more than 7 times per day (before meals, after meals, at bedtime, plus before and after exercise and when hypoglycemic). She uses a meter with memory but does not keep blood glucose records.

RO is 5 ft 4 in (163 cm) tall and weighs 140 lb (63 kg). She eats 3 meals daily plus afternoon and bedtime snacks. Her lunches are fast food and her afternoon snacks are from a vending machine. The amount of food that she eats varies greatly depending on where she is eating. She uses candy bars to treat hypoglycemia, and she usually eats more balanced, low-fat meals at home than when eating out.

RO's estimated daily calorie intake is 1500 to 2400 calories; her estimated daily calorie need for gradual weight loss is 1500 calories. Based on your assessment, the following macronutrient distribution has been recommended: 60% carbohydrate, 14% protein, 26% fat. The recommended distribution of carbohydrate is as follows: breakfast, 60 to 65 g; lunch, 50 to 55 g; afternoon snack, 15 g; dinner, 70 to 75 g; and bedtime snack, 25 to 30 g.

RO is a married college graduate and a sales representative for a large company. She travels frequently (about 1 out-of-town trip per week) to large metropolitan areas. Her finances are adequate.

She has been experiencing problems with midmorning and late-afternoon hypoglycemia. Safety factors are a concern since she spends 2 to 4 hours a day driving. She is also concerned about weight gain from treating insulin reactions. She recently switched from a split-mixed insulin regimen (NPH and regular twice a day) to the current MDI regimen. She is still not able to reach her blood glucose goals and continues to experience hypoglycemic reactions.

RO has been working on carbohydrate counting with her dietitian and has agreed to following a food/meal plan with specific carbohydrate goals for meals and snacks. RO has not kept 2 weeks of careful blood glucose levels, food intake, and activity records as requested. However, she states that she is interested in learning how to adjust insulin for varying amounts of food. She is also interested in getting an insulin pump, having learned from her medical team that it would promote euglycemia and help reduce hypoglycemic episodes. All of her preparation with MDI and insulin pump therapy will help in starting on an insulin pump.

## Questions for Discussion

**1** What level of carbohydrate counting is appropriate for RO's current skills?

**2** What carbohydrate counting skills or activities should RO work on prior to using carbohydrate-to-insulin ratios? Where should you start?

**3** How could you determine that RO is ready to learn carbohydrate-to-insulin ratios?

## Discussion

**1** RO needs flexibility with carbohydrate consumption at meals and snacks because her job involves frequent eating out and unpredictable meal times and locations. To achieve optimal glycemic control under these circumstances, she needs to learn how to adjust her premeal lispro insulin for varying amounts of carbohydrate. But first RO must establish a consistent carbohydrate intake around which insulin doses can be adjusted. She must proceed from basic or Level 1 carbohydrate counting through intermediate or Level 2 before she can develop accurate carbohydrate-to-insulin ratios.

**2** Nutrition and behavior change options that can be presented to RO include recording blood glucose levels before each meal, 2 hours after meals whenever possible, and at bedtime. In addition, for the first few days, she should test her blood glucose at 3 AM. She could test and record her blood glucose more frequently before driving and before and after exercise. Other options can include:

**A** Faxing her blood glucose records to her diabetes educator weekly so that they can discuss insulin adjustments and supplementation. She should follow her individualized food/meal plan, which consists of 3 meals and a bedtime snack with an optional additional snack for exercise. Her food/meal plan should include mutually agreed-upon carbohydrate goals for meals. She should focus on consistency of carbohydrate intake based on her target goals.

**B** Practicing portion control at home by weighing and measuring food for at least 2 weeks. She can buy a carbohydrate reference book that includes nutrition information about fast food and chain restaurants to help with making estimates when traveling.

**C** Keeping a food intake, blood glucose, and physical activity record for 2 weeks prior to her visit to the dietitian to learn carbohydrate-to-insulin ratios.

**D** Developing a carbohydrate-to-insulin ratio to use for adjusting insulin to anticipated food intake.

**3** RO is very quick to grasp the principles of carbohydrate counting, and with adequate motivation and cooperation she can probably proceed quickly through the basics of carbohydrate counting to carbohydrate-to-insulin ratios.

**4** At the initial visit and assessment (60 to 90 minutes), the dietitian and RO can develop a food/meal plan that includes food choices when eating away from home. The dietitian can explain the rationale for being disciplined about consistency in meal timing and carbohydrate portion sizes to facilitate insulin adjustments, emphasizing how these skills can lead to greater freedom and flexibility later when using carbohydrate-to-insulin ratios. The dietitian can also assess RO's skills in weighing, measuring, and estimating portion sizes by using measuring tools, food labels, and carbohydrate resources and references. The dietitian can emphasize that the possibility of developing carbohydrate-to-insulin ratios at the next visit depends on meeting carbohydrate goals and completeness of records. RO can send food records to the dietitian for feedback between visits.

**5** At a follow-up visit 2 to 3 weeks later, the dietitian and RO review food intake, physical activity, insulin, and blood glucose records. If insulin doses have been adjusted around consistent and accurate carbohydrate intake and target blood glucose levels are met, then they are ready to determine carbohydrate-to-insulin ratios. RO can practice with sample meals and snacks using carbohydrate-to-insulin ratios to make insulin dosage adjustments. Areas to discuss include glycemic effects of fat and fiber; any possible insulin adjustments needed for consuming large amounts of these nutrients; and continued need for portion control and control of fat intake to maintain weight control. The need for follow-up based on telephone contact to discuss records or additional visits for more practice needs to be determined based on the results of this visit.

**6** RO feels very comfortable with her C:I ratio. She has completed the paperwork for her medical insurance for receiving an insulin pump, it has been approved, and she has plans to receive it in 2 weeks. She is scheduled to start the pump initiation.

**7** RO goes through the insulin pump start (refer to the section on insulin pumps for details). She does very well with the mechanics of pump use and is able to use her C:I ratio and the carbohydrate counting training to manage her food, physical activity, and blood glucose levels.

# Carbohydrate Counting References

1  Hamet P, Abarca G, Lopez D, et al. Patient self-management of continuous subcutaneous insulin infusion. Diabetes Care. 1982;5:489-491.

2  Peters AL, Davidson MB. Protein and fat effects on glucose response and insulin requirements in subjects with insulin-dependent diabetes mellitus. Am J Clin Nutr. 1993;58:555-600.

3  Slama G, Klein JC, Delage A, et al. Correlation between the nature and amount of carbohydrate in meal intake and insulin delivery by the artificial pancreas in 24 insulin-dependent diabetics. Diabetes. 1981;30:101-105.

4  Rabasa-Lhoret R, Garon J, Langlier H, Poisson D, Chiasson J-L. Effects of meal carbohydrate on insulin requirements in type 1 diabetic patients treated intensively with the basal-bolus (Ultralente-regular) insulin regimen. Diabetes Care. 1999;22:667-673.

5  Lafrance L, Rabasa-Lhoret R, Poisson D, Ducros F, Chiasson J-L. The effects of different glycaemic index foods and dietary fibre on glycaemic control in type 1 diabetic patients on intensive insulin therapy. Diabetic Med. 1998;15:972-978.

6  Delahanty LM, Halford BN. The role of diet behaviors in achieving improved glycemic control in intensively treated patients in the Diabetes Control and Complications Trial. Diabetes Care. 1993;16:1453-1458.

7  Diabetes Control and Complications Trial Research Group. Nutrition interventions for intensive therapy in the Diabetes Control and Complications Trial. J Am Diet Assoc. 1993; 93:768-773.

8  Gillespie SJ, Kulkarni K, Daly AE. Using carbohydrate counting in diabetes clinical practice. J Am Diet Assoc. 1998;98:897-905.

9  Daly A, Barry B, Gillespie S, Kulkarni K, Richardson M. Carbohydrate Counting: Getting Started, Level 1; Moving On, Level 2; Using Carbohydrate/Insulin Ratios, Level 3. Alexandria, Va and Chicago: American Diabetes Association and American Dietetic Association; 1995.

10  Kulkarni K, Franz MJ. A dietitian's perspective on medical nutrition therapy for diabetes. In: Franz MJ, Bantle JP, eds. American Diabetes Association Guide to Medical Nutrition Therapy for Diabetes. Alexandria, Va: American Diabetes Association; 1999:3-17.

11  Geil PB. Complex and simple carbohydrates in diabetes therapy. In: Powers MA, ed. Handbook of Diabetes Medical Nutrition Therapy. Gaithersburg, Md: Aspen Publishers; 1996:303-319.

12  Kulkarni K, Tomky D. Influence of carbohydrate counting on blood glucose patterns in intensive insulin therapy. On the Cutting Edge [newsletter]. July 1996.

13  Daly A, Gillespie S, Kulkarni K. Carbohydrate counting: vignettes from the trenches. Diabetes Spectrum. 1996;9:114-117.

14  Strachan MWJ, Frier BM. Optimal time of administration of insulin lispro. Importance of meal composition. Diabetes Care. 1998;21:26-31.

15  Wursch P. Dietary fiber and unabsorbed carbohydrates. In: Gracey M, Kretchmer N, Rossi E, eds. Sugars in Nutrition. Vol 25. New York: Raven Press; 1991:153-168.

16  Ahren JA, Garcomb PM, Held NA, Pettit WA, Tamborlane WV. Exaggerated hyperglycemia after a pizza meal in well-controlled diabetes. Diabetes Care. 1993;16:578-580.

17  Vlachokosta FV, Piper CM, Gleason R, Kinzel L, Kahn CR. Dietary carbohydrate, a Big Mac, and insulin requirements in type I diabetes. Diabetes Care. 1988;11:330-336.

## Resources on Carbohydrate Counting

American Diabetes Association, American Dietetic Association. Exchange Lists for Meal Planning. Alexandria, Va: American Diabetes Association; 1995.

Franz MJ. Exchanges for All Occasions. 4th ed. Minneapolis: IDC Publishing; 1997.

Franz MJ. Fast Food Facts. 5th ed. Minneapolis: IDC Publishing; 1998.

Holzmeister LA. The Diabetes Carbohydrate and Fat Gram Guide, 2nd ed. Alexandria, Va and Chicago: American Diabetes Association and American Dietetic Association; 2000.

Kulkarni K, Fredrickson L, Graff M. Carbohydrate Counting. A Primer for Insulin Pump Users to Zero in on Good Control. Sylmar, Calif: MiniMed Technologies; 1999.

Monk A, Cooper N. Convenience Food Facts. 4th ed. Minneapolis: IDC Publishing; 1997.

Pennington JA. Bowes & Church's Food Values of Portions Commonly Used. 17th ed. Philadelphia: Lippincott; 1998.

Ross T, Geil P. Carbohydrate Counting Cookbook. New York: John Wiley & Sons; 1998.

Warshaw H. The ADA Guide to Healthy Restaurant Eating. Alexandria, Va: American Diabetes Association; 2000.

Warshaw H, Kulkarni K. The American Diabetes Association Complete Guide to Carbohydrate Counting. Alexandria, Va: American Diabetes Association; 2001.

# Learning Assessment: Post-Test Questions

## Insulin Pump Therapy and Carbohydrate Counting for Pump Therapy: Carbohydrate-to-Insulin Ratios

**6**

**1** Basal profiles usually are not adjusted to reflect:
**A** Decreased nocturnal insulin needs
**B** Increased early morning insulin resistance
**C** Mealtime insulin needs
**D** Exercise adjustments

**2** Red flags for potential insulin pump therapy failure include:
**A** Expectations that insulin pump therapy will "cure" diabetes
**B** Problems with glycemic control
**C** History of complications
**D** Problems with hypoglycemia

**3** Which of the following conditions may not be helped by insulin pump therapy?
**A** Pregnancy
**B** Hard-to-control diabetes in children
**C** Gastroparesis
**D** Severe depression

**4** How many basal profiles do most patients require?
**A** 10
**B** 2 or 3
**C** 1
**D** 5

**5** The infusion set may not be:
**A** Disconnected frequently
**B** Inserted with a device
**C** Placed in fatty tissue
**D** Changed every 2 to 3 days

**6** Mr. Jones has a correction factor of 40 and a target of 110 mg/dL. He needs 7 units of insulin to cover his lunch. His blood glucose is 190 mg/dL. How much insulin should he take as a bolus dose?
**A** 5 units
**B** 10 units
**C** 9 units
**D** 7 units

**7** The DCCT demonstrated that tighter control of diabetes with insulin pump therapy was associated with all of the following except:
**A** Decreased weight
**B** Decreased nephropathy
**C** Decreased retinopathy
**D** Increased patient satisfaction

**8** Benefits of insulin pump therapy include all of the following except:
**A** Improved insulin absorption
**B** Decreased insulin consumption
**C** Increased mealtime flexibility
**D** Reduced need for blood glucose testing

**9** Which of the following statements is true?
**A** Pump therapy makes diabetes less noticeable
**B** Pump therapy involves an accelerated learning curve
**C** Pump wearers are discouraged from participating in active sports
**D** Insulin pump therapy is appropriate for all type 1 patients

**10** What is the most important requirement for insulin pump success?
**A** Family support
**B** Fitness
**C** Motivation
**D** Proficiency in mathematics

**11** Carbohydrate counting does not involve (best answer):
**A** Weighing or measuring portions
**B** Carbohydrate-to-insulin ratios
**C** Making allowances for grams of fat and protein
**D** Reading food labels

*See next page for answer key.*

## Post-Test Answer Key

Insulin Pump Therapy and Carbohydrate Counting for
Pump Therapy: Carbohydrate-to-Insulin Ratios                    **6**

**1**  C

**2**  A

**3**  D

**4**  B

**5**  A

**6**  C

**7**  A

**8**  D

**9**  B

**10**  C

**11**  C

## Hypoglycemia 7

*Linda A. Gonder-Frederick, PhD*
*University of Virginia*
*Behavioral Medicine Center*
*Charlottesville, Virginia*

## Introduction

**1** It is extremely difficult to duplicate normal blood glucose metabolism with insulin therapies. Therefore, blood glucose levels in patients taking insulin tend to fluctuate between abnormally high *(hyperglycemia)* and abnormally low *(hypoglycemia)* levels due to under- and over-insulinization relative to food intake, physical activity, and metabolic needs.

**2** Almost every person using insulin therapy, especially those with type 1 diabetes, eventually experiences hypoglycemic episodes. Persons with type 2 diabetes using insulin or insulin secretagogues alone or in combinations are also at risk for hypoglycemia.

**3** Hypoglycemia tends to occur suddenly, and almost always requires immediate treatment to prevent blood glucose levels from continuing to fall to a dangerously low range.

**4** Hypoglycemia is associated with a number of negative consequences for the individual with diabetes:
  **A** Unpleasant physical symptoms
  **B** Impaired cognitive function
  **C** Embarrassment
  **D** Emotional trauma
  **E** Accidents
  **F** Bodily injury, including death

**5** The problem of hypoglycemia has become even more significant as patients strive to maintain their blood glucose levels in a near-normal range by using more intensive insulin therapies as recommended by the Diabetes Control and Complications Trial (DCCT).[1] As blood glucose levels are lowered toward normal, the frequency of hypoglycemic episodes increases. For this reason, hypoglycemia has been called the major barrier to optimal control of type 1 diabetes.[2]

## Objectives

Upon completion of this chapter, the learner will be able to

**1** Define and describe mild and severe hypoglycemic episodes, including the symptoms associated with varying levels of severity.

**2** Explain the physiological changes that occur with hypoglycemia.

**3** Describe hypoglycemic symptomatology, the effects of hypoglycemia on emotions and behavior, and factors underlying symptom idiosyncrasy.

**4** Identify causes of hypoglycemia and possible risk factors for individual patients.

**5** Explain the treatment for different levels of hypoglycemia, including guidelines for when the patient is unable to self-treat due to a severe hypoglycemic episode.

**6** Identify psychosocial sequelae of hypoglycemia.

**7** Develop general education plans for teaching patients about hypoglycemia as well as more specific assessment and intervention plans for patients experiencing frequent or severe hypoglycemic episodes.

## Definition of Hypoglycemia

**1** *Hypoglycemia* can be conservatively defined as any blood glucose (BG) level of 70 mg/dL (3.9 mmol/L) or lower. However, hypoglycemic episodes vary greatly in their severity. Currently, severity of hypoglycemia is not defined by any particular blood glucose level per se, but rather is defined symptomatically.

**A** *Mild hypoglycemia* is characterized by symptoms such as sweating, trembling, difficulty concentrating, and lightheadedness. These symptoms are usually alleviated quickly by drinking or eating carbohydrates.

**B** *Severe hypoglycemia* is characterized by an inability to self-treat due to mental confusion, lethargy, or unconsciousness. Because the individual is unable to self-treat, others must provide treatment to raise the blood glucose level out of a dangerously low range.

**2** Absolute blood glucose levels cannot be used to describe the severity of hypoglycemic episodes because glycemic thresholds for the onset of symptoms, as well as symptom magnitude, differ greatly across individual patients and from episode to episode, depending on various mediating variables.

**A** Some individuals remain alert with only a few symptoms at a blood glucose level of 40 mg/dL (2.2 mmol/L), while others become stuporous at the same glucose concentration.

**B** An individual patient may tolerate a blood glucose level of 40 mg/dL (2.2 mmol/L) with few symptoms on one occasion, but become completely incapacitated at the same glucose concentration on another occasion.

**3** The classification of hypoglycemic episodes as previously stated is based exclusively on whether individuals can treat themselves. Thus, the term mild does not necessarily mean that the symptoms experienced by the individual are mild or easily tolerated. In fact, a individual can be quite symptomatic (eg, sweating profusely, nauseous, disoriented, and uncoordinated) and still manage to self-treat. Therefore, even mild hypoglycemic episodes can be aversive and distressing from the individual's perspective.

**4** Hypoglycemic episodes caused by insulin secretagogues are just as potentially dangerous as episodes caused by insulin.

**A** Although the frequency of severe hypoglycemia from the use of oral medications is lower than that from insulin, the mortality rate is significant (10%). In survivors of these episodes, there is a 5% rate of permanent brain damage.

**B** Different rates of hypoglycemia appear to be associated with different oral medications.

- The risk is highest with sulfonylureas.
- Of the sulfonylureas, the highest rates are found with glyburide and chlorpropamide.
- The half-life of sulfonylureas is quite long and, when hypoglycemia occurs, it can be quite significant and prolonged.
- Monotherapy with metformin, rosiglitazone, pioglitazone, miglitol, or acarbose is not associated with hypoglycemia.
- Meglitinides, especially repaglinide, may cause hypoglycemia.

**C** Factors that increase the risk for hypoglycemia in patients with type 2 diabetes include
- Advanced age
- Poor nutrition
- Hepatic or renal disease

## Hypoglycemic Symptoms

**1** Two biological mechanisms are responsible for most hypoglycemic symptoms.

    **A** Hormonal counterregulation involves autonomic symptoms caused by hormonal reactions that increase the glucose level to counteract hypoglycemia.

    **B** Neuroglycopenia involves disruptions in mental and motor function secondary to depletion of glucose that is available to the central nervous system.

**2** The symptoms that result from these biological mechanisms are typically the first warning signs that blood glucose levels are too low, and thus play a critical role in the treatment of hypoglycemia and the prevention of severe episodes.[3]

**3** Some of the most common hypoglycemic symptoms are shown in Table 7.1.

    **A** The autonomic symptoms are generally adrenergically based, although sweating appears to be cholinergic.

    **B** Because hypoglycemia causes such widespread physiological changes in hormonal and central nervous system (CNS) function, many different symptoms can occur; the list presented in Table 7.1 is not intended to be exhaustive.

    **C** Hypoglycemic symptoms appear to be similar for type 1 and type 2 diabetes patients.

**4** Autonomic symptoms provide early warning signs of hypoglycemia.

    **A** In the nondiabetic person, the primary counterregulatory hormones are glucagon, which enhances the release of glucose that is stored in the liver, and epinephrine, which increases the liver's production of glucose and inhibits glucose utilization.[4]

    **B** After only a few years of diabetes duration (2 to 5 years), glucagon secretion is impaired in most type 1 patients and epinephrine secretion becomes the primary mechanism for raising low blood glucose levels.

    **C** If the epinephrine response to hypoglycemia is adequate, blood glucose levels will either stop falling or increase slightly before they become dangerously low. With prolonged hypoglycemia, growth hormone and cortisol may also play a role, although these hormones do not appear to contribute to early warning symptoms or early recovery.

    **D** Over the course of type 1 diabetes, defective hormonal counterregulation can cause the epinephrine response to hypoglycemia to be diminished or delayed.[5] The result is that epinephrine secretion may not occur until blood glucose levels are quite low or the amount of epinephrine released is inadequate to stop blood glucose levels from falling further.

    **E** Defects in hormonal counterregulation also delay or diminish the onset of autonomic symptoms, resulting in reduced hypoglycemic symptom awareness. Because the blood glucose level drops further before the patient recognizes that treatment is needed, the risk of becoming severely hypoglycemic increases greatly.

## Table 7.1.  Hypoglycemic Symptoms

| Type of Symptom | Symptom |
| --- | --- |
| *Autonomic* | • Trembling/shaking<br>• Sweating<br>• Pounding heart<br>• Fast pulse<br>• Changes in body temperature<br>• Tingling in extremities<br>• Heavy breathing |
| *Neuroglycopenic* | • Slow thinking<br>• Blurred vision<br>• Slurred speech<br>• Uncoordination<br>• Numbness<br>• Trouble concentrating<br>• Dizziness<br>• Fatigue/sleepiness |
| *Unknown Etiology* | • Hunger<br>• Nausea<br>• Weakness<br>• Headache<br>• General feeling of something not right |

**F** Hormonal counterregulation and autonomic symptoms can disappear almost completely, resulting in what is called *hypoglycemia unawareness.* This term is somewhat misleading because even patients with significantly reduced hypoglycemia awareness typically still have some symptoms such as those associated with neuroglycopenia.[6] However, the recognition of symptoms may occur too late to allow timely treatment before significant neuroglycopenia.

**G** Persons with reduced hypoglycemia awareness are at increased risk of severe hypoglycemia and should be encouraged to test their blood glucose more frequently, especially at times when blood glucose levels are likely to be low or when hypoglycemia may be especially dangerous, such as while driving a motor vehicle or operating machinery.

**H** Several clinical risk factors associated with defective hormonal counterregulation and reduced hypoglycemia awareness[7,8] are shown in Table 7.2; all appear to increase the frequency of hypoglycemia.

**I** The clinical risk factors listed in Table 7.2 result in what has been called *hypoglycemia-associated autonomic failure.*[9] Research suggests that this autonomic failure may be reversible. For example, when patients with defective counterregulation meticulously avoid low blood glucose fluctuations over a period of several weeks, epinephrine response improves and autonomic symptoms increase in magnitude.[10,11]

## Table 7.2.  Clinical Risk Factors That Increase the Frequency of Hypoglycemia

**1**  Use of intensive insulin therapies
**2**  Near-normal glycosylated hemoglobin level
**3**  Autonomic neuropathy
**4**  History of frequent/recurrent episodes of severe hypoglycemia

---

**J**  Research has shown that the occurrence of only 1 mildly low blood glucose episode can cause temporary deficits in epinephrine response and a reduction in autonomic symptoms for the next 24 hours.[12]

- If another low blood glucose episode occurs during the subsequent 24 hours, glucose levels will drop much lower before hormonal counterregulation and autonomic symptoms occur.
- Consequently, persons with diabetes need to be taught the importance of testing their blood glucose levels more frequently and monitoring themselves for symptoms more carefully for the next day or so after a hypoglycemic episode.

**5**  Neuroglycopenic symptoms provide early warning signs of hypoglycemia.

**A**  Traditionally, autonomic symptoms were considered to be the most reliable early warning signs of hypoglycemia.  Neuroglycopenic symptoms, in contrast, were believed to have little utility as early warning signs. These symptoms were assumed not to appear until blood glucose levels were quite low and the patient was too mentally compromised to recognize the low blood glucose level.

**B**  More recent research[3,5] has demonstrated that autonomic and neuroglycopenic symptoms occur at similar glycemic thresholds and that patients experience neuroglycopenic symptoms as frequently as other symptoms.

- The earliest signs of neuroglycopenia include a slowing down in performance and difficulty concentrating and reading.
- Subjectively, patients feel as if it takes more effort to perform routine tasks that are usually done easily.

**C**  As the blood glucose level drops further and neuroglycopenia progresses, the onset of the following symptoms occurs: frank mental confusion and disorientation, slurred or rambling speech, irrational or unusual behaviors, and extreme fatigue and lethargy.

- If the blood glucose level continues to fall, unconsciousness and seizures can occur.
- Neuroglycopenia is typically the cause of accidents and physical injuries that occur during hypoglycemic episodes.

**D**  Teach all patients that changes in their ability to do routine tasks can be a sign that blood glucose levels are too low.  Being alert for such changes is especially important for patients with reduced autonomic symptoms who are more likely to experience neuroglycopenic symptoms as the first sign of impending hypoglycemia.

**E**  Instruct patients to treat themselves as soon as possible when neuroglycopenic symptoms occur.  Failure to do so can cause patients to become so neuroglycopenic that they do not recognize that their blood glucose level is low.

**F**  Neuroglycopenia during hypoglycemia can severely compromise decision-making and self-treatment behavior; it is common for patients to resist attempts by others to give them carbohydrates or even to become belligerent when others try to persuade them to drink or eat.

**G** Neuroglycopenia can also cause a number of changes in patients' emotional states and social behavior.[13]

- Some of the most common emotional changes, most of which are negative (eg, irritability and anxiety), are listed in Table 7.3. In children, these emotional changes may result in crying, argumentativeness, and misbehavior.[14]
- Some individuals may also display positive emotional changes, such as inappropriate giddiness or euphoria.

**H** The effects of hypoglycemia on emotions can be a source of significant distress to patients, who often are not aware that such effects are common and who may be too embarrassed to talk to healthcare professionals about their behavior. Emotional changes are also a source of distress for family members and significant others because they have to contend with sudden negative shifts in their loved one's mood.

## Table 7.3. Changes in Emotions and Social Behavior Associated With Hypoglycemia

| | | |
|---|---|---|
| *Negative Moods* | • Anxiety<br>• Nervousness<br>• Tension<br>• Irritation | • Frustration<br>• Anger<br>• Sadness<br>• Pessimism |
| *Positive Moods* | • Giddiness<br>• Euphoria<br>• Disinhibition | |
| *Behaviors* | • Arguing<br>• Crying<br>• Resisting treatment<br>• Aggressive acts<br>• Inappropriate social/sexual behaviors | |

**6** Symptoms of hypoglycemia can differ across individual patients and individual hypoglycemic episodes.

**A** Hypoglycemic symptomatology tends to be idiosyncratic.[3] Although a given individual often has similar symptoms during different hypoglycemic episodes, the most reliable warning symptoms for one patient may not be representative symptoms for another patient.

**B** It is important for individuals to learn to identify their own most reliable symptoms.

- This identification process can be done systematically using a symptom diary like the one shown in Figure 7.1. Individuals record their symptoms whenever they measure their blood glucose and then review the data to identify symptoms that occur reliably with hypoglycemia.

# Figure 7.1. Symptom Diary

| Date | Time | Symptoms/Cues | Blood Glucose Estimate | Actual | Missed Cues | Causes of Hypoglycemia |
|------|------|---------------|------------------------|--------|-------------|------------------------|
|      |      |               |                        |        |             |                        |
|      |      |               |                        |        |             |                        |
|      |      |               |                        |        |             |                        |
|      |      |               |                        |        |             |                        |
|      |      |               |                        |        |             |                        |
|      |      |               |                        |        |             |                        |
|      |      |               |                        |        |             |                        |
|      |      |               |                        |        |             |                        |
|      |      |               |                        |        |             |                        |
|      |      |               |                        |        |             |                        |
|      |      |               |                        |        |             |                        |
|      |      |               |                        |        |             |                        |
|      |      |               |                        |        |             |                        |
|      |      |               |                        |        |             |                        |
|      |      |               |                        |        |             |                        |

**Instructions:** (1) Fill in date and time. (2) Scan your body for symptoms. Also consider other blood glucose cues such as changes in your food, insulin, and exercise. Write down all of your symptoms and cues. (3) Based on your symptoms and cues, estimate your current blood glucose. Record this number in the "Estimate" column. (4) Measure and record your actual blood glucose. (5) If your actual blood glucose is <70 mg/dL, but your estimated blood glucose was >70 mg/dL, go back and scan your body for symptoms. List any symptoms you notice in the "Missed Cues" column. (6) Finally, if your blood glucose is <70 mg/dL, think about what might have caused it. For example, have you eaten less food, exercised more, or taken more insulin in the recent past?

- A symptom diary also can be used to help persons with reduced hypoglycemia awareness (eg, loss of personally familiar symptoms) identify current reliable symptoms of hypoglycemia that they may not be aware of, such as neuroglycopenic symptoms.

**C** Individuals also differ greatly in their ability to recognize and interpret symptoms accurately.[3] This variability among persons may be due to differences in physiological responses to hypoglycemia as well as differences in psychological factors such as a tendency to attend to somatic cues.

- Because persons who tend to become neuroglycopenic do not seem to manifest early warning autonomic symptoms, these individuals need to be instructed to monitor more carefully and frequently in order to detect mild levels of low blood glucose that, if untreated, may lead to severe hypoglycemia.

**D** The type and magnitude of symptoms also can differ for a given individual from one hypoglycemic episode to the next.

- One reason why hypoglycemia episodes may vary within the same individual is because of delayed or reduced autonomic symptoms following a recent low blood glucose event.[12]

**E** Foods and medications may influence autonomic symptoms.

- In some studies,[15] caffeine consumption has been found to increase autonomic symptoms.
- Alcohol consumption can diminish awareness of hypoglycemic symptoms and impede glycemic recovery by interfering with hepatic glucose production (gluconeogenesis).
- Some medications, such as propranolol, also can mask early warning autonomic symptoms.

## Causes of Hypoglycemia

**1** Certain regimen factors and self-treatment behaviors can increase the risk of hypoglycemia.

**A** All hypoglycemic episodes are caused by excess blood glucose lowering medications (insulin or insulin secretagogues) relative to food intake and activity level.

- The first step in determining what is causing frequent hypoglycemia is a careful examination of the individual's insulin regimen. Insulin excess and hypoglycemia are more likely to occur at those times of the day when insulin action is peaking.

**B** Hypoglycemia is also more likely when no food has been eaten for several hours or when physical activity increases significantly.

- Many diabetes self-management behaviors related to food intake and physical activity can increase risk of hypoglycemia especially if appropriate changes are not made in medication. Some of these behaviors are shown in Table 7.4.
- Alcohol consumption without food intake may result in hypoglycemia.

**C** More than 50% of all episodes of severe hypoglycemia occur during the night.

- Because individuals may not awake by early warning symptoms with nocturnal hypoglycemia, the risk of severe episodes is greatly increased, especially in persons with deficient counterregulation. For individuals with adequate counterregulation, it is not uncommon to sleep through episodes of nocturnal hypoglycemia.

## Table 7.4. Diabetes Self-Management Behaviors That Increase the Risk of Hypoglycemia

| | |
|---|---|
| *Insulin* | • Frequent insulin adjustments<br>• Irregular timing of insulin dosages<br>• Failure to decrease insulin when eating less<br>• Inaccurate preparation of insulin dose |
| *Food* | • Skipping meals/snacks<br>• Delaying meals/snacks<br>• Irregular timing of meals<br>• Irregular carbohydrate content<br>• Not carrying carbohydrate source |
| *Physical Activity* | • Failure to eat additional carbohydrates<br>• High degree of variability in daily/weekly activity schedule<br>• Failure to recognize significant increases in caloric demand |

- The most common symptom to awaken patients is sweating, although this symptom is absent in patients with hypoglycemic awareness. Partners may be awakened by the patient's moaning and thrashing if sweating is not present.
- Nocturnal hypoglycemia is often caused by exercise during the previous day or failure to eat a bedtime snack. After strenuous exercise, individuals should test blood glucose levels more frequently. Performing additional self-tests during the night (eg, 3 AM) after strenuous exercise may be needed to avoid nocturnal hypoglycemia in persons at high risk. An increase in carbohydrate, especially at the bedtime snack, may also be indicated to avoid hypoglycemia.

**D** Several factors contribute to nocturnal hypoglycemia:
- Predinner injections of intermediate-acting insulin (NPH, Lente) may peak in action during the night and cause relative hyperinsulinemia overnight.
- Insulin requirements also appear to decrease between midnight and 3 AM, compared with insulin requirements at dawn.

**E** Significant increases in physical activity, combined with failure to increase carbohydrate consumption and/or reduce the insulin dose, are one of the most common causes of both daytime and nocturnal hypoglycemia.[16]
- Teach patients that any increase in physical activity can cause low blood glucose levels, even if they are not formally exercising. Caloric expenditure from exercise does not necessarily cause hypoglycemia. Inappropriate adjustments for exercise, duration, timing, etc are more likely to be factors.
- Individuals may not understand that activities such as shoveling snow are just as demanding as jogging and require the same adjustments in diabetes self-management (eg, eating extra carbohydrate).

**F** By increasing glucose requirements and utilization by muscle tissues, very intense physical activity can have both an immediate and a prolonged effect of lowering blood glucose levels (see Chapter 2, Exercise, in Diabetes Management Therapies).
- Because of the depletion and need to replenish muscle glycogen stores, more carbohydrate may be required to raise blood glucose levels after prolonged strenuous exercise.

- Blood glucose levels may be lower or become hypoglycemic for as long as 12 to 24 hours after exercise, which often causes nocturnal hypoglycemia in patients who exercise during the day.[16]

**G** Concomitant use of sulfa antibiotics (such as TMP, Septia, Bactim) with a sulfonylurea can cause profound and refractory hypoglycemia. Persons with diabetes need to be instructed to tell their physician that they are also taking a sulfonylurea if a sulfa-type of antibiotic is prescribed.

**2** Other factors can increase the risk of hypoglycemia.

**A** Reproductive hormonal changes in women can affect blood glucose levels.

- The incidence of hypoglycemia increases significantly during the first trimester of pregnancy due to fetal demand for glucose and increased sensitivity to insulin. Frequent vomiting can also increase the risk of hypoglycemia.
- The risk and incidence of hypoglycemia decreases as pregnancy progresses, as increased levels of placental hormones result in an increase in peripheral insulin resistance (see Chapter 2, Pregnancy: Preconception to Postpartum, in Diabetes in the Life Cycle and Research, for more information).
- The incidence of hypoglycemia increases significantly during the postpartum period due to increased insulin sensitivity and, if breastfeeding, increased glucose use.
- Women using intensive treatment programs frequently report higher blood glucose levels just prior to menses, followed by a lowering of blood glucose levels after the start of menstrual flow.

**B** The delayed absorption of carbohydrates and delayed gastric emptying caused by gastroparesis can cause hypoglycemia.

**C** Insulin sensitivity can affect blood glucose levels.

- Leaner individuals tend to be more sensitive to insulin and have reduced insulin requirements.
- Physically fit persons also are more sensitive to insulin than those who have a more sedentary lifestyle.

**D** Decreased renal function in the elderly or renal insufficiency in persons with type 2 diabetes can extend the duration of the effects of sulfonylureas or insulin and cause hypoglycemia.

**E** Decreases in caloric intake for weight loss that are not accompanied by decreases in insulin or oral medications.

## Prevention of Hypoglycemia

**1** Avoidance of nearly all episodes of hypoglycemia is the ideal goal, but this is difficult to achieve in many persons. Avoidance of severe hypoglycemia, which is associated with significant risk for injury, is critical.

**2** The most powerful tool for preventing hypoglycemia is diabetes patient education.

**A** Because the majority of hypoglycemic episodes are caused by overinsulinization relative to food intake and physical activity, patients' knowledge about their diabetes treatment programs and the causes of hypoglycemia should be carefully assessed.

**B** Even well-educated and experienced individuals may have misunderstandings or inadequate knowledge about hypoglycemia. For example, many individuals do not know that high-fat foods have a delayed and depressed glycemic effect. Thus, eating a high-fat, low-carbohydrate meal after insulin injections or boluses can lead to hypoglycemia.

**C** Because knowledge does not always influence behavior, patients' self-management habits also need to be assessed.

**3** Until recently, frequent hypoglycemia was often regarded as a sign of good glycemic control, and many patients continue to hold this belief.

**A** It is now know that frequent episodes of mild hypoglycemia greatly increase the risk of an episode of severe hypoglycemia.

**B** Hypoglycemic episodes also have little or no effect on metabolic control, which is determined by the frequency of hyperglycemia.

- HbA1c values of 7.0% or less may be the result of wide high-low blood glucose fluctuations, which further emphasizes the importance of blood glucose record review.

**4** It is especially important to prevent nocturnal hypoglycemia because patients cannot rely on being awakened by early warning symptoms. Guidelines for preventing nocturnal hypoglycemia are provided in Table 7.5.

## Treatment of Hypoglycemia

**1** Recommended thresholds for treatment of hypoglycemia vary across different healthcare providers and individual patients. A conservative recommendation is to treat all blood glucose levels less than 70 mg/dL (3.9 mmol/L), based on the evidence that even very mild hypoglycemia can reduce early warning symptoms and counterregulation.[11]

**2** Treatment guidelines are relatively straightforward.

**A** Eat or drink 10 to 15 g of glucose per se or carbohydrate-containing foods or beverages, which should raise the blood glucose level 30 to 45 mg/dL (1.7 to 2.5 mmol/L). Ten grams of oral glucose raised plasma glucose levels from 60 mg/dL (3.3 mmol/L) to 97 mg/dL (5.4 mmol/L) over 30 minutes with levels starting to fall after 60 minutes. Twenty grams of oral glucose raised plasma glucose levels from 58 mg/dL (3.2 mmol/L) with a greater response at 15 minutes, and again the levels started to fall after 60 minutes.[17] Different foods and drinks that supply this amount of carbohydrate are listed in Table 7.6.

- Glucose or carbohydrates are used to treat hypoglycemia so that blood glucose levels rise quickly. Drinks/food that are high in fat content slow gastric emptying and absorption of carbohydrate and, therefore, take longer to raise blood glucose levels. Adding protein to the treatment of hypoglycemia does not raise blood glucose levels and does not prevent subsequent hypoglycemia.[18]

**B** If blood glucose levels are less than 50 mg/dL (2.8 mmol/L), 20 to 30 g of carbohydrate may be needed.

**C** If possible, test blood glucose before beginning treatment. If pretreatment testing is not possible and symptoms are present, proceed with the treatment.

**D** Test blood glucose 15 to 20 minutes after initiating treatment. If the blood glucose level is still low, repeat the treatment even if symptoms have disappeared.

**E** If the patient is not scheduled to eat a meal or snack within the next hour, they should be cautious about additional hypoglycemia. Patients should be instructed that their blood glucose may fall again if food is not eaten within the next hour. Blood glucose levels should be tested again and treated if low.

## Table 7.5. Guidelines for Preventing Nocturnal Hypoglycemia

- Do not skip presleep snacks.
- Measure presleep blood glucose levels regularly.
- If the bedtime blood glucose level is 120 mg/dL (6.7 mmol/L) or lower, increase the carbohydrate content of the snack.
- If daytime physical activity was increased, eat additional carbohydrate at the night snack.
- Move the predinner NPH or Lente to presleep rather than decreasing the predinner dose, which can lead to fasting hyperglycemia. Use of Ultralente or glargine insulin instead of NPH or Lente insulin may also be effective.
- Measure 3 AM blood glucose levels at least once a week or more frequently if recurrent nocturnal hypoglycemia is a problem.
- Measure 3 AM blood glucose levels when daytime physical activity or food consumption was atypical and when insulin doses are being adjusted.

## Table 7.6. Carbohydrate Sources (15 to 20 g) for Treating Hypoglycemia

| Source | Quantity |
| --- | --- |
| Glucose tablets | 3 to 4 |
| Lifesavers® candies | 8 to 10 |
| Brach's® hard candies | 8 to 10 |
| Raisins | 2 tablespoons |
| Nondiet soft drinks | 4 to 6 oz |
| Fruit juice | 4 to 6 oz |
| Milk (no fat or low fat) | 8 oz |

**F** Following very mild episodes of hypoglycemia, patients usually can resume normal activity fairly soon after treatment. With more significant hypoglycemia, recovery of mental and motor function lags behind glycemic recovery. When blood glucose levels fall to 45mg/dL (2:5 mmol/dL), cognitive recovery may take as long as 45 to 75 minutes.[19,20] Advise patients that it may not be safe to engage in any potentially risky activities (eg, driving) during this period.

**3** The following patient guidelines are recommended for self-treatment of hypoglycemia.

    **A** Do not keep eating after the initial treatment; wait 15 to 20 minutes, then test blood glucose to determine whether further treatment is needed.

    **B** Do not keep eating until symptoms disappear.

    **C** Avoid using high-fat foods for treatment (Table 7.7).

    **D** Always carry some type of carbohydrate.

       - Keep something at your bedside to treat nocturnal hypoglycemia.

## Table 7.7. Foods With High Fat Content That are Poor Choices for Treating Hypoglycemia

- Ice cream
- Doughnuts
- Candy bars
- Meat

- Pies, cakes
- Cheese
- Nuts
- Cookie dough

- Pizza
- French fries
- Milkshakes
- Potato chips

**E** Always wear diabetes identification.

**F** Overtreatment will cause posttreatment hyperglycemia.

- Overtreating hypoglycemia is relatively common and can be attributed to both physiological and psychological factors. Patients may eat until autonomic symptoms abate completely, rather than consuming the recommended amount of carbohydrate and waiting to see if symptoms subside or blood glucose increases.
- Other patients overtreat because of the fear of losing control due to neuroglycopenia. This fear is especially common in patients who live alone, care for small children, or have experienced a traumatic episode of severe hypoglycemia in the past.
- Using commercially available, portion-controlled glucose products may help patients avoid overtreatment.

**4** Appropriate treatment of hypoglycemia is also determined by such complicated psychological processes as decision-making and judgment.[21]

**A** These processes can be compromised by diminished cognitive ability and inaccurate risk appraisal, either due to neuroglycopenia or inaccurate beliefs about hypoglycemia.

**B** Once individuals know that their blood glucose level is low, they make several decisions based on the following questions:

- Treat immediately or wait?
- What to eat and how much?
- Stop current activity or continue?

**C** Deciding to delay treatment is relatively common and often leads to severe hypoglycemia.

- Reasons for delaying treatment include the desire to finish a task and embarrassment about eating when others are not.
- Some individuals may even deny they are becoming hypoglycemic because it is a reminder of their diabetes or perceived as an indication that they have made some mistake in diabetes management.

**D** It is important to assess individuals' attitudes and beliefs about hypoglycemia. Some persons believe there is no reason to treat low blood glucose levels unless they are below 50 mg/dL (2.8 mmol/L) or until they feel symptoms.

- Many individuals believe that their ability to function is not affected until blood glucose levels fall very low, which often is not the case. Research shows that measurable deficits in mental and motor task performance occur at blood glucose levels of 65 mg/dL (3.5 mmol/L).[22-24]

**5** Treatment of hypoglycemia often must be done by family members or significant others.

   **A** The hypoglycemic type 1 patient often has to be treated by others because of the effect of neuroglycopenia on judgment and behavior.

- Teach family members and significant others how to cope with episodes of severe hypoglycemia and what to expect in terms of the patient's behavior (eg, stupor or possible resistance). Some family members report that it is helpful to use favorite foods to coax the hypoglycemic individual to eat.
- Coworkers, friends, and teachers also need to know how to respond to symptoms of hypoglycemia, which can be a problem if individuals do not want to reveal their diabetes to others.

   **B** The following basic guidelines are recommended for treating severe hypoglycemia.

- Persons who are able to swallow without risk of aspiration may be coaxed into drinking juice or a soft drink. If this is not possible, place some glucose gel, honey, syrup, or jelly inside the patient's cheek.
- Persons who are unable to swallow without risk of aspiration can be given glucagon by subcutaneous or intramuscular injection. *Glucagon* is a hormone secreted by the pancreatic alpha cells that stimulates hepatic glucose production. It increases both glycogenolysis and gluconeogenesis and is less effective in patients with glycogen depletion.[20] It can produce substantial hyperglycemia, but as with oral glucose, the glycemic response is transient with glucose levels beginning to fall after approximately 1.5 hours.[25]
- Teach patients to keep glucagon in their homes at all times, and family members need to know how to administer it. Glucagon kits can be obtained by prescription. Patients also need to be aware of the expiration date on their glucagon.
- Glucagon can be injected subcutaneously or intramuscularly. Recommended doses are 1 mg for adults and older children, 0.5 mg for children <5 years old, and 0.25 mg for infants.[25]
- The glycemic effect of glucagon is quite short-lived, so as soon as the individual is able to swallow, carbohydrate liquid (eg, juice, soft drink, lowfat milk) should be administered to maintain normoglycemia (see Chapter 3, Pharmacologic Therapies, in Diabetes Management Therapies, for more information on glucagon).
- Nausea and vomiting often follows treatment of hypoglycemia with glucagon.[26]
- Frequent blood glucose monitoring is needed over the next several hours to detect blood glucose levels that are falling again or to detect hyperglycemia due to overtreatment.
- Instruct patients to notify their healthcare professional following episodes of severe hypoglycemia.

   **C** If episodes of severe hypoglycemia become frequent or recurrent, it is often helpful for the patient and team members to discuss how best to cope with these episodes. This discussion should only be attempted when the patient is not hypoglycemic.

## Psychosocial Impact

**1** Patients may develop emotional distress and fear of hypoglycemia after experiencing mild or severe hypoglycemia episodes.

   **A** Negative moods, social embarrassment, and potential danger associated with hypoglycemia can clearly cause emotional distress for patients. Results from the

DCCT[27] showed that the occurrence of severe hypoglycemia alone was not necessarily related to emotional distress, but recurrent episodes appeared to have a negative impact on quality of life.

**B** Patients may also develop significant anxiety about hypoglycemia and go to extreme measures to avoid its occurrence. The Hypoglycemia Fear Survey[28] is an assessment tool used to measure the extent to which patients worry about hypoglycemia and engage in behaviors to avoid hypoglycemia and its negative consequences. Patient groups at high risk for excessive fear of hypoglycemia are identified in Table 7.8.

**C** High levels of fear can contribute to inappropriate diabetes management, such as keeping blood glucose levels above the target range to avoid hypoglycemic episodes, or phobic avoidance of certain situations such as being alone or driving. Individuals may also be reluctant to make necessary increases in medications or insulin because of fear of hypoglycemia.

  • Conversely, low levels of fear can also contribute to inappropriate or high-risk behaviors, such as delaying treatment in response to symptoms.

  • Assess the possible psychological sequelae of hypoglycemia on a routine basis, especially after a patient experiences an episode of severe hypoglycemia.

---

### Table 7.8. Patient Groups at High Risk for Excessive Fear of Hypoglycemia

**Patient Characteristics**

• Have just begun taking blood glucose lowering medication
• Have little or no experience in coping effectively with episodes of hypoglycemia
• Have frequent and/or recurrent episodes of hypoglycemia
• Have experienced emotionally traumatic episodes of hypoglycemia
• Tend to be overly anxious
• Have ineffective coping skills
• Have visual impairment or other physical disabilities

---

**2** There are numerous aspects of hypoglycemia that contribute to conflicts between patients and significant others.

**A** The emotional changes associated with hypoglycemia (tension, irritation, and pessimistic thinking) can lead patients to become argumentative with others.

**B** When hypoglycemia is frequent or recurrent, patients may feel as if others blame them, so they become defensive and resentful; these behaviors can increase the likelihood of resisting treatment.

  • Similarly, family members can become angry and resentful if they believe their loved one is not exerting enough effort to prevent hypoglycemia or behaving in ways that increase the risk.

  • Spouses of persons with diabetes who experience frequent, severe hypoglycemia report increased rates of marital conflict about diabetes-related issues, including the prevention and treatment of hypoglycemia.[29]

**C** In some families, power struggles occur over the management of hypoglycemia; these struggles may reflect other areas of unresolved conflict. The educator can offer to refer these couples or families for counseling.

**3** Family members and significant others may experience similar emotional distress and fear of hypoglycemia similar to that of persons with diabetes.

  **A** Family members also can develop significant fear of hypoglycemia, especially if they have experienced episodes associated with very frightening or traumatic consequences for their loved one.
   • Spouses of patients who have experienced frequent, severe hypoglycemia show very high levels of fear compared with spouses of patients who have experienced only mild episodes.[29]
   • Parents of children with type 1 diabetes report very high levels of fear in general, but especially if their child has been unconscious or had a seizure while hypoglycemic.[30]

  **B** If nocturnal hypoglycemia has been a problem, family members may even develop sleep disorders such as insomnia or restless sleep if they feel they must remain vigilant during the night to recognize symptoms.[29]

## Assessment and Intervention

**1** Assessment of knowledge about hypoglycemia and individual risk factors is essential for developing effective educational and intervention plans.

  **A** Hypoglycemia risk, treatment, and prevention are determined by many different factors, both general and specific for each individual that may change over time. Therefore, education and intervention must be ongoing, individually tailored, and reassessed regularly to reflect changing patient needs.

  **B** The frequency and severity of hypoglycemic episodes can change over the course of diabetes due to a variety of factors:
   • Changes in diabetes treatment
   • Physiological changes (eg, insulin sensitivity, hormonal counterregulation)
   • Changes in symptoms
   • Lifestyle and schedule changes

  **C** Objectively assess knowledge about hypoglycemia whenever possible. Patients often are reluctant to ask questions or admit that they do not understand the information they receive. Knowledge assessment can be done verbally, and written instruments also are available, such as the Hypoglycemia Knowledge Questionnaire.[31]

  **D** In addition to basic knowledge, assess the patient's (or parents' if the patient is a child) personal habits and routine behaviors for treating and preventing hypoglycemia.
   • It is important to identify beliefs about hypoglycemia and its treatment. Sample questions that can be used to identify personal risk factors and beliefs about hypoglycemia are listed in Figure 7.2.
   • Include possible emotional and social barriers to hypoglycemia management and treatment in the assessment. For example, adolescents often dislike having to eat a morning snack during school because it makes them feel different from their peers. Young women who are overly concerned about weight gain may be at increased risk of hypoglycemia due to low carbohydrate intake, even when blood glucose levels are low (see Chapter 6, Psychological Disorders, in Diabetes Education and Program Management, for more information).

## Figure 7.2. Sample Questions to Determine Patient Risk Factors and Beliefs About Hypoglycemia

| To what extent do you: | Not At All | | Somewhat | | A Great Deal |
|---|---|---|---|---|---|
| 1 Always carry some type of food or drink with sugar? | 1 | 2 | 3 | 4 | 5 |
| 2 Skip meals? | 1 | 2 | 3 | 4 | 5 |
| 3 Skip snacks? | 1 | 2 | 3 | 4 | 5 |
| 4 Worry about hypoglycemia? | 1 | 2 | 3 | 4 | 5 |
| 5 Try to keep your BG levels below 100 mg/dL? | 1 | 2 | 3 | 4 | 5 |
| 6 Delay eating when trying to finish a task? | 1 | 2 | 3 | 4 | 5 |
| 7 Think having low BG is a sign of good control? | 1 | 2 | 3 | 4 | 5 |
| 8 Eat extra food when you're going to be more active? | 1 | 2 | 3 | 4 | 5 |
| 9 Recognize low BG symptoms? | 1 | 2 | 3 | 4 | 5 |
| 10 Eat as little as possible to avoid gaining weight? | 1 | 2 | 3 | 4 | 5 |
| 11 Increase your insulin whenever your blood glucose is too high? | 1 | 2 | 3 | 4 | 5 |
| 12 Wait until you feel strong symptoms to treat a low BG? | 1 | 2 | 3 | 4 | 5 |
| 13 Only treat very low BG levels (between 40 and 50 mg/dL)? | 1 | 2 | 3 | 4 | 5 |
| 14 Believe you can function fine when your BG is below 50 mg/dL? | 1 | 2 | 3 | 4 | 5 |

**E** Some aspects of hypoglycemia management can be assessed directly. For example, patients can be asked to show the educator their diabetes identification and the emergency glucose they are carrying.

**F** Symptoms and the ability to recognize low blood glucose levels should be assessed on a regular basis. Changes in symptoms (eg, loss of autonomic symptoms) and decreased ability to tell when blood glucose is low require additional education and intervention.

**G** At each routine visit, ask patients if any hypoglycemic episodes have occurred since their last appointment. If so, a structured interview can be given to evaluate the following factors. This type of structured evaluation is especially important after episodes of severe hypoglycemia to help identify specific risk factors and problem areas for individual patients.
- Date, time, and location of the hypoglycemic episode
- Severity of the episode
- Possible causes of the episode (eg, events during preceding 24 hours)
- Degree of symptomatology and ability to recognize the need for treatment

- Ability to self-treat and/or respond to attempts by others to provide treatment
- Decisions made about when and how to treat
- Barriers to treatment (eg, no available food/drink)
- Type and amount of food eaten
- Negative consequences of the episode (eg, distress, accidents, or embarrassment)

**H** After severe, distressing, or traumatic episodes of hypoglycemia, patients need to be assessed for possible negative psychosocial sequelae. Objective measures of distress, such as the Hypoglycemia Fear Survey,[28] can be used. This assessment can also be accomplished by asking patients questions such as the following about the negative emotional and social effects of their hypoglycemic episode:

- How upsetting was the episode for you?
- How worried are you about another episode like that happening again?
- Have you changed your diabetes management to avoid another episode?
- Did the episode cause any problems between you and other people?

**2** The core intervention for hypoglycemia management and treatment is effective education, although behavioral interventions may be needed when patients have a solid knowledge and understanding of hypoglycemia, yet continue to have problems.

**A** Goal setting and contracting can be used by patients to make specific behavioral changes.

**B** Teaching patients problem-solving techniques also can be effective for dealing with barriers to hypoglycemia management.

**C** When reduced hypoglycemic awareness is a problem, patients can use a diary to improve their ability to recognize and avoid hypoglycemia (Figure 7.1). Using a diary provides important benefits:

- Increased awareness of hypoglycemic symptoms and other predictors of low blood glucose levels
- Objective assessment of symptoms that are reliable signs of low blood glucose levels
- Objective assessment of how accurately low blood glucose is recognized
- Means of identifying patterns in hypoglycemic episodes (eg, causes, time of day)

**D** When frequent and/or severe hypoglycemic episodes continue in spite of medical, educational, and behavioral interventions, patients need referral to a mental health specialist who has experience working with diabetes-related psychosocial issues (see Chapter 6, Psychological Disorders, in Diabetes Education and Program Management, for more information).

- Patients who remain rather unconcerned or refuse to change their behavior, even after potentially dangerous episodes, also need referral for a psychological assessment.
- Referrals for counseling or psychotherapy also are appropriate when patients are experiencing emotional problems due to hypoglycemia, such as anxiety, phobias, or marital conflict.

**E** Currently, one psychoeducational intervention, Blood Glucose Awareness Training (BGAT)[32,33] has been demonstrated empirically to improve ability to recognize low blood glucose levels, reduce the frequency of low blood glucose levels, and reduce the incidence of severe hypoglycemia without jeopardizing diabetes control.

- BGAT involves 8 weekly sessions using a manual with 8 chapters (1 per week) that provides training in recognizing hypoglycemic symptoms and predicting low blood glucose levels due to changes in insulin, food, and physical activity.

• Each chapter also provides exercises (eg, symptom diary) to be done during the rest of the week to increase awareness of hypoglycemia.

## Key Educational Considerations

**1** Provide persons with type 1 diabetes basic information about hypoglycemia at diagnosis. This initial education includes

**A** An explanation of hypoglycemia and its causes

**B** A description of hypoglycemic symptoms

**C** Guidelines for treatment

**D** Preventive measures

**2** At diagnosis, patients and their families are attempting to assimilate new information and are likely to process only a fraction of what they are taught.

**A** For this reason, give patients written materials such as handouts and articles about hypoglycemia for later review.

**B** Ask newly diagnosed patients and their families to call back soon after the first hypoglycemic episode occurs to determine how they managed the episode and to receive further education.

**3** Teach patients and their families that hypoglycemic symptoms are idiosyncratic and that patients need to learn to recognize how they feel when their blood glucose is low.

**A** They need to know that hypoglycemic symptoms can sometimes be difficult to recognize and distinguish from other types of symptoms (eg, nervousness, sweating due to exertion).

**B** Describe the emotional and behavioral changes that can occur with hypoglycemia as biologically based and a normal manifestation of hypoglycemia.

**4** In spite of the initial information overload, patients' families need to be taught immediately how to administer glucagon when severe hypoglycemia occurs. This information must be repeated and reinforced on subsequent visits because families who have not had to use glucagon may forget how to use it, forget where they have placed it, or fail to check the expiration date.

**5** Persons with type 2 diabetes who are taking blood glucose-lowering medication also need to be taught about hypoglycemia, even though they appear to be at less risk for severe hypoglycemia.

**A** Patients who are changing from oral medications to insulin may have considerable fears and concerns about hypoglycemia and need to be taught to monitor themselves for warning symptoms, especially at those times of the day when they are at most risk (eg, just before lunch). These patients may also need to increase the frequency of self-blood glucose monitoring.

**B** Many type 2 patients are not adequately educated about hypoglycemia when they begin taking sulfonylureas or repaglinide and are not aware of the risks that hypoglycemia can impose. Knowledge about hypoglycemia, including warning symptoms, needs to be assessed even in patients who have been taking medication for a long period of time.

**C** Hypoglycemia is treated by carbohydrate consumption, following the guidelines prescribed for patients with type 1 diabetes. However, glucagon is not appropriate for type 2 diabetes because it stimulates insulin secretion.

**D** Sulfonylurea-induced hypoglycemia can be quite prolonged and can recur. For this reason, hospitalization may be necessary.

**E** While more research is needed, persons with type 2 diabetes requiring insulin may have the same risk for hypoglycemia as persons with type 1 diabetes.

**6** Education about hypoglycemia is an ongoing process.

**A** After diagnosis and initial education, the next important step in the learning process occurs when patients experience their first episode of hypoglycemia. Every hypoglycemic episode can be an opportunity for increasing knowledge.

**B** Use of the structured interview procedure can help teach patients about diabetes management behaviors that lead to lower blood glucose levels, their symptoms, and treatment decisions that increase the risk of severe episodes.

**C** Evaluation of specific episodes also provides an opportunity to give patients positive feedback when they have used their knowledge and judgment to avoid more severe problems with hypoglycemia.

**7** Initial education about hypoglycemia provides an opportunity to instill treatment habits such as using commercially packaged glucose tablets and consuming carbohydrates immediately when blood glucose is low.

**8** Ask patients and their families to describe their concerns about hypoglycemia; their input provides focus and direction for the educational efforts. Because areas of concern differ greatly across different patient groups and developmental stages, educational priorities are based on the personal needs of individual patients.

**A** Parents of infants with type 1 diabetes may justifiably worry about the negative long-term effects of hypoglycemia on their child's intellectual abilities; provide this group with more intensive diabetes education aimed at prevention.

**B** The lifestyle changes and attitudes of adolescent patients often place them at increased risk of hypoglycemia. For example, adolescents will try alcohol and periodically skip meals or eat inappropriate foods. Adolescents need to be reminded frequently about the effects of alcohol and drug use, increased exercise, dietary indiscretion, and other risky behaviors on blood glucose levels.

**9** Patients and their families need to be instructed about the risks of hypoglycemia and driving.

**A** These risks include automobile accidents and injury as well as being mistakenly arrested for driving while intoxicated, which can happen when an individual is not wearing diabetes identification.

**B** At each visit, ask patients if they keep some kind of emergency carbohydrate in their car and, if so, what kind of food/drink they carry. They can also be asked to show their
- Diabetes identification
- Emergency carbohydrate they carry at all times in their purse pocket.

**C** Assess patients' beliefs about driving and hypoglycemia.
- Ask how low they believe their blood glucose needs to be before they will not drive.

- Many patients believe that they can continue to drive safely with blood glucose levels quite low.[34]
- Patients should be instructed not to drive when their blood glucose is <70 mg/dL because they may have motor impairments they do not recognize and because their blood glucose can quickly become lower while they are driving.[35]

**D** Teach patients about the importance of checking their blood glucose before driving. This is especially important for patients who have previously experienced problems with hypoglycemia while driving or who have hypoglycemia unawareness.

## Self-Review Questions

**1** Define the different levels of hypoglycemia.

**2** List 10 symptoms associated with hypoglycemia and name the physiological basis for each of the symptoms.

**3** State 3 reasons why hypoglycemic symptoms can vary across individual patients and different episodes.

**4** Explain what reduced hypoglycemic awareness is and what causes it.

**5** Describe emotional and behavioral changes that can occur with hypoglycemia.

**6** List 3 of the most common causes of hypoglycemia.

**7** Describe the reason prolonged, vigorous exercises have a delayed effect on blood glucose levels.

**8** Describe the guidelines for treating a patient with a BG between 50 and 70 mg/dL (2.8 to 3.9 mmol/L); with a BG lower than 50 mg/dL (2.8 mmol/L).

**9** Name 3 foods that are not as effective for treating hypoglycemia and explain why these foods are inappropriate choices.

**10** Describe 2 beliefs about hypoglycemia that can lead patients to risky treatment behaviors such as delaying treatment.

**11** Describe fear of hypoglycemia and the types of patients who are most likely to exhibit it.

**12** Name 3 possible effects that hypoglycemia can have on family members and significant others.

## Learning Assessment: Case Study 1

LE is a 23-year-old female who has had type 1 diabetes for 12 years. Her metabolic control was fair during her adolescent and college years. LE currently is working full-time and living in an apartment with a roommate. For the last year, her glycemic control has been improving with regular insulin and NPH injections before breakfast and before dinner. She measures her BG before each insulin injection and sometimes before lunch. Because her fasting BG levels have been high, she has recently increased her predinner NPH. For weight control, LE jogs 3 miles after dinner several times each week and she only eats a bedtime snack if she feels hungry. At a routine office visit, LE reports that she is having 2 or 3 episodes of nocturnal hypoglycemia per week. In addition, she had many BG measurements during the day that were less than 50 mg/dL (2.8 mmol/L) and she felt no symptoms at all. LE also reports that during a recent episode, her roommate had to force jelly into her mouth to treat her.

## Questions for Discussion

**1** What clinical and behavioral factors increase LE's risk of hypoglycemia?

**2** What steps can be taken by LE and her diabetes care team to reduce the frequency of LE's nocturnal hypoglycemic episodes without jeopardizing her improved metabolic control?

## Discussion

**1** Several factors are contributing to LE's increased hypoglycemic risk:

  **A** Increase in predinner NPH dose

  **B** Failure to decrease predinner regular and/or NPH insulin dose before postdinner vigorous exercise

  **C** Failure to eat regular bedtime snacks and larger snacks after evening exercise

  **D** Failure to test bedtime BG levels

  **E** Reduction in hypoglycemic symptoms due to deficient and/or delayed hormonal counterregulation

**2** Ask LE to identify her concerns regarding hypoglycemia. Problem-solve with her about strategies to reduce nocturnal hypoglycemia. She can also make these behavioral goals.

**3** Strategies she might identify are

  **A** Consistently eat a bedtime snack. Check BG levels before eating the snack and make appropriate increases in the size of the snack depending on physical activity and BG level.

  **B** If nocturnal hypoglycemia continues despite these interventions, LE could move her predinner NPH to bedtime and her predinner regular insulin could be adjusted. She also could switch to a regimen of Ultralente twice a day, with preprandial lispro insulin. The effect of insulin regimen changes should be assessed after a few days, with additional dose changes implemented, if necessary. Frequent contact with the healthcare provider is critical while insulin adjustments are being made.

  **C** Because of her reduced hypoglycemia awareness, LE could do more frequent blood glucose monitoring and keep a blood glucose awareness diary. She should be taught to measure her blood glucose before driving or engaging in any other potentially risky activities.

  **D** Provide LE with a prescription for glucagon. LE can teach her roommate how to use it and place it where her roommate can easily find it.

## Learning Assessment: Case Study 2

MJ is a 66-year-old man who is overweight and was diagnosed with type 2 diabetes 4 years ago. His blood glucose has been poorly controlled using a meal plan and exercise program, so glyburide each morning before breakfast was added. MJ was instructed that it was critical that he eat breakfast soon after taking his medication. He said that this would be no problem, describing himself as an old-fashioned, meat-and-potatoes man who always has a hearty breakfast. When MJ returned to the clinic for his 3-month checkup, his blood glucose records showed that most of his fasting and predinner levels were in a normal range. However, MJ reported that his medication was causing unpleasant side effects. He described feeling shaky, dizzy, and nauseous during the mid- to late-morning hours. While these symptoms seemed to eventually subside on their own, MJ found them to be quite aversive and disruptive to his work. He indicated that he wanted to stop taking the medication and attempt again to control his blood glucose levels with a meal plan and exercise.

## Questions for Discussion

**1** What is the likely cause of MJ's unpleasant symptoms?

**2** What can be done to help MJ continue to take his oral medications?

**3** What food/meal factors would you want to assess as possible contributors to MJ's problem?

## Discussion

**1** Although it seems almost certain that MJ is experiencing midmorning hypoglycemia, this suspicion should be confirmed with daily midmorning BG measurements and additional measurements when symptoms occur.

**2** Because MJ appears to be confused by his symptoms, additional education is needed about:

**A** Causes, warning symptoms, and treatment of hypoglycemia

**B** Importance of carrying carbohydrate at all times, including having food or drink at the office and in the car for quick treatment

**3** MJ's meal pattern, especially breakfast foods, needs careful evaluation.

**A** He may eat a large breakfast that consists of high-fat, low-carbohydrate foods such as eggs, bacon, and milk. Consequently, his postmeal blood glucose levels may be lower than usual, causing him to become hypoglycemic.

**B** MJ should be given further nutritional education. Point out that by increasing his carbohydrate intake at breakfast he may prevent hypoglycemia.

**C** Another of his options is to eat a midmorning snack on a routine basis.

**4** If MJ continues to have problems with hypoglycemia in spite of these interventions, his morning dose of glyburide may need to be decreased, or he may need to switch to an oral agent that does not increase the risk for low blood glucose levels.

# References

1  The Diabetes Control and Complications Trial Research Group. The effect of intensive treatment of diabetes on the development and progression of long-term complications in insulin-dependent diabetes mellitus. N Engl J Med. 1993;329:977-986.

2  Cryer PE. Hypoglycemia: the limiting factor in the management of IDDM. Diabetes. 1994;43:1378-1389.

3  Cox DJ, Gonder-Frederick L, Antoun B, Cryer PE, Clarke WL. Perceived symptoms in the recognition of hypoglycemia. Diabetes Care. 1993;6:519-527.

4  Santiago JV, Clarke WL, Shah SD, Cryer PE. Epinephrine, norepinephrine, glucagon and growth hormone release in association with physiological decrements in the plasma glucose concentration in normal and diabetic man. J Clin Endocrinol Metab. 1980; 51:877-883.

5  Clarke WL, Gonder-Frederick LA, Richards E, Cryer PE. Multifactorial origin of hypoglycemic symptom unawareness in IDDM: association with defective glucose counterregulation and better glycemic control. Diabetes. 1991;40:680-685.

6  Clarke WL, Cox DJ, Gonder-Frederick LA, Julian D, Schlundt D, Polonsky W. Reduced awareness of hypoglycemia in adults with IDDM. A prospective study of hypoglycemic frequency and associated symptoms. Diabetes Care. 1995;18:517-522.

7  Amiel SA, Sherwin RS, Simonson DC, Tamborlane WV. Effect of intensive insulin therapy on glycemic thresholds for counterregulatory hormone release. Diabetes. 1988;37:901-907.

8  Amiel SA, Tamborlane WV, Simonson DC, Sherwin RS. Defective glucose counterregulation after strict glycemic control of insulin-dependent diabetes mellitus. N Engl J Med. 1987;316:1376-1383.

9  Cryer PE. Iatrogenic hypoglycemia as a cause of hypoglycemia-associated autonomic failure in IDDM. A vicious cycle. Diabetes. 1992;41:255-260.

10 Cranston I, Lomas J, Maran A, MacDonald I, Amiel SA. Restoration of hypoglycaemia awareness in patients with long-duration insulin-dependent diabetes. Lancet. 1994;344:283-287.

11 Fanelli CG, Epifano L, Rambotti AM, et al. Meticulous prevention of hypoglycemia normalizes the glycemia thresholds and magnitude of most neuroendocrine responses to, symptoms of, and cognitive function during hypoglycemia in intensively treated patients with short-term IDDM. Diabetes. 1993;42:1683-1689.

12 Heller SR, Cryer PE. Reduced neuroendocrine and symptomatic responses to subsequent hypoglycemia after 1 episode of hypoglycemia in nondiabetic humans. Diabetes. 1991;40:223-226.

13 Gonder-Frederick LA, Cox DJ, Bobbitt SA, Pennebaker JW. Mood changes associated with blood glucose fluctuations in insulin-dependent diabetes mellitus. Health Psychol. 1989;8:45-59.

14 McCrimmon RJ, Gold AE, Deary IJ, Kelnar CJ, Frier BM. Symptoms of hypoglycemia in children with IDDM. Diabetes Care. 1995;18:858-861.

15 Kerr D, Sherwin RS, Pavalkis F, et al. Effect of caffeine on the recognition of and responses to hypoglycemia in humans. Ann Intern Med. 1993;119:799-804.

16 MacDonald MJ. Postexercise late-onset hypoglycemia in insulin-dependent diabetic patients. Diabetes Care. 1987;10:584-588.

17 Wiethop BV, Cryer PE. Alanine and terbutaline in the treatment of hypoglycemia in IDDM. Diabetes Care. 1993;16:1131-1136.

**18** Gray RO, Butler PC, Beers TR, Kryshak EJ, Rizza RA. Comparison of the ability of bread versus bread plus meat to treat and prevent subsequent hypoglycemia in patients with insulin-dependent diabetes mellitus. J Clin Endocrinol Metab. 1996;81:1508-1511.

**19** Blackman JD, Towle VL, Sturis J, Lewis GF, Spire JP, Polonsky KS. Hypoglycemic thresholds for cognitive dysfunction in IDDM. Diabetes Care. 1992;41:392-399.

**20** Evans ML, Pernet A, Lomas J, Jones J, Amiel SA. Delay in onset of awareness of acute hypoglycemia and of restoration of cognitive performance during recovery. Diabetes Care. 2000;23:893-897.

**21** Gonder-Frederick L, Cox D, Kovatchev B, Schlundt D, Clarke W. A biopsychobehavioral model of risk of severe hypoglycemia. Diabetes Care. 1997;20:661-669.

**22** Gonder-Frederick LA, Cox DJ, Driesen NR, Ryan CM, Clarke WL. Individual differences in neurobehavioral disruption during mild and moderate hypoglycemia in adults with IDDM. Diabetes. 1994;43:1407-1412.

**23** Driesen NR, Cox DJ, Gonder-Frederick LA, Clarke WL. Reaction time impairment in insulin-dependent diabetes: Task complexity, blood glucose levels, and individual differences. Neuropsychology. 1995;9:246-254.

**24** Ryan CM, Atchison J, Puczynski S, Puczynski M, Arslanian S, Becker D. Mild hypoglycemia associated with deterioration of mental efficiency in children with insulin-dependent diabetes mellitus. J Pediatr. 1990;117:32-38.

**25** Cryer PE, Fisher JN, Shamoon H. Hypoglycemia (technical review). Diabetes Care. 1994;17:734-755.

**26** Collier A, Steedman DJ, Patrick AW, et al. Comparison of intravenous glucagon and dextrose in treatment of severe hypoglycemia in an accident and emergency department. Diabetes Care. 1987;10:712-715.

**27** The Diabetes Control and Complications Trial Research Group. Influence of intensive diabetes treatment on quality-of-life outcomes in the diabetes control and complications trial. Diabetes Care. 1996;19:195-203.

**28** Irvine A, Cox D, Gonder-Frederick L. The fear of hypoglycemia scale. In: Bradley C, ed. Handbook of Psychology and Diabetes. Switzerland: Hardwood Academic Publishers; 1994:133-155.

**29** Gonder-Frederick L, Cox D, Kovatchev B, Julian D, Clarke W. The psychosocial impact of severe hypoglycemic episodes on spouses of patients with IDDM. Diabetes Care. 1997;20:1543-1546.

**30** Clarke WL, Gonder-Frederick LA, Miller S, Richardson T, Snyder A. Maternal fear of hypoglycemia in their children with insulin-dependent diabetes mellitus. J Pediatr Endocrinol Metab. 1998;11:189-194.

**31** Drass JA, Feldman RH. Knowledge about hypoglycemia in young women with type I diabetes and their supportive others. Diabetes Educ. 1996;22:34-38.

**32** Cox D, Gonder-Frederick L, Polonsky W, Schlundt D, Julian D, Clarke W. A multicenter evaluation of blood glucose awareness training—II. Diabetes Care. 1995;18:523-528.

**33** Gonder-Frederick LA, Cox DJ, Clarke WL, Julian DM. Blood glucose awareness training. In: Snoek FJ, Skinner TC, eds. Psychology in Diabetes Care. Chichester, England: John Wiley & Sons; 2000:169-206.

**34** Clarke WL, Cox DJ, Gonder-Frederick LA Kovatchev B. Hypoglycemia and the decision to drive a motor vehicle by persons with diabetes. JAMA. 1999;282:750-754.

**35** Cox DJ, Gonder-Frederick LA, Kovatchev BP, Julian DM, Clarke WL. Progressive hypoglycemia's impact on driving simulation performance. Diabetes Care. 2000;23:163-170.

## Suggested Readings

Clarke WL, Cox DJ, Gonder-Frederick L, Julian D, Kovatchev B, Young-Hyman D. Biopsychobehavioral model of risk of severe hypoglycemia. Diabetes Care. 1999;22:580-584.

Cox DJ, Gonder-Frederick L, Clarke WL. Helping patients reduce severe hypoglycemia. In: Anderson BJ, Rubin RR, eds. Practical Psychology for Diabetes Clinicians. Alexandria, Va: American Diabetes Association; 1996:93-102.

Cryer, PE. Hypoglycemia: Pathophysiology, Diagnosis and Treatment. New York: Oxford University Press; 1997.

Gonder-Frederick L, Clarke WL, Cox DJ. The emotional, social, and behavioral implications of insulin-induced hypoglycemia. Semin Clin Neuropsychiatry. 1997;2:57-65.

Gonder-Frederick L, Cox DJ, Clarke WL. Helping patients understand and recognize hypoglycemia. In: Anderson BJ, Rubin RR, eds. Practical Psychology for Diabetes Clinicians. Alexandria, Va: American Diabetes Association; 1996:83-92.

Ter Braak EWMT, Appelman AMMF, van de Laak MF, Stolk RP, van Haeften TW, Erkelens DW. Clinical characteristics of type 1 diabetic patients with and without severe hypoglycemia. Diabetes Care. 2000;23:1467-1471.

### Other Resources

Blood Glucose Awareness Training was developed at the University of Virginia and is currently being used throughout the US, Canada, and Europe. Information about BGAT can be obtained by writing: The BGAT Institute, 555 Gillums Ridge Road, Charlottesville, VA 22901.

# Learning Assessment: Post-Test Questions

## Hypoglycemia                                                    7

1   When a patient with type 1 diabetes of
    10 years suddenly begins trembling,
    shaking, and experiencing other symp-
    toms indicating a hypoglycemic reaction,
    the body responds by releasing:
    A  Acetylcholine
    B  Epinephrine
    C  Hydrocortisone
    D  Glucagon

2   Neuroglycopenic symptoms now have
    been shown to:
    A  Occur before autonomic symptoms
    B  Occur later than autonomic symp-
       toms
    C  Be cholinergic in origin
    D  Occur at about the same time as
       autonomic symptoms

3   Which of the following is not a symptom
    of neuroglycopenia?
    A  Extremely high energy and excitation
    B  Slurred or rambling speech
    C  Mental confusion and disorientation
    D  Irrational or unusual behavior

4   When neuroglycopenic symptoms first
    occur, patients should:
    A  Wait for help from a healthcare pro-
       fessional
    B  Not treat themselves because of the
       possibility of an accident
    C  Treat themselves immediately
    D  Wait before any treatment because
       their symptoms may eventually disap-
       pear

5   Consumption of coffee may:
    A  Be a first aid treatment for hypo-
       glycemia
    B  Increase autonomic symptoms
    C  Enhance neuroglycopenia
    D  Interfere with gluconeogenesis

6   Hypoglycemia can be defined as any
    blood glucose level of:
    A  85 mg/dL or lower
    B  80 mg/dL of lower
    C  75 mg/dL or lower
    D  70 mg/dL or lower

7   Physical activity by the person with dia-
    betes:
    A  May require an increase in carbohy-
       drate consumption and/or insulin
       reduction
    B  May be beneficial to prevent hypo-
       glycemia
    C  Has no effect on hypoglycemia
    D  May require an increase in the insulin
       dose

8   Over the course of type 1 diabetes,
    defective hormonal counterregulation
    can cause:
    A  Neuroglycopenic symptoms to
       diminish
    B  Decreased epinephrine secretion
       leading to a diminished or delayed
       onset of symptoms
    C  Decreased glucagon secretion leading
       to a diminished or delayed onset of
       symptoms
    D  Fewer or delayed symptoms because
       of diminished cortisol secretion

9   Persons with type 1 diabetes and their
    families/significant others:
    A  Should not be given information con-
       cerning hypoglycemia on diagnosis
       because it increases their anxiety level
    B  Should be given written materials on
       hypoglycemia and instruction on
       administering glucagon
    C  Should be given written material, but
       no instruction on glucagon adminis-
       tration, because it is dangerous for a
       nonprofessional to administer
    D  Should be given instructions in
       glucagon administration but not on
       hypoglycemia to avoid information
       overload

**10** Patients with type 2 diabetes who are taking sulfonylureas and meglitinides:

**A** Do not require instruction in hypoglycemia because they are less at risk due to a maintenance of integrity of hormonal counterregulation

**B** Have an increased risk of hypoglycemia because of a lack of hormonal counterregulation

**C** Need to be taught about hypoglycemia, although they appear to be at less risk for severe hypoglycemia

**D** May experience occasional hypoglycemic attacks, but these are mild and never require corrective measures

**11** Problems with hypoglycemia:

**A** Are minimal for persons with type 2 diabetes receiving combination therapy

**B** Are more significant because of current treatment approaches and blood glucose goals

**C** Are less problematic as a result of the more intensive insulin therapies

**D** Only occur with patients using insulin therapy

**12** Symptoms associated with hypoglycemia:

**A** May vary for a person from one hypoglycemic episode to the next

**B** Are well-documented and occur consistently in patients with diabetes

**C** Are less likely to be affected by physiological or psychological factors

**D** Are only slightly affected by food, alcohol, or medications

**13** Most hypoglycemic episodes:

**A** Occur within 2 hours after taking intermediate-acting insulin

**B** Are likely to occur during the night

**C** Occur despite a consistent carbohydrate consumption and regularly scheduled meals

**D** Are unrelated or unaffected by physical activity

**14** Physical activity can have immediate and prolonged effects on blood glucose levels. One of these effects is:

**A** Increased glucose utilization combined with decreased glucose production

**B** Decreased glucose utilization by muscle tissue

**C** Delayed insulin absorption

**D** Accelerated glycogenolysis by the liver during exercise

*See next page for answer key.*

# Post-Test Answer Key

## Hypoglycemia 7

| | | | | |
|---|---|---|---|---|
| **1** | B | | **8** | B |
| **2** | D | | **9** | B |
| **3** | A | | **10** | C |
| **4** | C | | **11** | B |
| **5** | B | | **12** | A |
| **6** | D | | **13** | B |
| **7** | A | | **14** | A |

*Elaine Boswell King, MSN, RN, CS, CDE*
*Vanderbilt Diabetes Research and Training Center*
*Nashville, Tennessee*

*Janie Lipps, MSN, RN, CS, CDE*
*Vanderbilt Diabetes Research and Training Center*
*Nashville, Tennessee*

## Introduction

**1** This chapter will address the knowledge and skills needed by healthcare professionals and patients to manage diabetes during illness and surgery.

**2** Illness can cause problems when managing diabetes. During times of illness, the body releases stress hormones that oppose the action of insulin and contribute to hyperglycemia and the formation and accumulation of ketones. If appropriate action is not taken, dehydration and ketosis or a hyperosmolar hyperglycemic state (HHS) can result, requiring hospitalization.

**3** Surgical conditions can impact diabetes control. Persons with diabetes may require usual surgical interventions as well as surgery for associated complications of diabetes such as coronary artery disease, peripheral vascular disease, neuropathic ulcers, kidney disease, and proliferative retinopathy.

 **A** Patients' usual treatment programs are affected when surgery is performed; typical adjustments involve medical nutrition therapy, medications, and mobility.

 **B** Surgery can place persons with diabetes at risk for infections if their blood glucose remains above normal levels.

 **C** The perioperative management of persons with type 1 and type 2 diabetes can differ.

**4** An understanding of normal physiology is necessary to provide adequate support to the person with diabetes who is experiencing an illness or undergoing a surgical procedure. Special care is needed to achieve and maintain euglycemia, maintain fluid and electrolyte balance, provide adequate nutrition, and prevent further complications.

## Objectives

Upon completion of this chapter, the learner will be able to

**1** Describe the physiological effects of illness and surgery on blood glucose levels, ketone levels, and fluid and electrolyte balance.

**2** Describe specific guidelines that healthcare professionals can follow when managing the care of patients with intercurrent illnesses.

**3** Identify sick-day situations that require evaluation and possible treatment in an office, emergency room, or hospital setting.

**4** Identify assessment information needed preoperatively.

**5** Describe methods of insulin/glucose management for the surgical patient.

**6** Explain the importance of euglycemia during the perioperative period.

**7** Explain postoperative concerns.

## Physiologic and Clinical Effects of Illness and Surgery on Blood Glucose Levels, Ketone Levels, and Fluid/Electrolyte Balance

**1** Metabolic homeostasis is maintained by the balance of the anabolic hormone insulin and the major catabolic hormones glucagon, catecholamines, cortisol, and growth hormone. *[handwritten: not catabolic]* A major role of insulin is to lower glucose levels. Physiological stress caused by intercurrent illnesses, surgery, infection, injury, emotional trauma, or medications can disrupt homeostasis and cause hyperglycemia and ketosis.

**2** During illness and surgery, there is an increase in the secretion of counterregulatory hormones, including cortisol, catecholamines (epinephrine and norepinephrine), growth hormone, and glucagon.[1,2]

**A** Catecholamines cause an increase in heart rate, increase blood pressure, and dilate the bronchi to maximize the amount of oxygen that is supplied to the body tissues. Blood is diverted from the vulnerable surface of the body to the core to supply the vital organs with essential oxygen. Since blood is diverted from the skin and subcutaneous fat, injected insulin may not be absorbed.

**B** Epinephrine decreases the uptake of glucose by the muscle tissue and inhibits the release of endogenous insulin.

**3** In type 1 diabetes, counterregulatory hormones enhance the following metabolic changes: glycogenolysis, gluconeogenesis, lipolysis, and ketogenesis.[3,4]

**A** Counterregulatory hormones contribute to the release of glucose from the liver and oppose the action of insulin.

**B** Catecholamines and cortisol raise blood glucose levels by
- Causing glycogen that is stored in the liver to break down into glucose (*glycogenolysis*) and be released into the bloodstream.
- Causing the liver to create additional glucose (*gluconeogenesis*) from amino acids (alanine), glycerol, and lactate.
- Increasing peripheral insulin resistance.

**C** Catecholamines also suppress insulin release.

**D** Cortisol inhibits the uptake of glucose by the muscle tissue.

**4** With hyperglycemia, urine volume is increased due to osmotic diuresis; fluid requirements also increase.

**A** Signs and symptoms related to increased fluid requirements include polydipsia, polyuria, thirst, and dry mouth.

**B** If hyperglycemia persists without fluid and electrolyte replacement, dehydration can occur. Adequate insulin replacement must be given to lower glucose, correct the osmotic diuresis, and prevent diabetic ketoacidosis (DKA).

**C** Signs and symptoms resulting from dehydration include muscle weakness and fatigue related to loss of sodium, potassium, phosphorus, and magnesium.

**5** Ketogenesis and lipolysis are caused by an inadequate carbohydrate intake and/or insufficient insulin. Ketonuria and/or ketonemia are clinical manifestations of lipolysis and ketogenesis.

**A** Symptoms of ketosis include nausea and anorexia. If ketosis goes untreated, acidosis can result.

**B** Warning signals of ketoacidosis include fruity acidic breath, abdominal pain, and/or rapid, labored breathing (Kussmaul respiration) (see Chapter 2, Hyperglycemia, in Diabetes and Complications, for more information on DKA).

**C** Hospitalization is appropriate for DKA when the plasma glucose is >250 mg/dL (>13.9 mmol/L) with arterial pH <7.30 and serum bicarbonate level is <15 mEq/L in the presence of moderate ketonuria and/or ketonemia.[5]

**6** In type 2 diabetes, hyperosmolar hyperglycemic state (HHS) can occur as a manifestation of severe metabolic decompensation and dehydration. Although DKA and HHS are often discussed as distinct entities, they may overlap in a spectrum of decompensation.

**A** HHS is differentiated from DKA by the absence of significant ketosis. In HHS, volume depletion and dehydration result, but ketogenesis usually is suppressed because of levels of insulin high enough to prevent ketosis but not hyperglycemia.

**B** HHS is characterized by severe hyperglycemia (eg, plasma glucose >600 mg/dL (>33.3 mmol/L) and hyperosmolarity (eg, >320 mOsm/kg (>320 mmol/kg).[5,6]

**C** HHS is seen most often in the elderly, who have poor fluid intake or a diminished thirst mechanism.[7,8]

**D** If undetected or inadequately treated, lethargy, impaired mental status, or coma may result.[9]

**E** Recommendations for prevention and early treatment are similar to those for diabetic ketoacidosis. (See Chapter 2, Hyperglycemia, in Diabetes and Complications, for more information on HHS.)

## Guidelines for Sick-Day Management

**1** Maintain adequate hydration because of the risk of dehydration from decreased fluid intake, polyuria, vomiting, diarrhea, and evaporative losses from fever.

**A** Instruct patients to drink at least 8 oz (240 mL) of calorie-free fluids every hour while they are awake. Examples of calorie-free liquids include diet soft drinks, water, broth, and sugar-free Kool-Aid® soft drink. Because caffeine acts as a diuretic, the fluids consumed should be caffeine-free. Bouillon, consommé, and canned clear soups provide sodium and electrolytes as well as fluids and at least 8 oz should be consumed every third hour. A major cause of persistent ketoacidosis is inadequate sodium intake.

**B** If the patient is unable to tolerate fluids by mouth, antiemetic suppositories or intravenous fluids may be required. Vomiting that cannot be suppressed may require emergency room care.

**2** Increase the frequency of blood glucose monitoring and initiate ketone monitoring during suspected or acute illness.

**A** The signs and symptoms of a developing acute illness can be preceded by elevated blood glucose levels and ketone levels.

**B** More frequent monitoring is indicated when the person experiences unusual physical symptoms such as malaise, fever, anorexia, and/or nausea or when blood glucose levels rise. These symptoms may disappear or may develop into an identifiable illness.

**C** The frequency of blood glucose monitoring may need to be increased to every 2 to 4 hours while glucose levels are elevated and/or until symptoms subside. Blood or urine ketone levels also need to be tested every 4 hours until negative results are obtained. Monitoring is performed at times when decisions regarding the insulin dose are needed.

**D** Instruct patients to record their monitoring results and response to treatment adjustments in order to more readily provide this information to the healthcare professional over the telephone, if needed.

**3** Adjust medications during illness.

**A** Insulin and/or most oral agents are still needed during illness even when the patient is unable to eat. Omission of insulin is a common cause of ketosis.

- Continue the routine dose of intermediate- or long-acting insulin (NPH, Lente, Ultralente).
- The full dose of daily insulin usually is required.
- Individuals using insulin pump therapy should continue their basal insulin and may need to increase their basal rate. The pump should not be removed unless an adequate amount of insulin is administered via injections. Pump infusion site problems may result in hyperglycemia and ketoacidosis. Pump users should be instructed to change the infusion site in response to any unexpected metabolic decompensation. This is recommended even if the site has recently been changed, as the first sign of a site problem may be the development of hyperglycemia and ketosis.
- Metformin should be stopped during a serious illness and insulin treatment may be initiated. Lactic acidosis is a rare but potential adverse effect in metformin-treated patients when an illness causes hypotension and decreases tissue perfusion.[10]

**B** Supplemental doses of rapid-acting or short-acting insulins also may be required for continuously rising or persistently elevated blood glucose levels, large ketones, or persistent ketones.[11] Teach patients to call the healthcare professional for instructions on taking extra insulin if they have not previously been given an insulin algorithm for sick days.

- Rapid-acting or short-acting insulins may be given every 1 to 4 hours.
- The doses of rapid- and short-acting insulin depend on the severity of the illness. During most illnesses, 10% of the total daily dose can be given safely as a supplemental dose of rapid-acting or short-acting insulin. If the blood glucose level is higher than 300 mg/dL (16.7 mmol/L) with large ketones, 20% of the routine dose may be given as a supplement. There are a variety of alternative approaches to the acute treatment of hyperglycemia.
- In the rare event that hypoglycemia exists, the rapid-acting or short-acting insulin doses can be decreased while maintaining the usual intermediate-acting or long-acting insulin doses. Hypoglycemia may occur with nausea and vomiting of short duration without systemic involvement such as fever.

**C** Over-the-counter and prescription medications may contribute to hyperglycemia or hypoglycemia (see Chapter 3, Pharmacologic Therapies, in Diabetes Management Therapies, for more information).

**4** Substitute liquids or soft foods if patients are unable to tolerate usual foods at meal times because of nausea or anorexia.

**A** In general, oral ingestion of approximately 200 g of carbohydrate per day in evenly divided doses (45 to 50 g, or 3 or 4 carbohydrate choices, every 3 to 4 h) should be sufficient, along with medication adjustments, to prevent starvation ketosis. If regular foods are not tolerated, liquid or soft carbohydrate-containing foods, such as regular soft drinks, juices, soups, and ice cream, can be eaten.[12,13]

**B** The foods and beverages shown in Table 8.1 contain approximately 15 g of carbohydrate and are appropriate for sick-day use.

**5** Teach patients when to call their healthcare provider.

**A** Some patients hesitate to telephone the healthcare team because they are concerned that their call might be a bother. Encourage patients to call anytime when questions and problems arise.

**B** Instruct patients to call a healthcare professional immediately if any of the conditions in Table 8.2 develop.

---

## Table 8.1. Foods That Contain 15 g of Carbohydrate

- ½ cup apple juice
- ½ cup regular soft drink (not diet, caffeine-free)
- 1 Popsicle® stick
- 5 Lifesavers® candies
- 1 slice dry toast
- ½ cup cooked cereal
- 6 saltines
- ⅓ cup frozen yogurt
- 1 cup Gatorade® (replaces electrolytes) sports drink
- ½ cup regular ice cream
- ¼ cup sherbet
- ¼ cup regular pudding
- ½ cup regular gelatin/Jell-O®
- 1 cup yogurt (not frozen) artificially sweetened or plain
- Milkshake (⅓ cup lowfat milk and ¼ cup ice cream)

---

## Table 8.2. Conditions That Require Immediate Contact With a Healthcare Professional

- Vomiting more than once
- Diarrhea more than 5 times or for longer than 6 hours
- Difficulty breathing
- Blood glucose levels higher than 300 mg/dL (16.7 mmol/L) on 2 consecutive measurements that are unresponsive to increased insulin and fluids
- Moderate or large urine ketones or blood ketones above 0.6 mmol/L

---

## Table 8.3. Signs and Symptoms That Require Clinic or Hospital Treatment by a Healthcare Professional

- Persistent vomiting or an inability to tolerate fluids by mouth
- Persistent diarrhea and progressive weakness
- Orthostasis
- Difficulty breathing, rapid and labored respirations
- Blood or urine ketones that do not improve
- Change in mental status

## Sick-Day Situations That Require Examination and Possible Treatment by a Healthcare Professional

1 The healthcare professional can determine whether telephone management is possible or if an assessment and evaluation in the clinic or emergency room is indicated.

2 Teach patients the signs and symptoms listed in Table 8.3 since they indicate a need for examination, treatment, and possible hospital care.

## Perioperative Treatment for Patients With Diabetes

1 The goals of therapy during the perioperative period are prevention of hypoglycemia, excessive hyperglycemia, lipolysis, protein catabolism, and electrolyte disturbance.
   A Hyperglycemia has been associated with problems such as decreased effectiveness of leukocytes, increased risk of platelet aggregation, and increased rigidity of the red blood cell. This results in decreased circulation through the small vessels and deprivation of oxygen and nutrients.
   B Ketosis and ketoacidosis may ensue with persistent hyperglycemia, leading to a drop in pH. Patients with type 1 diabetes undergoing surgery are more prone to developing acidosis even with moderate hyperglycemia.[14]
   C All patients with glucose intolerance are susceptible to electrolyte abnormalities and volume depletion from osmotic diuresis.
   D Unrecognized and untreated hypoglycemia may endanger the life of the surgical patient. Because hypoglycemia in the anesthetized patient can be difficult to identify, frequent perioperative blood glucose monitoring is imperative.

2 Theoretically, enhanced healing depends on establishing and maintaining homeostasis. Normal glucose levels are essential for the normal protein synthesis that is required for wound healing without infection.[15] For maximum healing the blood glucose level should be less than 200 mg/dL (11.1 mmol/L).[16]

## General Preoperative Assessment and Preparation for Surgery

1 Preoperative care includes a thorough history and physical examination.

2 Include the following information on the admission history:
   A Date of diabetes diagnosis
   B Any current signs and symptoms including those of uncontrolled diabetes
   C Medications, including type, dosage, and timing of insulin and/or oral agents
   D Over-the-counter medications
   E Assessment of metabolic control using home blood glucose records and HbA1c if available
   F Current weight and maximum weight
   G Previous hospital admissions for surgery and other illnesses
   H For women, the last menstrual period and childbearing history
   I Allergies
   J Previous episodes of ketoacidosis, HHS, and severe hypoglycemia

**3** Diagnostic laboratory data should be reviewed prior to admission for surgery with special consideration given to electrolyte balance and blood count.

**A** An elevated HbA1c may indicate that the patient has been in poor control, is dehydrated, and may have a greater risk for ketoacidosis. A glycosylated albumin or fructosamine test may help determine the most recent level of glucose control.

**B** Just prior to surgery, a complete blood count and electrolyte profile should be performed to assess for any metabolic derangements. Patients who have been hyperglycemic may be dehydrated. Patients with diabetic nephropathy may need monitoring to avoid fluid overload and hyperkalemia. An elevated white blood cell count (WBC) may indicate an underlying infection that would impede postoperative recovery.

**4** Special considerations need to be given to the patient's cardiovascular, cerebrovascular, peripheral vascular, respiratory, neurological, and renal systems.

**A** Certain cardiovascular assessments and considerations are necessary.

- A thorough assessment is performed of any past cardiac problems and any cardiovascular symptoms. Cardiac problems are the leading cause of death in persons with diabetes. The presence of carotid bruits or transient ischemia attacks (TIAs) prior to surgery may indicate cerebrovascular disease. Metabolic and hemodynamic stresses may compromise the cardiovascular system and lead to myocardial infarction, congestive heart failure, cerebral vascular accidents, or acute renal failure. Anesthesia agents can depress heart muscle function and may induce rhythm disturbances. Several events during surgery can place additional stress on the myocardium: bleeding may result in hypovolemia, hypotension, tachycardia, or bradycardia; volume overload, fever, and shivering all may put additional stress on the myocardium. Patients with diabetes are also at risk for developing postoperative myocardial ischemia.[14]

- If there is a history consistent with atherosclerotic cerebrovascular disease, the patient needs a vascular evaluation. All patients need, at minimum, auscultation of the carotids.

- Preoperative and postoperative electrocardiograms should be obtained as well as measurements of cardiovascular enzyme activity, when indicated.

- Blood pressure needs to be carefully monitored; antihypertensive medications should be reinstituted promptly after surgery.

- It is important that a patient with a history of congestive heart failure (CHF) be assessed for fluid status. Caution is needed to prevent overhydration. The patient with CHF or hypertension may be at risk for hypokalemia due to previous diuretic therapy.

**B** Certain neurological assessments and considerations are necessary.

- If the patient has had recent TIAs, a neurological evaluation may be indicated.

- The presence of some manifestations of neuropathy may affect recovery from the operation. Orthostatic hypotension, neurogenic bladder, hyperesthesia or hypoesthesia, and gastroparesis (including a history of early satiety) are some manifestations of diabetic neuropathies. Physical assessment needed to identify these problems includes lying and standing blood pressure readings, reflex and light touch assessment of the feet, and determination of residual urine, if there is any suggestion of autonomic neuropathy.

**C** Certain renal assessments and considerations are necessary.

- The presence of renal disease may alter the types and amounts of fluid infused and medication dosages. As part of the general assessment to guide diabetes management, measurement of urine protein and creatinine clearance may be indicated if the patient's diabetes has been diagnosed for more than 5 years and the tests have not been performed recently. If there is inadequate time to perform a 12- or 24-hour urine collection for a quantitative evaluation, random dipstick for proteinuria may be used for screening. A serum creatinine should be included in the electrolyte screen.

- Arteriography procedures using radiocontrast material (nephrotoxic) need to be undertaken with caution in the patient with renal disease. The use of low osmolar dyes may be indicated; adequate hydration is essential and as small a dose as possible should be utilized.

## Perioperative Concerns for Patients With Type 1 Diabetes

**1** Several protocols for insulin management of the surgical patient with diabetes are available and effective. Ideally, a diabetologist or endocrinologist will be consulted for insulin and fluid management. In all insulin protocols, however, the usual insulin dosage is altered for the day of surgery and adequate glucose is supplied.

**A** A glucose and insulin infusion regimen is the best option for providing optimal glucose control during surgery and the immediate postoperative period.

- Rapid-acting or short-acting insulin is mixed in a normal saline solution and infused intravenously using an infusion pump. An initial rate of 0.5 to 1.5 units per hour may be used. Beginning a dose at the low range is a safe way to start. Dose adjustments may be made frequently based on blood glucose monitoring.

- Most protocols use a 5% or 10% glucose solution in a separate bag from the insulin solution. The glucose solution is administered in a piggyback fashion with the insulin solution. This method allows the insulin dose to be adjusted as needed while also allowing adjustment of the glucose infusion.

- Hourly capillary blood glucose measurements are used to determine the dose of insulin based on an algorithm.[16]

**B** Insulin is usually given subcutaneously with brief surgical procedures when the patient will be able to eat lunch.

- Subcutaneous rapid-acting insulin may be given with a 5% or 10% glucose intravenous solution to maintain the target glucose levels. Numerous methods have been used to calculate the dosage, from unit per kilogram body weight to present total daily dose. The rate of insulin given usually varies from 0.5 to 5.0 units per hour.[11]

- Another approach is to withhold the morning rapid- or short-acting insulin and give one half to all of the morning intermediate-acting insulin. This method can lead to unpredictable glycemic excursions due to the variable absorption times of intermediate-acting insulin and the decreased peripheral perfusion during surgical procedures. However, if coverage is provided for basal insulin needs during a brief surgical procedure, rapid- or short-acting insulin can be given as needed based on bedside glucose monitoring.

**C** Persons wearing an insulin infusion pump may continue wearing the pump during surgery and be given additional intravenous insulin if needed.

**2** Sufficient glucose to prevent hypoglycemia and to provide the basal energy requirement is administered during surgery in the insulinopenic patient. Administering 150 g of glucose over 24 hours (ie, 5 g per hour) will avoid ketosis.[16]

**3** Electrolytes may be given as needed and added to the glucose solution.[16]

**4** Persons who must be on fluid restrictions due to renal failure or heart failure may receive higher concentrations of glucose in smaller volumes of fluid using a central venous line.[16]

**5** Surgery or tests that require the patient to have nothing by mouth (NPO) should be scheduled early in the morning whenever possible to prevent long periods of fasting. If the test or procedure is scheduled mid-to-late morning or in the afternoon, intravenous fluids and insulin should be initiated on the morning of the procedure to prevent hyperglycemia, hypoglycemia, and ketosis. For testing that requires an overnight fast in a person using an insulin pump or on an intensive insulin regimen, the basal insulin or intermediate insulin may be continued. Frequent blood glucose monitoring is needed to provide the information to make treatment decisions.

**6** Frequent blood glucose and urine ketone monitoring are necessary to evaluate the adequacy of the insulin dose and calorie replacement.
  **A** Urine ketone accumulation should be monitored every 4 to 6 hours, or anytime the blood glucose level is greater than 240 mg/dL (13.3 mmol/L).
  **B** The ease of obtaining and testing capillary samples using a blood glucose meter makes frequent blood glucose testing feasible with less expense. At minimum, blood glucose levels need to be checked preoperatively and postoperatively and before insulin administration. If the patient is receiving intravenous insulin, it is essential to monitor the blood glucose every hour if the patient is unstable or changes have been made in the insulin dose. Intraoperative blood glucose levels should be checked every 30 to 60 minutes.

## Perioperative Concerns for Persons With Type 2 Diabetes

**1** Type 2 patients who undergo surgery may be using insulin to manage their diabetes.
  **A** These patients may respond metabolically like type 1 patients so the treatment approach may be the same.
  **B** The main determinants for therapy in type 2 patients are the magnitude of the procedure and the metabolic state of the patient on the day of surgery.[16]

**2** Patients whose diabetes is well controlled with medical nutrition therapy (MNT) or MNT plus oral antidiabetes agents do not require specific therapy. Patients with fasting blood glucose levels lower than 140 mg/dL (7.8 mmol/L) treated with an oral agent can be given their medication and started on a glucose infusion the morning of surgery; however, it is sometimes suggested to stop the oral agent the evening before surgery. Discontinue the longer acting chlorpropamide 48 to 72 hours prior to the surgical procedure. Discontinue metformin the morning of the surgery. Metformin should not be resumed postoperatively until the patient has resumed a regular diet and has normal renal function.

**3** Type 2 patients who are poorly controlled on oral agents may need insulin during their perioperative period using the same regimens as type 1 patients.[16] Aggressive treatment of hyperglycemia and maintaining adequate hydration can prevent HHS, infection, and improve wound healing.

## Postoperative Care

**1** Impaired wound healing can occur when the blood glucose level is greater than 200 mg/dL (11.1 mmol/L).[16]

   **A** The wound needs to be observed carefully for any signs of inflammatory changes or drainage, and alterations in the patient's temperature noted. Meticulous wound care is essential to prevent infection.

   **B** Maintaining and improving circulation to promote wound healing is particularly important for the person with diabetes who may have peripheral vascular disease.

**2** Continue monitoring of blood glucose and electrolytes in the postoperative period. Hypoglycemia is a particular concern because the blood glucose level and insulin dose may decrease dramatically as the stress of surgery declines or as an infection is treated.

**3** Postoperative nutritional management consists of 2 phases. Involvement of a registered dietitian will help to ensure a successful transition through these phases and reinitiation of medication that are essential for a successful outcome.

   **A** The first phase of nutritional management is the initial catabolic phase that extends from the period just before surgery into the period immediately following the operation. The second phase is the transition time during which the patient moves from NPO status to the usual meal plan.

   **B** During the reintroduction of foods such as clear liquids, it is preferable to continue a low-maintenance dose of intravenous or subcutaneous rapid-acting or short-acting insulin along with fluids to maintain target blood glucose levels.

   **C** Returning to the usual meal plan as soon as possible will promote healing and reestablish homeostasis. Adequate carbohydrate is needed daily to prevent ketosis due to starvation. Solid foods can be started as soon as tolerated.

**4** Once food tolerance is established, the intravenous insulin infusion is stopped and a new treatment program is planned, considering such elements as infection, pain, steroids, or total parenteral nutrition (TPN). For patients treated with oral agents, the usual dose may be given with supplements of rapid-acting or short-acting insulin. For insulin-treated patients, a combination of intermediate-acting and rapid-acting or short-acting insulin may be given. When using only rapid-acting or short-acting insulin, care must be taken not to leave insulinopenic patients without basal insulin.

**5** It is very important to note that subcutaneous insulin needs to be given at least 30 minutes prior to the discontinuation of any intravenous insulin infusion to prevent hyperglycemia.

**6** Capillary blood glucose monitoring is needed a minimum of 4 times per day, usually before meals and at bedtime to determine the effectiveness of the therapy.

**7** Pain can cause the release of counterregulatory hormones that can increase the blood glucose level. Adequate pain management will help relieve this response. Because pain medication can make the patient drowsy, frequent assessment is necessary to recognize hypoglycemia. Hyperglycemia may heighten the perception of pain.

**8** Peripheral neuropathy and peripheral vascular disease increase the risk of ulcerations. Careful monitoring of pressure areas and ambulation as soon as possible will help reduce the risk of these postoperative complications.

**9** Written instructions are mandatory for postsurgical home care, with instructions for insulin, other medications, meal planning, physical activity, and wound care, if applicable.

## Emergency Surgery

**1** In situations that require emergency surgery, diabetes management will depend upon the metabolic condition of the patient. Surgical emergencies, particularly if there is underlying infection, can cause rapid metabolic decompensation, with dehydration and hyperglycemia, and ultimately ketoacidosis in the patient with type 1 diabetes. If the patient is in early or established DKA, the first priority is metabolic management.

**2** If the patient is without severe metabolic disturbance, the initial diabetes management can involve intravenous insulin infusion. If the patient is dehydrated, normal saline is used for fluid replacement.[17]

## Surgery in Children

**1** Few published guidelines exist for the surgical management of diabetes in children. In general, adult regimens have been adapted for use.[17]

**2** Caution needs to be taken in calculating fluid and insulin requirements. Consult a pediatric endocrinologist, if available.

## Key Educational Considerations

**1** Sick-day management is a survival skill and should be taught at an appropriate level to all patients with diabetes.

**A** Sick-day instruction and reinforcement are a priority before a hospital discharge; before starting day care, school, or college; before the flu season; when administering the flu vaccine; and before overnight travel away from home.

**B** Learning is reinforced and retained when it is applied immediately. Because sick-day guidelines usually are taught when patients are healthy, evaluation needs to include assessing the patient's immediate and long-term recall of knowledge about sick-day management.

**C** Give patients written instructions as reinforcement, keeping the guidelines as simple as possible.

• If appropriate, ask the patient if it will help to copy the guidelines or highlight notes on a provided handout to enhance retention and personalize the written instruction.

- Ask the patient where the guidelines will be posted or placed for easy access when needed.
- Suggest that the patient pack a sick-day box with supplies and nonperishable items that can be stored for use during illness. Acknowledge that the patient may not be accustomed to keeping glucose-containing products such as Jell-O® gelatin, regular soft drinks, or regular sports drinks at home. Review the rationale for keeping these items on hand for sick days and determine if the patient is willing to prepare this kit. Ask about the site for storage or placement.

**D** Evaluate patient's actual skills during and following an intercurrent illness.

- During telephone contact and/or clinic visits on sick days, ask the patient to describe action taken during illness and assess results.
- Ask the patient to describe how the sick-day plan worked and identify what changes are needed to make the plan work better.
- During follow-up visits, props and simulations can be used for reinforcement and to assist the patient in recalling sick-day guidelines. For example, props such as rapid-acting or short-acting insulin vials, blood glucose and ketone testing materials, and an 8-oz plastic glass can be used to emphasize sick-day care. Simulations such as telephone call role-playing, review of blood glucose records, and actions to take may help to evaluate patient recall.

**E** During an illness, many patients experience malaise, fatigue, and sleepiness, making self-care more difficult. Therefore, family members or significant others need to be familiar with sick-day guidelines and know where sick-day supplies and instructions are kept. Discuss a plan for their role and participation prior to an illness. They also need to know when to call a healthcare professional.

**2** The preoperative assessment may provide insight into the educational needs of the patient and significant other(s). Assessing the patient's knowledge will help provide direction for preoperative and postoperative diabetes teaching. Include family members or significant others in the preoperative teaching, so they understand the postoperative recovery care needed.

**A** Explain to the patient how the insulin dose will be administered and adjusted during surgery. Many patients are fearful of giving others the decision-making responsibility for insulin adjustment.

**B** Explain the need for dextrose in the intravenous solution. Many patients know that dextrose raises the blood glucose level and they are concerned that an error may be made.

**C** Explain to patients with type 2 diabetes who are treated with oral agents that they may need insulin just for the time before, during, and immediately after surgery. Many patients are concerned that insulin therapy may permanently replace their previous treatment.

**D** Prepare the patient for frequent capillary blood glucose and urine ketone testing. Blood glucose levels may be checked every 1 to 2 hours.

**3** Provide written discharge instructions for any medications, including insulin (if applicable), meal plan, physical activity, and surgical and medical follow-up. Work with the significant other(s) to plan menus for the first few days at home. Prior to discharge, provide updated information about medical nutritional therapy.

## Self-Review Questions

1 Describe the physiologic effects of illness and surgery on blood glucose levels, ketone levels, and fluid and electrolyte balance.

2 Discuss specific guidelines that healthcare professionals may use when managing an intercurrent illness.

3 List situations that require examination and possible treatment in an office, emergency room, or hospital setting during an illness.

4 Describe the effects of surgery on the cardiovascular system.

5 State the reason why the prevention of hyperglycemia is important to the surgical patient with diabetes.

6 List methods to prevent hyperglycemia in the surgical patient.

7 Describe what should be included in preoperative management.

8 List 2 alternatives for insulin therapy intraoperatively and immediately postoperatively. Discuss advantages and disadvantages of these alternatives.

9 List 4 potential postoperative problems that may be more common in the person with diabetes.

10 State which oral agent should be discontinued the morning of surgery.

## Learning Assessment: Case Study 1

RS is a 32-year-old sales representative who was diagnosed with type 1 diabetes 1 year ago. He manages his diabetes with multiple daily injections of insulin consisting of long- and rapid-acting insulin before breakfast, rapid-acting insulin before lunch, and long-acting and rapid-acting insulin before dinner. He monitors his blood glucose 4 times per day, counts carbohydrates, and strives for consistency. RS has been instructed on the recognition and treatment of hypoglycemia, ketone testing, and sick-day management. He returns to the clinic for follow-up once every 2 to 3 months.

This morning RS calls you to report that he is feeling nauseated. He states that his blood glucose level before breakfast was 233 mg/dL, he administered his usual dose of insulin using his insulin algorithm, and then he was only able to drink one small glass of apple juice before becoming nauseated. It is now noon and he is still nauseated and does not feel like eating lunch or going to the office. RS reports that he vaguely recalls being instructed on sick-day management, but he is unsure what he should do because this is his first episode of being sick since his diagnosis.

## Questions for Discussion

1 What additional assessment data would you obtain at this point?

2 What instruction and/or advice might be given?

## Discussion

1 Gather information to determine if the patient's condition is stable.

   A Assess whether the patient has been vomiting or experiencing diarrhea, how often, and for how many hours.

**B** Listen for symptoms of respiratory distress and ask whether the patient has had difficulty breathing.

**C** RS reported no vomiting, diarrhea, or respiratory distress.

**2** Once acute distress is ruled out, recent blood glucose and blood or urine ketone results are needed. Although diabetic ketoacidosis usually develops over hours, hyperglycemia and ketosis could be present yet unknown if self-monitoring of blood glucose and ketone testing is not performed or if testing is performed incorrectly.

**A** RS had not tested his blood glucose since before breakfast and had not checked for ketones. He was asked to obtain blood glucose and blood or urine ketone measurements.

**B** Depending on the circumstances, the healthcare professional may wait for the patient to report the testing results or ask the patient to call back immediately with the results.

**C** RS reported a blood glucose value of 363 mg/dL (20.2 mmol/L) and a small amount of ketones.

**3** Assess fluid and food intake.

**A** Fluid intake was assessed and RS reported that he had been sipping on a diet soft drink during the morning because of thirst; because of nausea he had consumed only a total of approximately 8 oz.

**B** He reported eating no solid foods.

**C** The concept of avoiding dehydration by consuming adequate fluids was explained.

**D** Because his blood glucose was 363 mg/dL, he agreed to have bouillon (a source of sodium and fluid) and a diet soft drink for lunch – both items were on hand and choices he likes. He also agreed to drink 8 oz of calorie-free, caffeine-free fluids hourly during the afternoon and evening, drinking in sips if necessary.

**4** Reinforce the rationale for not omitting insulin doses.

**A** RS was given reassurance that administering his morning dose of insulin was appropriate.

**B** He then was instructed to use his insulin algorithm and administer his pre-lunch dose of rapid-acting insulin immediately after the telephone conversation.

**5** Review plan of care and when to call.

**A** RS was instructed to retest his blood glucose and blood or urine ketone levels in 3 hours, pre-supper (7 PM), and at bedtime.

**B** He was reminded to call if his blood glucose values were higher than 300 mg/dL (16.7 mmol/L) and if he had moderate or large ketones.

**C** RS was encouraged to telephone the clinic immediately if vomiting occurred more than once, if he experienced more than 5 episodes of diarrhea, or if he had difficulty breathing.

---

## Learning Assessment: Case Study 2

CB is a 42-year-old female who was diagnosed with type 1 diabetes at age 17 years. She is being admitted for an elective cholecystectomy with general anesthesia. CB is hypertensive and being treated with ACE inhibitors. She also has background diabetic retinopathy and proteinuria.

CB monitors her blood glucose 3 to 4 times per day and injects 15 units of Ultralente with 6 units of a lispro insulin before breakfast, 4 units of lispro before lunch, 8 units of lispro before dinner, and 15 units of Ultralente at bedtime.

In a team meeting the day before CB's admission for surgery, the resident suggests the following plan:

**1** Based on CB's blood glucose level, make the following adjustments in insulin:
- <150 mg/dL (8.3 mmol/L) = no insulin
- 151 to 200 mg/dL (8.4 to 11.1 mmol/L) = 4 units
- 201 to 250 mg/dL (11.2 to 13.9 mmol/L) = 6 units
- 251 to 350 mg/dL (14.0 to 19.4 mmol/L) = 8 units

*? Lispro*

**2** CB will be advised to take her usual Ultralente dose on the morning of surgery.

**3** Capillary blood glucose readings are ordered every 4 hours and she will be given lispro insulin using a sliding scale.

## Questions for Discussion
**1** What problems do you see with the resident's plan?
**2** What other options can be considered?
**3** What pre- and post-operative teaching needs can you identify for CB and her family?

## Discussion
**1** Use of an insulin/glucose infusion would be optimal.
   **A** Use of an intermediate-acting or long-acting insulin prior to a lengthy surgical procedure could lead to difficulties with hypoglycemia or hyperglycemia.
   **B** Subcutaneous insulin is not given during surgery due to unpredictable absorption from changes in body temperature, varying blood volumes, and anesthesia. Subcutaneous insulin pump use is discontinued during surgery when the insulin/glucose infusion method is used. The basal rate insulin of the pump or the intermediate- or long-acting insulin should be given 1 to 2 hours before discontinuing intravenous insulin. Rapid-acting or short-acting insulin given intravenously has a very short half-life.
   **C** Intravenous fluids will be discontinued after CB is able to tolerate food.
   **D** A patient with proteinuria may tolerate only small amounts of intravenous fluid. When necessary to meet the caloric needs of a patient with end-stage renal disease during surgery, a more concentrated dextrose solution may be used.

**2** Blood glucose monitoring should be increased during the perioperative period.
   **A** Blood glucose monitoring should be done every 30 to 60 minutes during surgery and until CB awakens from the anesthesia.
   **B** Blood glucose monitoring should be done every 1 to 2 hours as long as CB receives intravenous insulin.

**3** The ACE inhibitor could be given after surgery when CB fully awakens.

**4** Both CB and her family have educational needs.

  **A** Preoperative teaching should include information about the frequency of glucose monitoring, the surgical procedure, and postoperative care.

  **B** CB will be discharged as soon as possible from the hospital with written instruction. Discharge instructions to CB and her family include wound care, assessment of her wound for infection, frequency of monitoring, safety issues related to the use of pain medication, when to call for assistance, and when to return for follow-up. When using narcotics, family members will need to ascertain that the patient has followed her diabetes self-care plan (eg, taken correct insulin dose, has eaten), and monitor her glucose for hypoglycemia.

## References

**1** Rosenbloom AL, Hanas R. Diabetic ketoacidosis (DKA): treatment guidelines. Clin Pediatr. 1996;35:261-266.

**2** Schade DS, Eaton RP. Pathogenesis of diabetic ketoacidosis: a reappraisal. Diabetes Care. 1979;2:296-306.

**3** Alberti KG. Role of glucagon and other hormones in development of diabetic ketoacidosis. Lancet. 1975;1:1307-1311.

**4** Keller U, Schnell H, Girard J, Stauffacher W. Effect of physiological elevation of plasma growth hormone levels on ketone body kinetics and lipolysis in normal and acutely insulin-deficient men. Diabetologia. 1984;26:103-108.

**5** American Diabetes Association. Hospital admission guidelines for diabetes mellitus. Diabetes Care. 2001;24(suppl 1):S91.

**6** Genuth S. Diabetic ketoacidosis and hyperosmolar hyperglycemic nonketotic syndrome in adults. In: Lebovitz HE, DeFronzo RA, Genuth S, Kreisberg RA, Pfeifer MA, Tamborlane WV, eds. Therapy for Diabetes Mellitus and Related Disorders. 3rd ed. Alexandria, Va: American Diabetes Association; 1998:83-96.

**7** Ennis ED, Kreisberg RA. Diabetic ketoacidosis and the hyperglycemic hyperosmolar syndrome. In: LeRoith D, Taylor SI, Olesky JM, eds. Diabetes Mellitus: A Fundamental and Clinical Text. Philadelphia: Lippincott-Raven Publishers; 1996:276-286.

**8** Matz R. Hyperosmolar nonacidotic diabetes (HNAD). In: Porte D Jr, Sherwin RS, eds. Ellenberg & Rifkin's Diabetes Mellitus. 5th ed. Stamford, Conn: Appleton & Lange; 1997:845-860.

**9** Minaker KL. What diabetologists should know about elderly patients. Diabetes Care. 1990;13(suppl 2):34-46.

**10** Bailey CJ, Turner RC. Drug therapy: metformin. N Engl J Med. 1996;334:574-579.

**11** Travaglini MT, Garg SK, Chase HP. Use of insulin lispro in the outpatient management of ketonuria. Arch Pediatr Adolesc Med. 1998;152:672-675.

**12** American Diabetes Association. Translation of the diabetes nutrition recommendations for health care institutions. Diabetes Care. 2001;24(suppl 1):S49.

**13** Schafer RG, Bohannon B, Franz M, et al. Translation of the diabetes nutrition recommendations for health care institutions. Diabetes Care. 1997;20:96-105.

**14** Gaare-Porcari JM, O'Sullivan-Maillet JM. Care for persons with diabetes during surgery. In: Powers MA, ed. Handbook of Diabetes Medical Nutrition Therapy. Gaithersburg, Md. Aspen Publishers; 1996:601-615.

**15** Palmisano J. Surgery and diabetes. In: Kahn R, Weir G, eds. Joslin's Diabetes Mellitus. 13th ed. Philadelphia: Lea & Febiger; 1994:955-961.

**16** Golden SH, Kao WHL, Peart-Vigilance C, Brancati FL. Perioperative glycemic control and the risk of infectious complications in a cohort of adults with diabetes. Diabetes Care. 1999;22:1408-1414.

**17** Alberti KGMM. Diabetes and surgery. In: Rifkin H, Porte D Jr, eds. Ellenberg & Rifkin's Diabetes Mellitus: Theory and Practice. 4th ed. New York: Elsevier, 1990:626-633.

## Suggested Readings

Avilés-Santa L, Raskin P. Surgery and anesthesia. In: Lebovitz H, ed. Therapy for Diabetes Mellitus and Related Disorders. 3rd ed. Alexandria, Va: American Diabetes Association; 1998;224-233.

Hirsch IB, Paauw DS. Diabetes management in special situations. Endocrinol Metab Clin North Am. 1997;3:631-645.

Illness: Plan ahead for under the weather days. Available on the Internet at: *http://www.diabetes.org/ada/c30l.asp*. Accessed October 2000.

Irons MJ. Fighting colds and flu. Diabetes Self-Management. 1998 Jan/Feb;47-52. Also available on the Internet at: *www.diabetes-self-mgmt.com/jf98art.html*. Accessed October 2000.

Kaufman FR, Dergan S, Roe TF, Costin G. Perioperative management with prolonged intravenous insulin infusion versus subcutaneous insulin in children with type 1 diabetes mellitus. J Diabetes Complications. 1996;10:6-11.

Lorber DM. Surgical management of the patient with diabetes. Pract Diabetology. 1996;15(2):2-4.

White NH, Henry DN. Special issues in diabetes mellitus. In: Haire-Joshu D, ed. Management of Diabetes Mellitus: Perspectives of Care Across the Life Span. 2nd ed. St. Louis. Mosby; 1996:378-384.

# Learning Assessment: Post-Test Questions

## Illness and Surgery

**3**

**1** Which of the following is a sick-day management guideline?
  **A** Omit insulin dose when vomiting occurs
  **B** Increase frequency of blood glucose monitoring
  **C** Drink large amounts of carbohydrate containing liquids
  **D** Only call healthcare professionals if urine ketones are positive

**2** Increased ketone levels in a postsurgical patient are most likely to be caused by:
  **A** Insufficient insulin and/or carbohydrate intake
  **B** Decreased lipolysis and/or carbohydrate intake
  **C** Decreased protein catabolism and/or carbohydrate intake
  **D** Increased protein anabolism and/or carbohydrate intake

**3** In addition to completing an admission history, reviewing laboratory data, and performing a physical exam, what additional information would be most useful in a preoperative assessment of a 42-year-old patient with type 2 diabetes and no cardiovascular risk factors?
  **A** Medical records from previous hospital admission
  **B** Cardiovascular enzyme activity laboratory data
  **C** Information about the patient's cognitive and affective needs
  **D** Postoperative glucose and insulin protocol of hospital

**4** Cardiac problems can be serious, even fatal, in a person with diabetes and should be assessed prior to surgery. During surgery, which of the following could occur?
  **A** Anesthesia agents could stimulate heart muscle function
  **B** Hyperglycemia could cause excessive bleeding
  **C** Patients risk hypotension, hypovolemia, and rhythm disturbances
  **D** Metabolic stresses cause carotid bruits to develop

**5** A particular postoperative concern for a patient with diabetes whose blood glucose level is higher than 200 mg/dL is:
  **A** Fluid restrictions
  **B** Discontinuation of oral hypoglycemic agents
  **C** Peripheral vascular disease
  **D** Impaired wound healing

**6** To maintain adequate hydration, caffeine-free, calorie-free liquids should be used. The reason such liquids should be caffeine-free when used by a patient with diabetes during 'sick days' is because:
  **A** Caffeine is a stimulant and causes insomnia
  **B** Caffeine is a diuretic
  **C** Caffeine in small amounts will raise blood glucose levels
  **D** Caffeine will decrease blood glucose levels

**7** Surgical patients with type 2 diabetes who are taking antidiabetes agents:
  **A** Will not need insulin before surgery
  **B** Will need to take insulin after surgery as a permanent replacement of their previous treatment
  **C** Should be informed that they may need insulin before, during, and immediately after their surgery
  **D** Should not be told that their insulin may be adjusted during surgery because they may become fearful of giving others decision-making responsibility for insulin adjustment

**8** On discharge from a hospital, patients with diabetes need:
  **A** Oral instructions on sick-day management of their disease sufficient to avoid medical emergencies
  **B** To be told to contact healthcare providers only at certain times of the day so that proper attention can be given to their condition
  **C** Not be given any instructions on discharge since they will be too overwhelmed by all the procedures to grasp the meaning
  **D** Survival skills that include written instructions on sick-day management

**9** When patients with diabetes are too sick to eat or tolerate large volumes of fluids, they are advised to consume something that contains 15 g of carbohydrate every 1 to 2 hours. An example of this would be:
**A** 1 cup Gatorade® sports drink
**B** 1 can diet Coca Cola® soft drink
**C** ½ cup of sugar-free Jello-O® gelatin
**D** 2 Popsicle® sticks

**10** Which guideline is important during postoperative care?
**A** Meticulous wound care
**B** Frequent monitoring of blood glucose
**C** Adequate pain management
**D** All of the above are important

*See next page for answer key.*

# Post-Test Answer Key

## Illness and Surgery

3

| 1 | B | 6 | B |
|---|---|---|---|
| 2 | A | 7 | C |
| 3 | A | 8 | D |
| 4 | C | 9 | A |
| 5 | D | 10 | D |

# A Core Curriculum for Diabetes Education
Diabetes Management Therapies

## Index

Acarbose, 111, 114, 126-128, 138
    food interactions, 132
    interactions, 116, 118
Acesulfame, 15
Acetoacetate, 161-162, 171, 172
Acetone, 161
Acidifiers, urinary, 119
Activity, see Exercise
Actos, see Pioglitazone
Adolescents
    calorie requirements, 27
    hypoglycemia and, 250
    lipoprotein values, 5
    My Food Plan for Kids & Teens, 30
    nutrition plans, 22-23
Adrenergic antagonists, 116
Aging
    exercise considerations, 57, 71-72
    glucose self-monitoring, 158
    hyperosmolar hyperglycemic state, 265
Albumin, glycosylated, 160, 162, 178, 269
Albuminuria, 162
Alcohol
    diabetes management and, 20-21
    hypoglycemia and, 238
    sulfonylureas and, 138
Alertness, see Mental states
Algorithm approach, see Insulin
Allopurinol, 116
Alpha-glucosidase inhibitors, 111, 114, 118, 126-128, 179
Alpha-1 antagonists, 133
Amaryl, see Glimepiride
American Diabetes Association
    "ADA diet" not appropriate term, 29
    nutrition recommendations, 3
Amylin agonists, 128
Anabolic steroids, 116
Androgens, 116
Animas pump, 208
Anticholinergic medications, 133
Anticoagulants, 116
Antidiabetes agents, oral, 111-128
    review (educational exercises), 137-143, 148-150
Antihistamines, 133
Anti-inflammatory agents, 118, 133

Antioxidants, 20
Asparaginase I, 116
Aspart, see Insulin preparations
Aspartame, 14-15
Aspirin, 116
Atherosclerosis, 269
Automobile drivers, 250-251
Autonomic nervous system, hypoglycemic symptoms, 233-235
Avandia, see Rosiglitazone
Basal profile (background) rate, see Insulin
Benzoic acid derivative, 111, 114, 120
3-beta-hydroxybutyrate, 161-162
Beta-adrenergic antagonists, 116
Beta-blockers
    adverse effects, 133
    exercise and, 67
Bibliography
    blood glucose pattern management, 196-197
    carbohydrate counting, 225
    exercise, 85
    hypoglycemia, 256
    insulin pump therapy, 215
    monitoring, 169
    nutrition publications, resources, 30-31, 50-51
    pharmacologic therapies, 147
    sick-day management, 279
    surgery, 279
Biguanides, 111, 114, 123-124
Blood
    count, preoperative assessment, 269
    ketones, 267
    plasma insulin concentration, 61
Blood glucose, see Glucose; Hyperglycemia; Hypoglycemia
Blood Glucose Awareness Training, 248
Blood pressure, preoperative assessment, 269
Body
    exercise and weight, 58
    mass index, 8, 9
    weight assessment, children, 163
    weight control, 7
Breathing difficulties, see Respiratory difficulties
C-peptide, 92, 93

Calcium, 19
Calcium-channel blockers, 113, 116
Carbohydrate counting, 30, 31-34, 41, 51
    choices (exchanges), 26, 218, 219
    choices, servings, 32
    insulin pump therapy, 207, 216-223, 227-228
Carbohydrate Counting (booklets), 30
Carbohydrates, see also Carbohydrate counting
    cakes and frosting, 39
    choices (exchanges), 26, 218, 219
    choices, servings, 32
    diabetes food/meal plan, 13-15
    diabetes type 1, 6
    diabetes type 2, 8, 10
    exchange list, 26
    food labels, 38
    health facility meal plans, 29
    hypoglycemia treatment, 241, 242
    insulin ratios, 33, 39
    insulin ratios (pump therapy), 209, 216-223
    intolerance, 19
    replacement and exercise, 64-65
    sick-day management, 266, 267
    types of, 11
Cardiovascular system
    disease risk and lipoproteins, 5
    exercise benefits, 57, 58
    exercise considerations, 63
    exercise programs, 67-68
    hypertension and exercise, 73
    macrovascular disease and fat, 16-17
    preoperative assessment, 269
Catecholamines, 264
Central nervous system, drug adverse effects, 134
Cerebrovascular disease, preoperative assessment, 269
Charcot's foot, 74
Chemotherapy, adverse effects, 133
Children
    glucose self-monitoring, 158-159

growth, weight assessment, 163

infants and hypoglycemia, 250

insulin pump therapy, 207

lipoprotein values, 5

*My Food Plan for Kids & Teens*, 30

nutrition plans, 22-23

nutritional education, 29

oral antidiabetes agents not recommended, 111

surgery, 273

Chloramphenicol, 116

Chloroquine, 116

Chlorpropamide, 113

discontinuance and surgery, 271

hypoglycemia risk, 232

Cholesterol

dietary fat and, 10

drug adverse effects, 135

fat, diet and, 17-18

lipoprotein values, 5

Cholestyramine, 116

Chromatography, 159-160

Chromium, 19, 20

Cimetidine, 117

Clofibrate, 117

Clonidine, 133

Codeine, 133

Cold, see Weather

Colorimetric assay, 159-160

Complications of diabetes, 63, 73-76; see also Ketoacidosis, diabetic; Nephropathy, diabetic; Neuropathy, diabetic; Retinopathy, diabetic

Continuous subcutaneous insulin infusion, see Pump therapy

Contraceptives, 118, 139

Coronary artery disease, 58, 74

Corticosteroids, 117

Cortisol

counterregulatory hormones, 94

during illness and surgery, 264

hormonal response, metabolic effects during exercise, 60

Costs

glucose monitoring, 164

insulin pump therapy, 205, 207

Counterregulatory hormones, see Hormones

D-phenylalanine derivative, 111, 114, 120

Dahedi pump, 208

Dehydration, 263

Dextrose, 274

DiaBeta, see Glyburide

Diabetes, see also Diabetes complications; Diabetes mellitus, type 1; Diabetes mellitus, type 2; Glucose; Glucose control; Glucose monitoring; Hyperglycemia; Hypoglycemia; Insulin; Patient education; Self-management

medical nutrition therapy goals, 4-6

monitoring, 153-172

personal identification information, 66, 243

secondary, insulin requirement, 94

Diabetes complications, 63, 73-76; see also Ketoacidosis, diabetic; Nephropathy, diabetic; Neuropathy, diabetic; Retinopathy, diabetic

Diabetes education, see Patient education

Diabetes, gestational, see Pregnancy

Diabetes mellitus, type 1

counterregulatory hormones and metabolic changes, 264

exercise and, 58, 61, 62

exercise recommendations, 69

hypoglycemia, 61, 231, 233, 249

insulin dosage, 138-139

insulin requirements, 94, 103

ketone tests, 161

medical nutrition therapy goals, 6-7

oral antidiabetes agents, 111

pattern management, problem-solving practice, 186, 188, 189

perioperative concerns, 270-271

protein intake, 15

surgery and, 268

youth and nutrition, 6

Diabetes mellitus, type 2

changing drugs, 138

drug therapy, 140-141

exercise and, 58, 69

fat intake, 18

hyperosmolar hyperglycemic state, 264-265

hypoglycemia, 233, 249-250, 252-253

insulin requirements, 94, 103, 138

nutrition, therapy, goals, 7-10, 40-43

oral antidiabetes agents, 111, 138

pattern management, problem-solving practice, 187, 190, 191

perioperative concerns, 271-272

protein intake, 15

surgical patients, 272

youth and nutrition, 6

Diabetes nutrition therapy, see Nutrition

Diabetes patient education, see Patient education

Diabetes patient self-care, see Self-management

Diabetic ketoacidosis, see Ketoacidosis, diabetic

Diabetic nephropathy, see Nephropathy, diabetic

Diabetic neuropathy, see Neuropathy, diabetic

Diabetic retinopathy, see Retinopathy, diabetic

Diabinese, see Chlorpropamide

Diaport system, 211

Diaries, 236-238, 248

Diarrhea, see Gastrointestinal system

Diazoxide, 117

Dicumarol, 116, 117

Diet, see Nutrition

*Dietary Guidelines for Americans*, 5, 30

Dietitians, 22, 38

Disaccharides, 11

Disetronic pumps, 208

Disopyramide, 117

Diuretics, 117, 133

Doxazosin, 133

Driving, see Automobiles

Drugs, see also names of specific drugs and treatments, eg, Antidiabetes agents; Insulin alertness impairment in diabetes self-management, 131

antidiabetes, combinations listed, 112

combination therapies, 179

during illness, 266

interaction, 137

interactions, agents other than antihyperglycemics, 130-136

interactions with antidiabetes agents, 116-119

mimicking diabetes warning signs, 131

oral antidiabetes agents, 111-128

pharmacologic therapies, 91-150

review (educational exercises), 137-143, 148-150

Eating habits, see Nutrition

Elderly, see Aging

Electrolytes
balance during illness, surgery, 263
surgery and, 268, 269, 271

Emergency services
conditions requiring immediate contact, 267, 268
surgery, 273

Epinephrine
counterregulatory hormones, 94
during illness and surgery, 264
hormonal response, metabolic effects during exercise, 60
hypoglycemic symptoms, 233, 235

Equipment, see Injection devices; Needles; Pump therapy; Syringes

Estrogen products, 117

Ethanol, 117

Ethnic groups, food choices, 36, 38

Exchange Lists for Meal Planning, 30

Exercise, 57-88
aerobic, 67, 72, 73, 80
anaerobic, 67
benefits, 57-58
diabetes complications, 63, 73-76

educational considerations, review, 78-80, 87-88

equipment, clothing, warm-ups, cool-downs, 66

hyperglycemia induced by, 63, 66

hypoglycemia induced by, 61-62, 64-66, 239-240

increasing, maintaining, 76-78

insulin pump therapy, 205

ketosis and, 63

meal planning and, 72

physiology (individuals with diabetes), 60-62

physiology (individuals without diabetes), 58-60

programs, schedule, 67-71, 73

recommendations summarized, 69

strength (resistance training), 69-71

suggested readings, 85

tolerance test, 67

walking and peripheral vascular disease, 73-74

Eye, see also Vision impairment
drug adverse effects, 135
retinopathy and exercise, 74, 75, 78-80
retinopathy and resistance/weight training, 71

Facilitating Lifestyle Change: A Resource Manual, 30

Family (impact of hypo-glycemia), 244-246

Fat
carbohydrate counting, 31
content and hypoglycemia, 243
diabetes food/meal plan, 16-19
diabetes type 2, 10
exchange list, 26
nutrition and, 12
saturated, polyunsaturated, 17-18
substitutes, 18-19
types of dietary fats, 17

Fatty acids, free, 12

Fiber, 11, 13

Fibrinolysis, exercise and, 58

The First Step in Diabetes Meal Planning, 5, 30

Fish, 18

Fluconazole, 118

Fluids
balance during illness, surgery, 263
exercise and hydration, 67
requirements during illness and surgery, 264
sick-day management, 265

Fluoxetine, 118

Folate, 19

Food, see Nutrition

Food Guide Pyramid, 5, 30

Fructosamine, 160, 178, 269

Fructose, 14

Fruit, exchange list, 26

Gastrointestinal system, 134, 267

Gastroparesis, 240

Gemfibrozil, 118

Genitourinary system
drug adverse effects, 134
urinary tract infections, 141-143

Gestational diabetes, see Pregnancy

Glargine, see Insulin preparations

Glimepiride, 113

Glipizide, 113, 187, 191

Glitazones, 111, 124-126

Glucagon
administration, 249
counterregulatory hormones, 94
during illness and surgery, 264
hormonal response, metabolic effects during exercise, 60
hypoglycemic symptoms, 233
injection for severe hypoglycemia, 128-130

Gluconeogenesis, 11
alcohol and, 20
diabetes type 1, 264
insulin's effects, 92

Glucophage, see Metformin

Glucose, see also Glucose control; Glucose monitoring; Hyperglycemia; Hypoglycemia
absorption-delaying agents, 111, 128
alcohol and, 20
conversion of proteins (misinterpretations), 15-16
data analysis, pattern management, 175, 177

data analysis, problem-
solving practice, 185-191
data uses, 156
exercise effects, 60-61, 62
fluctuations, 231
homeostasis and healing, 268
hypoglycemia causes,
238-240
hypoglycemia treatment, 241
illness and surgery, 273-278,
280-281, 283
insulin effects (glycogenesis,
glycogenolysis,
gluconeogenesis), 92
levels and hypoglycemic
episodes, no direct
correlation, 232
levels and medical nutrition
therapy, 4
levels during illness, 267
management of surgical
patients, 270, 271
sensors, 211
surgical wound healing, 272
testing and nutrition, 10
urine testing, 162-163
Glucose control
conversion of proteins
(misinterpretations), 15-16
data analysis, problem-
solving practice, 185-191
data uses, 156
during illness, surgery,
263-264, 267
exercise and, 58
fluctuations, 231
glycosylated hemoglobin,
159-161
homeostasis and healing, 268
hypoglycemia treatment, 241
levels during illness, 267
meal planning, 38
medical nutrition therapy, 4
pattern management,
175-200
Glucose meters, 153-159,
163-167
Glucose monitoring
accuracy, errors, 154-155,
170, 171, 172
exercise and, 64, 66
objective summary
assessments, 178
postmeal, pattern
management, 182-184
premeal, pattern
management, 180-181

quality assurance, 158
self-monitoring, 153-159,
163-167, 170-172
sick days, 265
surgical patients, 271
testing and nutrition, 10
timing of, 176-177
urine testing, 162-163
Glucotrol, see Glipizide
Glucovance, see Glyburide/
metformin
Glyburide, 113, 232
Glyburide/metformin, 123-124
Glycemic control, see Glucose
control
Glycemic index, 14
Glycogenesis, 92
Glycogenolysis, 11, 92, 264
Glycosylation, 159-161, 165,
170, 172, 178
Glynase Prestabs, see Glyburide
Glyset, see Miglitol
Growth, see Children
Growth hormone
counterregulatory hormones,
94
during illness and surgery,
264
metabolic effects during
exercise, 60
Guanethidine, interactions with
antidiabetic agents, 118
H-2 antagonists, 117
HbA1c, see Hemoglobin,
glycosylated
HCTZ, see Hydrochlorothiazide
Healing period, see Surgery
Healthcare facilities, see
Hospitals
Healthy Eating for People with
Diabetes, 30
Healthy Food Choices, 30
Heart failure, congestive, preop-
erative assessment, 269
Heart rate, exercise and, 68, 73
Heat, see Weather
Height, body mass index and, 9
Hemoglobin, glycosylated, 21,
159-161, 165, 170, 172,
178, 269
Herbal medicines, 20
History-taking, 268
Home care, postoperative, 273
Homocysteine, 19
Hormones
counterregulatory, 94, 264
growth, 60, 94, 264

response to exercise, 60
stress, 263
Hospitals
bedside glucose monitoring,
158
diabetes nutrition
recommendations, 29
surgery, 263, 268, 270-273
Hydration, see Fluids
Hydrochlorothiazide, 140-141
3-beta-hydroxybutyrate, 161-
162
Hyperglycemia, see also
Glucose; Glucose control
early morning, 106
exercise and, 63, 66
overtreatment of
hypoglycemia, 243
perioperative period, 268
preoperative assessment, 269
prevention and nutrition, 37
stress hormones and, 263
urine volume, fluid
requirements, 264
Hyperinsulinemia, reduced, with
exercise, 58
Hyperosmolar hyperglycemic
state
diabetes type 2, 264-265
elderly and, 265
insulin requirement, 94
stress hormones and, 263
Hypersensitivity, insulin, 101
Hypertension, 58, 73
Hypoglycemia, 231-260
autonomic failure, 234
causes, 238-240
common symptoms, 234
definition, description,
232-233
diary-keeping, 248
driving and, 250-251
drug adverse effects, 135
educational considerations,
review, 249-253, 258-260
episodes, 232, 241, 247-248
exercise and, 61-62, 64-66
exercise-induced, 58, 206
frequency, risk factors for
increased, 235
glucose monitoring, testing,
153, 156, 177
high-fat foods, poor treatment choices, 243
insulin's effects, 92, 94

knowledge assessment, intervention plans, 246-249
mild, 232, 242
nocturnal, 106, 166-167, 238-239, 241, 246, 252
nocturnal, minimization with pump therapy, 204, 206
nocturnal, prevention, 242
patient fears, 245
perioperative period, 268
post-exercise, late-onset, 61-62, 65-66
prevention and treatment, 240-244, 246
protein and, 15-16
psychosocial impact, 244-246
seizure, monitoring, 166-167
severe, 232, 243, 244
symptom diary, 236, 237, 238
symptoms, 233-238
teaching about recognition, treatment of, 137
treatment by family, friends, 244
unawareness, 234
Hypotension, orthostatic, and surgery, 267, 269
IDDM (insulin-dependent diabetes mellitus), see Diabetes mellitus, type 1
Identification tags, see Patient identification
Illness, 263
sick-day management, 265-267
sick-day management (review, educational exercises), 273-278, 280-281, 283
Inhaled insulin, see Insulin
Injection devices, 100
Insulin 91-150; see also Diabetes mellitus, type 1; Diabetes mellitus, type 2; Insulin preparations; Pump therapy
administration and storage guidelines, 99-101
algorithm approach to therapy, 178
allergies, 101
basal profile (background) rate, 210
biochemical formation from proinsulin, 93
carbohydrate ratio, 33, 39

combinations, 95, 97
concentrations, 99
counterregulatory hormones and, 94
decreased need with exercise, 60
dosing, schedules, regimen, 102-111
during illness, 264, 265-266
effects, usage, 92-94
endogenous, defined, 94
endogenous, time action, 103
exercise and hypoglycemia, 62, 63, 65, 66
exogenous, defined, 94
food interactions, 132
gestational diabetes and, 94, 104
glucose and, 92
hormonal response, metabolic effects during exercise, 60
human insulin analogue, 95
human-source, 96
hyperosmolar hyperglycemic state and, 94
hypoglycemia, 92, 94
impurity, purity, 98, 101
inhaled, 110-111
injection frequency, 104-110
injection routine, technique, 100-101
insufficient, consequences, 62
intensive therapy, 105
intermediate-acting, 95, 97, 105, 106, 108
ketoacidosis and, 94
ketogenesis, 92
lipogenesis and lipolysis, 92
long-acting, 95, 97 108
long-acting, during illness, 266
management of surgical patients, 270
meal timing, frequency, 6-7
mixing, 101-102
nutrition and, 11
"oral," confusion about sulfonylureas, 137
parenteral nutrition and, 94
pattern management, glucose analysis, problem-solving practice, 185-191
plasma, concentration, 61
postmeal monitoring, pattern management, 182-184
postoperative care, 272

premeal monitoring, pattern management, 180-181
preparations (eg, species/ source, type, action), 94-99
pulmonary, 110-111
pump therapy, 203-228
rapid-acting, 95, 97, 106 107, 108, 109
rapid-acting, during illness, 266
regimen and medical nutrition therapy, 4, 23
reuse of syringes, needles, 100
review (educational exercises), 137-143, 148-150
secretagogues, 111
sensitivity and exercise, 58
sensitivity and hypoglycemia, 240
sensitivity and pump therapy, 206
sensitizers, 111
short-acting, 95, 97, 106, 107, 108, 109
short-acting, during illness, 266
sliding-scale approach, 179
split-mixed regimen, 104
stress hormones and illness, 263
surgery and, 264
syringes, needles, injection devices, pumps, 100
time action, 103, 105-110
Insulin-dependent diabetes mellitus, see Diabetes mellitus, type 1
Insulin preparations
administration and storage guidelines, 99-101
algorithm approach to therapy, 178
aspart, 96, 97-98, 180-184
biochemical formation from proinsulin, 93
bovine (beef-source), 95, 96
combinations, 95, 97
concentrations, 99
dosing, schedules, regimen, 102-111
glargine, 96, 97, 98, 102, 180-181, 184
human insulin analogue, 95
human-source, 96
impurity, purity, 98, 101
inhaled, 110-111

injection frequency, 104-110
injection routine, technique, 100-101
intermediate-acting, 95, 97, 105, 106, 108
Lente, 96, 97, 102, 105, 106, 107, 109
Lente, during illness, 266
lipogenesis and lipolysis, 92
lispro, 96, 97, 102, 106, 107, 108, 109, 110, 180-184, 186, 189
long-acting, 95, 97, 108
long-acting, during illness, 266
mixing, 101-102
NPH, 96, 97, 98, 102, 105, 106, 107, 108, 109, 180-182, 186, 188
NPH, during illness, 266
pattern management, glucose analysis, problem-solving practice, 185-191
porcine (pork-source), 95, 96
postmeal monitoring, pattern management, 182-184
premeal monitoring, pattern management, 180-181
pulmonary, 110-111
rapid-acting, 95, 97, 106 107, 108, 109
rapid-acting, during illness, 266
review (educational exercises), 137-143, 148-150
short-acting, 95, 97, 106, 107, 108, 109
short-acting, during illness, 266
species/source, type, action, etc, 94-99
split-mixed regimen, 104
syringes, needles, injection devices, pumps, 100
time action, 103, 105-110
time action profiles, glargine vs NPH, 98
Ultralente, 96, 97, 102, 107, 108, 181, 184, 189
Ultralente, during illness, 266
Insulin pumps, see Pump therapy
Insurance coverage, see Costs; Pump therapy
Islam (human insulin preferences), 96
Isoniazid, 118

Judaism (human insulin preferences), 96
Ketoacidosis, diabetic
insulin requirement, 94
perioperative period, 268
pump therapy, 210
warning signals, 264
Ketoconazole, 118
Ketogenesis, 92, 264
Ketonemia, 264
Ketones
formation and illness, 263
monitoring, sick days, 265
tests, 161-162
urine and blood, 267
urine monitoring, surgical patients, 271
Ketonuria, 264
Ketosis, 263
exercise and, 63
insulin pump therapy and, 205
perioperative period, 268
starvation, 266
symptoms, 264
Kidney, see also Nephropathy, diabetic
drug adverse effects, 134
insufficiency and hypoglycemia, 240
preoperative assessment, 269-270
Kussmaul respiration, 264
Laboratory testing, preoperative assessment, 269
Lancets, 164
Lente, see Insulin preparations
Lifestyle, see also Nutrition; Self-management
continuing nutritional education, 28
*Facilitating Lifestyle Change: A Resource Manual*, 30
insulin pump therapy, 205, 206
Lipids, cardiovascular disease risk, 5
Lipodystrophies, 101
Lipogenesis and lipolysis, 92, 264
Lipoprotein lipase, 12
Lipoproteins, 5
Lispro, see Insulin preparations
Liver, gluconeogenesis, 264
Long-term care, nutritional plans, 29

Macrovascular disease, see Cardiovascular system
Magnesium, 19
Meat
carbohydrate counting, 31
exchange list, 26
Medical nutrition therapy, see Nutrition
Medical records, history-taking, 268
Meglitinides
analogues, 111, 116-119, 120-122
exercise and, 66
hypoglycemia risk, 232
interactions (drug-disease and drug-drug), 116-119
Mental states
alertness decreases, hypoglycemia, 235
changes in, immediate treatment, 267
unconsciousness, 235
Metabolism
goals, in type 2 diabetes, 7-8
homeostasis during illness, surgery, 263
long-term monitoring, 159-161
medical nutrition therapy goals, 4-5
normal, goals, 11
Metformin, 111, 114, 123-124, 138
combination therapies, 179
discontinuance and surgery, 271
during illness, 266
food interactions, 132
interactions, 117
interactions with antidiabetic agents, 118
pattern management, problem-solving practice, 187, 191, 194
Microalbuminuria, 162
Micronase, see Glyburide
Miglitol, 111, 114, 126-128
food interactions, 132
interactions, 118
Milk, exchange list, 26
Minerals, 12, 19-20
Mini-Med 508 pump, 208
Monitoring, see Carbohydrate counting; Glucose monitoring; Self-management

Monoamine oxidase inhibitors, 118

Monosaccharides, 11

Moslems, see Islam

Muscles
   mass and aging, 71
   strength (resistance training), 69-71
   weight loss and, 72

Muslims, see Islam

*My Food Plan*, 30

*My Food Plan for Kids & Teens*, 30

Nateglinide, 111, 114, 120, 121-122
   combination therapies, 179
   food interactions, 132

Needles, 100

Nephropathy, diabetic
   exercise and, 74
   preoperative assessment, 2 69-270
   resistance/weight training, 71

Nervous system complications, see Neuropathy, diabetic

Neuroglycopenia, 233, 234, 235-236, 244

Neuropathy, diabetic
   autonomic, and exercise, 75-76
   peripheral, and exercise, 74-75
   peripheral, postoperative care, 273
   preoperative assessment, 269

Niacin, 118

Nicotinic acid, 118

NIDDM (noninsulin-dependent diabetes mellitus), see Diabetes mellitus, type 2

Nitroprusside, 161-162, 171, 172

Noninsulin-dependent diabetes mellitus), see Diabetes mellitus, type 2

Norepinephrine, 60, 94, 264

NPH, see Insulin preparations

NSAIDS, see Anti-inflammatory drugs

Nutrition, 3-54; see also
   Carbohydrates
   "ADA diet" not appropriate term, 29
   American Diabetes Association recommendations, 3

carbohydrate counting, 30, 31-34

carbohydrate counting and specific foods, 220

diabetes daily record, 34

diabetes medication interactions with food, 132

diabetes type 1 and, 6-7

diabetes type 2 and, 7-10, 40-43

ethnic and cultural differences, 36

exchange lists, 22, 26, 30

exercise and meal planning, 72

fasting (nothing by mouth) and surgery, 271

food diaries, 23, 27

food label meanings, 35

food labeling, 35-36, 38, 39

food/meal planning teaching methods, 29-31

*Food Guide Pyramid*, 5, 30

glucose levels and food, 164

glucose monitoring and food decisions, 156

high-fat foods, poor treatment choices for hypoglycemia, 243

history, 22

history form, 24, 25

hospitals, health facilities, 29

hypoglycemia and, 238, 240-241

insulin pump therapy, 205

insulin regimen and, 4, 23, 103-110

key educational considerations, 37-39

lifestyle, changes, 3, 5, 10

maintenance calories, 26

meal frequency, 10

meal planning, spacing, frequency, 10, 29-31, 37

medical nutrition therapy goals, 4-6

medical nutrition therapy (preferred term), 3

new foods, 39

parenteral, insulin requirement, 94

pattern management, problem-solving practice, 185-191

portion skills, 39

postoperative care, 272

premeal monitoring, pattern management, 180-181

publications, resources, 30-31, 50-51

review (educational exercises), 39-43, 52-54

self-management, individual plan development, 21-29

sick-day management, 266

travel adaptations, 36-37

youth calorie requirements, 27

Obesity (exercise considerations), 72-73

Octreotide, 118

Orinase, see Tolbutamide

Pain management, surgical patients, 273

Pancreatic enzymes, 118

Pancrelipase, 118

Parenteral nutrition, see under Nutrition

Patient education, see also
   Self-management
   avoidance, barriers in glucose monitoring, 165-166
   Blood Glucose Awareness Training, 248
   carbohydrate counting, 30, 31-34
   carbohydrate counting for pump therapy, 216-223
   continuing, and in-depth nutritional skills, 28, 29
   exercise, 78-80, 87-88
   food/meal planning teaching methods, 29-31
   glucose meters, 157
   glucose self-monitoring, 156-157, 163-167, 170-172
   hypoglycemia, 249-253, 258-260
   hypoglycemia knowledge assessment, intervention plans, 246-249
   hypoglycemia prevention, 240-241
   hypoglycemia treatment, 242-243
   insulin administration and storage, 99-101
   insulin/antidiabetes agents, 137-143, 148-150
   insulin pump therapy, 211-214
   insulin pump therapy learning curve, 205, 207, 209-211

insulin pump troubleshooting, 210-211

mental, emotional changes and hypoglycemia, 235-236, 238

nutrition publications, resources, 30-31, 50-51

nutrition therapy, 23, 26, 28, 29, 37-39

nutritional considerations, 37-43, 52-54

patient-centered, empowerment approach, 23, 26

pattern management, 175-176, 192-194

severe hypoglycemia, 244

sick-day management, 273-278, 280-281, 283

surgery, 273-278, 280-281, 283

Patient identification, 66, 243

Patient psychology, see Mental states; Psychology

Patient self-management, see Self-management

Pattern management, see Glucose

Pentamidine, 118

Peptide, C-, 92, 93

Perioperative period, see Surgery

Peripheral vascular disease

drug adverse effects, 135

exercise and, 73-74

postoperative care, 273

Pharmacologic therapies, see Drugs; Insulin

Phenothiazines, 119

Phenylalanine, D-, derivative, 111, 120

Phenytoin, 119

Pioglitazone, 111, 114, 124-126

interactions, 118

pattern management, problem-solving practice, 190

Polysaccharides, 11

Polyunsaturated fats, see Fat

Potassium, 19

Prandin, see Repaglinide

Prazosin, 133

Precose, see Acarbose

Pregnancy

glycosylated albumin testing, 178

hypoglycemia and, 240

insulin and gestational diabetes, 94

insulin pump therapy, 206, 213-214

insulin requirements, 103-104

ketone tests, 161

nonnutritive (low-calorie) sweeteners, 15

nutrition and, 6

oral antidiabetes agents not recommended, 111

Preoperative assessment, see Surgery

Probenecid, 119

Proinsulin, 93

Propranolol, 140-141

Protamine, 101

Protease inhibitors, 119

Protein

diabetes food/meal plan, 15-16

exchange list, 26

glucose conversion (misinterpretations), 15-16

hypoglycemia and, 15-16

nutritional considerations, 12

Psychology

alertness, mental, emotional changes, 235-236, 238, 243, 267

glucose monitoring, meter accuracy, 165-166

hypoglycemia fears, 245

hypoglycemic episodes, 235-236, 238, 243, 244-246, 248

insulin pump therapy contraindications, 207-208

pump therapy and motivation, 207

Publications, see Bibliography

Pulmonary insulin, see Insulin

Pump therapy, 100, 110, 203-228

basal profile (background) rate, 210

carbohydrate counting, 220-223, 227-228

carbohydrate-to-insulin ratio, 209, 216-223

correction, sensitivity factor, 209

cost, insurance considerations, 205, 207, 208, 209

educational exercises, reviews, 211-214

failure rates, 208

glucose self-monitoring, 177

indications, candidates, contraindications, 206-208, 212-214

infusion site, set, 210, 227, 228

number of users, 204

patient motivation, 207

safety, 204-205

selecting, obtaining pumps, 208-209

starting, 209-211

therapy, benefits, limitations described, 204-205

troubleshooting, 210-211

Reading lists, see Bibliography

Reagents, strips, 154-155, 170, 172

Religious beliefs (human insulin preferences), 96

Repaglinide, 111, 114, 120-121, 194

combination therapies, 179

food interactions, 132

hypoglycemia risk, 232

Resistance training, see Exercise

Respiratory difficulties, 267

Retinopathy, diabetic, see also Vision impairment

exercise and, 74, 75, 78-80

proliferative, 74, 75

resistance/weight training, 71

Rifampin, interactions with antidiabetic agents, 119

Rosiglitazone, 111, 114, 124-126

interactions, 116, 118

Saccharin, 15

Safety, see Pump therapy

Salicylates, 119

Saturated fats, see Fat

Scheduling, see Insulin

Seizures, 235

Self-management, see also Patient education

alertness, mental, emotional changes, 235-236, 238, 243

avoidance, barriers in glucose monitoring, 165-166

carbohydrate counting, 30, 31-34

continuing nutritional education, 28, 29

diabetes daily record, 34

drug impairment of alertness, 131

drugs mimicking diabetes warning signs, 131
exercise participation, 76-78
food diaries, 23
glucose pattern management, 175-200
hypoglycemia effects, treatment, 235-236, 238, 242-243
insulin dosing, schedules, regimen, 102-111
insulin pump therapy, 203-228
ketone tests, 161-162
monitoring, 153-172
nutritional recommendations, individual plan development, 21-29
patient-centered, empowerment approach, 23, 26
sick-day management, 263, 265-267, 273-278, 280-281, 283
Serum levels, see Blood; Glucose; Glucose control
Single-Topic Diabetes Resources, 30
Skin-drug adverse effects, 134
Sliding-scale approach, see Insulin
Sodium, 19
Sorbitol, 134
Starch
    carbohydrate types, 11
    exchange list, 26
Starlix, see Nateglinide
Steroids, anabolic, 116
Sucralose, 15
Sucrose, 13, 38-38
Sugars
    alcohols, 14
    carbohydrate types, 11
    sweeteners, 14-15
Sulfa antibiotics, 240
Sulfonamides, 119
Sulfonylureas, 111, 112, 113, 115, 120
    alcohol and, 138
    combination therapies, 179
    exercise and, 66
    food interactions, 132
    hypoglycemia causes, 240
    hypoglycemia risk, 232
    interactions (drug-disease and drug-drug), 116-119
    "oral insulin," confusion, 137

Surgery
    children, 273
    diabetes treatment programs and, 263
    diabetes type 1 and, 270-271
    diabetes type 2 and, 271-272
    emergency, 273
    fasting (nothing by mouth) and, 271
    glucose management, 270, 271
    healing (postoperative) period, 272-273
    healing, 268
    infection risk, 263
    insulin management, 270
    perioperative period, 268, 270-272
    postoperative care, 272-273
    preoperative assessment, 268-270
    review (educational exercises), 273-278, 280-281, 283
Sweeteners, 14-15
Sympathomimetics, adverse effects, 134
Syringes, 100
Tacrolimus, 119
Terazosin, 133
Terminology, medical nutrition therapy, 3
Thiazolidinediones, 111, 114, 124-126, 194
    combination therapies, 179
    food interactions, 132
3-beta-hydroxybutyrate, 161-162
Thyroid product interaction with antidiabetic agents, 119
Time action of insulin, see Insulin
Tolazamide, 113
Tolbutamide, 113
Tolinase, see Tolazamide
Transient ischemic attacks, 269
Travel, 177
    adaptations, 36-37
    insulin pump therapy, 206
Triglycerides, 12
    drug adverse effects, 135
    lipoprotein values, 5
    lowering, 18
    dietary fat and, 10
Type 1 diabetes, see Diabetes mellitus, type 1

Type 2 diabetes, see Diabetes mellitus, type 2
TZDs, see Thiazolidinediones
Ultralente, see Insulin preparations
Unconsciousness, see Mental states
Urinary acidifiers, 119
Urinary tract infections, see Genitourinary system
Urine
    glucose testing, 162-163
    ketone monitoring, surgical patients, 271
    ketones, 267
    tests, 162-163
    tests, preoperative assessment, 270
    volume, 264
Vegetables, exchange list, 26
Vegetarians, human insulin for, 96
Vision impairment
    exercise and, 75
    glucose self-monitoring, 159
Vitamins, 12, 19-20
Vomiting, 267
Walking, see Exercise
Water, 12
Weather extremes and exercise, 66
Weight
    assessment, children, 163
    body mass index and, 9
    control, 7
    exercise and, 58
Weight lifting, 69-71
Weight loss, 37, 38
    aerobic exercise, 73
    glucose control and, 194
    hypoglycemia and, 240
    ketone tests, 161
    muscle mass, 72
    type 2 diabetes, 8
Wound healing, see Surgery
Zinc, 19, 101